Holistic Bodywork

Blending Modern and Ancient Bodywork Principles

JAMES PULCIANI, CMT, LAc

PEARSON

Boston   Columbus   Indianapolis   New York   San Francisco   Upper Saddle River

Amsterdam   Cape Town   Dubai   London   Madrid   Milan   Munich   Paris   Montreal   Toronto

Delhi   Mexico City   Sao Paulo   Sydney   Hong Kong   Seoul   Singapore   Taipei   Tokyo

Library of Congress Cataloging-in-Publication Data

Pulciani, James.
  Holistic bodywork / James Pulciani.—1st ed.
    p. ; cm.
  Includes bibliographical references and index.
  ISBN-13: 978-0-13-513895-3
  ISBN-10: 0-13-513895-7
  1. Massage therapy. 2. Holistic medicine. I. Title.
  [DNLM: 1. Massage. 2. Holistic Health. WB 537]
  RM721.P87 2012
  615.8'22--dc22

          2011000690

Notice: The author and the publisher of this volume have taken care that the information and technical recommendations contained herein are based on research and expert consultation, and are accurate and compatible with the standards generally accepted at the time of publication. Nevertheless, as new information becomes available, changes in clinical and technical practices become necessary. The reader is advised to carefully consult manufacturers' instructions and information material for all supplies and equipment before use, and to consult with a health care professional as necessary. This advice is especially important when using new supplies or equipment for clinical purposes. The author and publisher disclaim all responsibility for any liability, loss, injury, or damage incurred as a consequence, directly or indirectly, of the use and application of any of the contents of this volume.

Publisher: Julie Levin Alexander
Assistant to Publisher: Regina Bruno
Editor-in-Chief: Mark Cohen
Executive Editor: John Goucher
Associate Editor: Melissa Kerian
Assistant Editor: Nicole Ragonese
Editorial Assistant: Rosalie Hawley
Senior Media Editor: Amy Peltier
Media Project Manager: Lorena Cerisano
Managing Production Editor: Patrick Walsh
Production Liaison: Yagnesh Jani
Production Editor: Bruce Hobart, Laserwords Maine
Manufacturing Manager: Ilene Sanford
Manufacturing Buyer: Alan Fischer

Senior Art Director: Maria Guglielmo
Photographer: Michael Rieger
Cover Designer: Jayne Conte
Front Cover Image: Michael Rieger
Chapter Openers: Michael Rieger; Stephen Colburn/Shutterstock
Tab Icons: Maxstockphoto; Kristo-Gothard Hunor/Shutterstock; 3d Brained/Shutterstock
Director of Marketing: David Gesell
Executive Marketing Manager: Katrin Beacom
Marketing Specialist: Michael Sirinides
Composition: Laserwords, Maine
Printer/Binder: R. R. Donnelley/Willard
Cover Printer: Lehigh Phoenix Color/Hagerstown

10 9 8 7 6 5 4 3 2 1

www.pearsonhighered.com

PEARSON

ISBN-13: 978-0-13-513895-3
ISBN-10:   0-13-513895-7

Dedication

This book is dedicated to my family for all of their love and support
To my colleagues for their invaluable collaboration over the years
And especially to my students, past and present, for their enthusiasm
for learning and dedication to bodywork.

Brief Contents

Acknowledgments

First and foremost, I must extend a very heartfelt thank you to Megan Phillips. As contributing editor Megan has had an impact on every element of this book. Thank you for your creativity in developing so many of the pedagogical elements that make this book unique. Thank you for your dedication to making this book the very best that it could be. Thank you for your enthusiasm for research and, of course, for your attention to detail. Thank you for cheering me on and for toughing it out from start to finish. This book would not have been completed without your help and support. Last but not least, thank you for being my partner in life. I wouldn't want to do it without you.

I would also like to thank:

- Mike Rieger, our photographer, for his generosity and over 30 years of friendship and artistic collaboration.
- John and Lani Rieger for their hospitality in providing their home for our photo sessions and to Pam Phetsomphou for taking good care of us during the photo shoot.
- Mark Cohen for giving me this opportunity and for cheering me on through the process.
- Nicole Ragonese for her patience, guidance, and assistance getting me through the process of producing a textbook.
- Bruce Hobart for his organization and help in the critical final stages of production.
- Michelle Marie Livingston for catching all those little things in the copy edits.
- Our many reviewers whose comments, criticisms, and critiques helped shape this book into a much better resource.
- Willow Pulciani for her support and contributions to the bibliography.
- Duncan Pulciani for his support and help in running the household while I dedicated many extra hours to writing.
- D'Ette Carter for her keen eye and help during the final stages of editing and production.
- Our friends and families for their constant encouragement on this project, as well as their generosity in time and patience.
- All of my teachers—those from whom I've learned directly and those who have shared information through books, videos, and on-line resources. Thank you for sharing your knowledge.
- My colleagues throughout the years; thanks for walking the halls with me and sharing your handouts as well as your knowledge.
- All of my students through the years who have taught me much more than I could ever have taught them. Thank you for helping me grow personally and professionally.

Reviewers

Jennifer Barrett, BS, LMT
Queensborough Community College
Bayside, New York

Paul V. Berry Jr., LMT, NCTMB,
RHE, PTA
High Tech Institute
Marietta, Georgia

John Casbere
Alexandar School of Natural Therapeutics
Tacoma, Washington

Jackie Derby
Everest Institute
Grand Rapids, Michigan

Jo Ann DiFedele, LMBT
Greenville Technical College
Greenville, South Carolina

T.J. Ford, BS, LMT
East West College
Portland, Oregon

Cynthia Jaggers, MS, LMT, CNMT
Virginia College, School of Business
and Health
Chattanooga, Tennessee

Karen Mitchell Jackson, ACMT,
NCTMB, LMT
St. Louis College of Health Careers
Fenton, Missouri

Marsha Myers, BS, CMT
Ivy Tech Community College
Fort Wayne, Indiana

Teresa Patterson
Southwest Mississippi Community
College
Summit, Mississippi

Lou Peters, LMT, CNMT
American Institute of Alternative Medicine
Columbus, Ohio

Kristin Phillips, LMT, CNMT
Massage Therapy Training Institute
Kansas City, Missouri

Carolyn Talley Porter
Greenville Technical College
Greenville, South Carolina

Sonja Radinovich CMT, CST
San Joaquin Valley College
Salida, California

Dave Riedinger, BS, MS, LMT, NMT
American Institute of Alternative Medicine
Dublin, Ohio

Margie Schaeffer, M.Ed
Synergy Massage
Blue Ridge Summit, Pennsylvania

Victoria J. Stone, MA, NCMT
Blue Ridge School of Massage & Yoga
Blacksburg, Virginia

Pete Whitridge BA, LMT
Florida School of Massage
Gainesville, Florida

About the Author

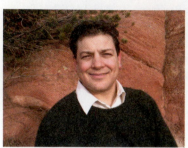

James began his studies at the University of Colorado where in 1991 he earned a bachelor's degree in secondary education. In addition to teaching, James had a long interest in healing and holistic therapies. This led him to continue his schooling and earn a diploma in therapeutic massage.

After maintaining a practice for a number of years James decided to expand his practice and began his master's degree study of traditional Chinese medicine. During the course of his studies James self-published his first book, a study guide for TCM national exams.

Upon graduation in 1998, James returned to Colorado to develop his practice. He blended his unique style of massage with the techniques of acupuncture, herbology, and exercise physiology to establish a specialty in treating physical injury. Specializing in physical medicine and injury care, James has had the opportunity to work with members of the Tampa Bay Buccaneers, the Colorado Rapids, and the Denver Nuggets.

Through the years James has had the opportunity to combine his love of animals with his skills in the healing arts by treating injured wild animals with a local wildlife rescue organization. More recently he has worked with trainers and veterinarians to apply his unique style of treatment to horses and other animals.

In the year 2000 James began the pursuit of his teaching aspirations as he moved forward in his career as an educator. James has spent the past decade teaching, developing curricula, and writing text materials for coursework in anatomy and physiology as well as massage and traditional Chinese medicine. James currently lives and teaches in Colorado, where he continues to expand his knowledge in the healing arts and share his passion for teaching with those around him.

Contents

PART 5   THE ACUPRESSURE APPROACH   275

Preface

GET THE MOST FROM THIS BOOK

This textbook is designed to create many opportunities for effective learning. Repetition is important for understanding and remembering information. To get the most from your reading, begin by going over the Chapter Objectives and Key Terms. Also skim through the headings and Quick Quizzes of the sections you'll be reading. This will prepare your mind to look for key concepts as you read the material.

Once you have finished a section, use the Chapter Summary to reinforce the main ideas that you've learned about. Answer the Discussion Questions to solidify your understanding and to review and reinforce any information that may have been challenging.

GET THE MOST OUT OF TEACHING FROM THIS BOOK

This textbook is designed to be flexible and easily adapted to various curricula. Each chapter can stand alone so that the chapters can be taught in any order. In some cases it is more practical to present portions of theoretical and "hands-on" information simultaneously. The information within chapters is broken down so that portions of each may be presented together.

This book is also designed to provide a variety of teaching opportunities. Quick Quizzes and Discussion Questions can be used for assignments or discussion topics to help your students review and retain information. Holistic Connections and Did You Know? boxes provide additional opportunities for discussion topics or independent investigation assignments. Sample protocols can be used as classroom hands-on exercises. The supplemental teacher materials offer further tools for using this text to its fullest.

A HOLISTIC APPROACH TO BODYWORK

Holistic means incorporating a wide range of possibilities into the practice of massage. It also means looking at each client as a whole person—at all times remembering that the client is more than the sum of his or her many parts.

Massage and bodywork is practiced in some form in almost every culture. There are ancient techniques as well as cutting-edge modern applications. The field is continuously evolving, changing, and reinventing itself.

It is therefore impossible to include every approach and idea within a single book. The core of this book is to provide an opportunity to learn the fundamentals of different representative methods. It is about keeping a broad perspective on massage and a clear focus on the overall well-being of the individual clients that we serve.

ABOUT THIS BOOK

Like many teachers in my field, I am also a practitioner of massage. I had practiced massage and traditional Chinese medicine for over 10 years before taking over a classroom. Over the years, I grew to appreciate the multitude of massage techniques and theories available to me. After a while I found that I had integrated the techniques and approaches so much that I was challenged when presented with the task of teaching the basics individually. My task as an instructor was to find a way to teach the basic concepts and techniques separately and still lead the student toward a holistic perspective.

As I developed lessons and materials for my classes, I realized that each approach to bodywork could be defined through the unique scientific, historical, and theoretical perspectives that influenced it. This became the basis for my classroom and eventually for this book.

This text examines four approaches to bodywork that provide a representative sample of ideas and which create a strong foundation of basic techniques (deep tissue massage, neuromuscular therapy, myofascial therapy, and acupressure). In organizing the information for this text, I asked four basic questions about each of the core approaches:

What Is the Physiology Behind the Approach?

- Exploring the anatomy and physiology as defined by each major approach gives a deeper understanding of the effects the techniques have on the tissues.

What Are the Major Theories Behind the Approach?

- Viewing the history, the major thinkers, and the theories that helped define each approach is meant to take the study of massage to a high level.

What Are the Fundamental Techniques of the Approach?

- Boiling down the multitude of available techniques to a few that best represent a broad spectrum of options allows the student to work with a few simple principles and develop them into their own blend and style.

How Are the Techniques Applied in Practice for Effective Therapy?

Learning to organize and combine techniques and theories becomes easier with demonstration and practice.

Answering these questions provided the basic framework for presenting material about these massage modalities.

It can be said that the difference between a "beginning" and "advanced" level of ability is having a more practiced understanding of the basics. This book is designed to develop the basics and to provide the opportunity to rehearse the skills toward developing advanced abilities.

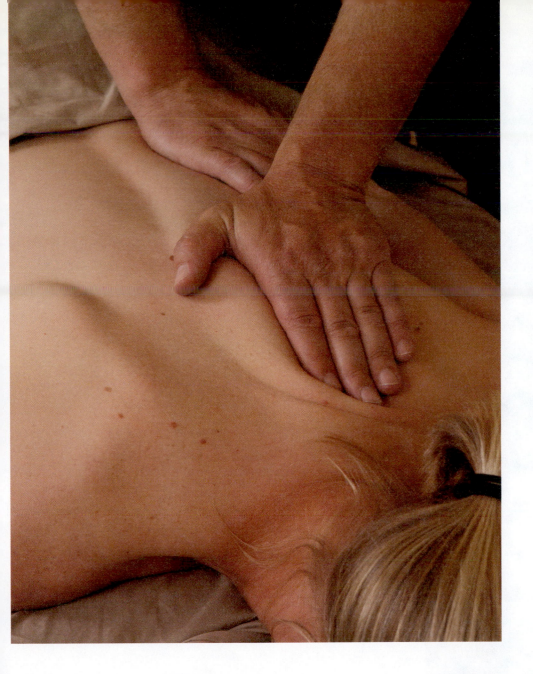

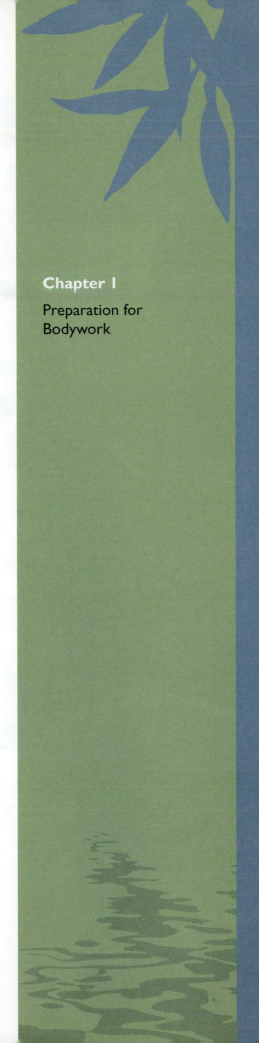

PART

1

Getting Started

1 Preparation for Bodywork

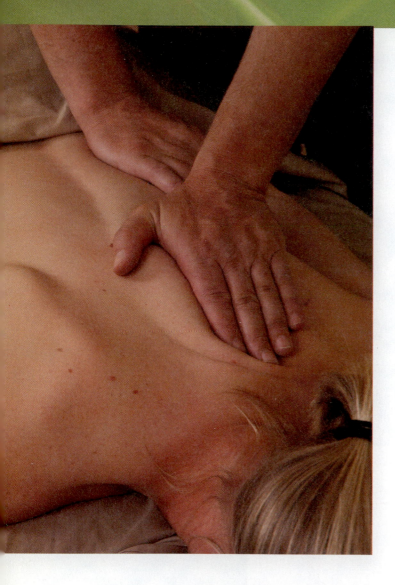

CHAPTER HIGHLIGHTS

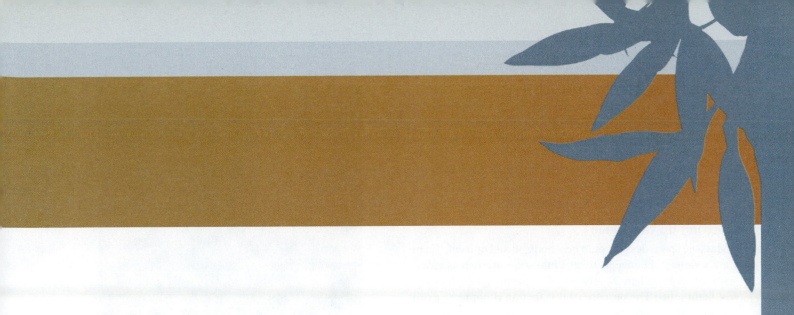

CHAPTER OBJECTIVES

- Identify key details in preparing a massage space
- Explore the components of a therapist's preparation for bodywork
- Learn the basics of postural analysis

- Establish planning and record-keeping basics for therapeutic massage practice
- Understand the proper preparation for massage clients
- Consider the best areas and methods for starting a massage

KEY TERMS

BEFORE PERFORMING BODYWORK

Bodywork is a healing art that requires preparation on all levels. How you prepare for a therapy session is just as important as how you apply the specific techniques. To lay the groundwork for success, it is important to consider preparations for the space, the therapist, and the client. Preparation is the foundation upon which the application is built.

Setting Up the Space

Massage space design could be a book, in and of itself. There are a variety of concepts to take into account, such as accessibility, color schemes, artwork placement, and the location of bathrooms. The purpose of this section is not to be a full discourse on massage settings, but rather a simple discussion of the basic elements needed to effectively perform professional massage therapy.

Constant communication between the client and therapist is essential to good bodywork. Therefore, the room must be free of noisy distractions. The room should be clean and tidy. The lighting should be soft and indirect, to prevent it from shining in the client's eyes.

Bodywork relies on your body posture and footwork in order to apply the techniques. The proper stance can be very wide; therefore, you must make sure there is enough room around the table to stand in a deep lunge without bumping into furniture. Make sure the floor is clear of debris. Be sure you can move about unencumbered. This will help you flow from movement to movement, which is especially important during stretching techniques.

The table height should be at or below the tips of your fingers when you are standing next to the table with your arms at your sides (see Figure 1.1 ■). This may seem very low at first, but you will find, after practicing the proper body mechanics, that a low table actually lends itself to preventing stress on your body.

Because bodywork affects the body on many levels, and because clients are at rest, they will often respond with chills. Make sure the room is at a comfortable temperature, and keep extra towels, sheets, or a light blanket handy to cover clients and warm them up. I have used a heating pad on the table to keep the client warm while I keep the room cooler for my comfort. Some practitioners use heated rice bags on the hands and feet to help keep the client relaxed and warm.

Preparing Yourself

GATHERING INFORMATION

The very first level of personal preparation is to obtain the necessary knowledge. A therapist should first gain a working knowledge of the muscular structures. You should not only know what muscles are affected, but also the origin, insertion, action, and the primary direction of fibers for each. Also know the major nerves and nerve roots that feed each muscle. This is important because proper bodywork impacts both mechanical and neurological structures. When treating uncommon or complicated areas, review reference materi-

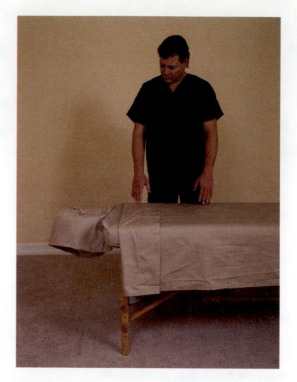

FIGURE 1.1

The Proper Table Height for Good Leverage

als, such as muscle charts, before the session. Make sure you are familiar with the muscles upon which you will be working. This is especially important when the situation is complicated by injury or surgery.

Be sure to understand the physiology and principles behind the techniques you will be using. It is critical to thoroughly comprehend the proper application of the techniques you plan to use. Review reference materials when you plan to include a method that you don't use very often.

These techniques should be well practiced on healthy individuals before attempting to work on clients with pathology. Plenty of practice on relatively healthy clients will develop the necessary sensitivity of touch, without the risk of exacerbating an injured client's condition.

Body workers must consistently keep abreast of new information regarding massage techniques and theory, as well as new information about anatomy and physiology. Seek out current books and periodicals. Continuing education programs are also an excellent way to expand knowledge in the field of bodywork.

PREPARING YOUR BODY

Gaining the proper knowledge is only the first step in personal preparation. The next step is to prepare your body for the physical nature of bodywork. Mechanics maintain their equipment to ensure that it will work for a long time. Massage therapists must also take care of their equipment—their bodies. The physical body needs maintenance to be able to apply the techniques effectively and to avoid being overtaxed.

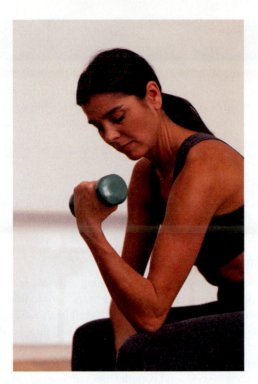

FIGURE 1.2

Weight Training Is Important to Build Strength and Stamina

Athletes must work out their muscles to prepare for competition. Their training session is usually more rigorous than the actual contest. They train harder than they compete because it makes their bodies perform at a higher level and it helps their bodies become more resistant to injuries. Massage therapists should follow this same principle (see Figure 1.2 ■).

Strengthening   Massage therapy is a very physical career. Each massage is a performance for which the body must be prepared. Because it is strenuous, there is a tendency to allow the bodywork to be the only form of exercise. This is likely to be a recipe for injury. You should exercise as an athlete does, by working out above and beyond what is required for the performance. Treatment sessions will be easier to perform, because you are prepared for a higher level of stress. Training the body is the most effective way to reduce the negative impact massage can have over time. Important as it is to exercise, don't overdo it. Moderation is the key. Use simple routines that stress multiple muscle groups in a moderate way. The exercise regime should include activities that stimulate both the muscles and the cardiopulmonary system (i.e. heart and lungs). Yoga and Pilates are great ways to achieve these basic goals. Even a simple activity, such as walking with hand weights, is an easy way to work the muscles with resistance while aerobically challenging the heart and lungs. It is a good idea to include some specific resistance work on the muscles of the shoulders and arms. These structures receive the most repetitive strain during massage.

Flexibility   In addition to resistance exercise, stretching is extremely important to preventing injury. Flexible tissues adjust more easily to the rigors of massage. Before stretching, it is important to warm up first. (Light jogging in place for a few minutes will do.) Then begin to systematically stretch all muscle groups in the body. Try to stretch at least twice per day. A good practice is to stretch all muscle groups at the beginning of the day and at the end of the day. In the morning you prepare your body for the day by stretching, and in the evening you stretch out any tension you accumulated during the day. This schedule makes it easy to remember to incorporate stretching in your daily routine (see Figure 1.3 ■).

It is also recommended to take a couple of minutes before each massage to gently stretch and loosen the major muscle groups. Often this can be done while the client is getting undressed and onto the table. This ensures that you are fully relaxed and prepared for the work to follow.

Nutrition   Along with exercise and stretching, it is important to provide proper nutritional support to the muscles, bones, and joints. The body needs the basic building blocks (proteins, vitamins, minerals, enzymes, etc.) in order to maintain and rebuild tissues. A balanced diet that contains lots of raw or slightly cooked vegetables will go a long way toward contributing to good health and a long career.

Rest and Recovery   Just as nutrition is important to recovery, so is sleep. It is important to get enough sleep so the body can recover from the day's work. During sleep the body recuperates

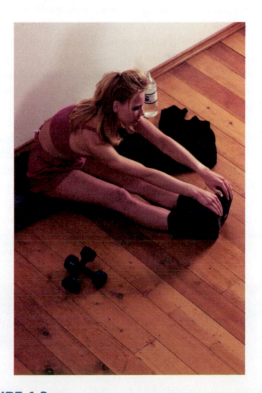

FIGURE 1.3

Yoga and Other Practices That Promote Flexibility Will Contribute to a Healthy Body

HOLISTIC CONNECTION

As a massage therapist you will be able to further the effectiveness of your treatments by assigning appropriate stretches and exercises for your clients to perform at home. By practicing stretches and exercises yourself, you will understand their benefits more fully. This will strengthen your ability to provide appropriate stretching and exercise recommendations to your clients.

and does a lot of healing. It is very difficult to muster the focus and the energy for a proper bodywork session without having enough rest.

PREPARING YOUR MIND

Focus is the key to the proper application of bodywork. It is easier to tune in to the client's experience when you are relaxed and clear-minded. This can be difficult, as it requires leaving personal problems outside of the treatment space. If you are distracted by personal affairs, the subtle clues that the client's body is sending will go unnoticed. Furthermore, the releases in the tissues may also go unnoticed. I recommend placing aside personal mental issues during the few minutes of stretching before each treatment. While stretching, take all personal thoughts, problems, and issues and place them in a mental envelope. Then, mentally file it. The mental file can be reopened after the treatment session. This type of preparation clears the head and allows for proper focus on the client.

Concentrate on relaxing by slowing down the breath rate. The breath rate is intimately coupled to both the *sympathetic* and the *parasympathetic* divisions of the nervous system. It is possible to switch from one system to the other just by increasing or decreasing the breath rate. When you increase the rate of your breaths you will stimulate the sympathetic division, which is associated with a stress response called "fight or flight." When your body is under sympathetic control, your organs slow down and your muscles become tense. If you decrease the rate of your breath, your parasympathetic division will be stimulated. This is associated with organ function and physical and mental relaxation. It is most desirable to be in the parasympathetic division.

Whenever tension seems to be building up in your body and mind, simply concentrate and slow your breath rate to encourage relaxation. It is especially important to maintain

a slow breath rate during bodywork as it helps to maintain good posture and encourages relaxation for both the therapist and the client.

PREPARING A TREATMENT PLAN

Assessing, Planning, and Record Keeping   Before performing any type of massage on a client, it is important to first obtain a proper assessment of the client's overall health and specific conditions. Using this information, you will then be able to prepare a treatment plan.

Within the field of massage there tends to be a great deal of variation in styles and completeness of assessment as well as record keeping. It is very common that formal history, assessment, and treatment planning is minimized or even bypassed. This is often because in many massage therapy settings there is an allotted time for sessions, and that time is to be spent performing massage. Therefore the assessment is performed at the same time that therapy is being applied (i.e., palpation occurs during the warm-up of tissues). Essentially, a therapist performs these tasks "on the fly" during treatment. This makes it difficult to formulate a proper plan as well as keep good records of the assessment and treatment session.

Taking a few minutes before the therapy to assess the client and record the findings will greatly improve the therapy session. You will have a much clearer picture of the problems the client is experiencing and a system for developing a treatment plan to address the client's specific needs. Documenting the session is a very important element to this process. When the information is written in an organized format, it is easier to see the pathological patterns as well as keep track of the assessment process.

As massage has become more widely applied in clinical and medical settings, it has become more important to achieve higher standards of documentation and records management. Specifically, there is a need to be in line with proper medical record-keeping techniques. These records are legal documents as well as a way for you to track and develop treatment plans. In fact, insurance companies often require copies of your records to review as "proof of reasonable and necessary care" in order to reimburse you for treatment. Furthermore, in many states you are required by law to keep proper records of your therapy sessions.

No matter the setting in which you will be performing massage, it is important to be skilled in performing proper assessment, planning, and record-keeping techniques.

DID YOU KNOW

In my practice, I perform four or five slow deep breaths before entering the room to massage. This clears my mind, energizes my body, and gets me focused.

The **SOAP** method is one of the most common ways in which an assessment and treatment plan are organized and documented. Each letter stands for a section in the assessment and planning process. This helps to keep the information organized and provides a simple acronym to help you remember all of the components that are needed for a proper assessment. (See Appendix 1 for sample SOAP notes forms.)

- The **S** stands for *subjective information*. Information reported by the client is placed in this section. This is the health survey described below.
- The **O** stands for *objective information*. Information gained from the physical evaluation (including postural analysis, palpation, and range of motion) is placed in this section.
- The **A** stands for *assessment*. Use the information from the subjective and objective analyses to formulate an assessment of the client's condition (S + O = A).
- The **P** stands for *plan*. In this section, a plan is developed to treat the pathologies.

Health Survey (Subjective Information)

General Health Information

A good client history should include a **health survey** to review the client's general health. Their present physical condition is a result of a huge variety of circumstances, including past history of injury, as well as environment, nutritional habits, thoughts, and emotions. This information will give insight into the client's current complaints and will also help reveal which, if any, types of therapies are *contraindicated* at this time.

Information Specific to the Client's Complaint

Clients are the best source of information about their conditions. Ask the client exactly how the injury occurred or how the pathology developed. Understanding the process of how the situation developed often helps isolate the specific structures involved.

In addition to the development of the pathology, here are a few other general questions to ask the client about their symptoms:

1. When did you first notice your symptoms?
2. What makes it worse/better?
3. Does rest or exercise make it better or worse?
4. Do you notice it is worse when you are stressed or upset?
5. Was there any significant change of environment at the time of onset?
6. Did you get a new chair at work, a new bed, etc.?

Listen carefully to your client, and pay attention to any emotions or thoughts patterns that are associated with the condition. This will help you as you tailor your plan to the client's emotional as well as physical needs.

It is also important to determine whether the client is receiving care from a physician. If so, it is generally helpful to work with the client's physician to develop a massage treatment strategy. In some cases it may be necessary to have a doctor's permission before providing treatment. Be aware of the regulations in your licensing area. In addition to consulting with the client's physician it is important to obtain a list of medications the client is currently taking. Familiarize yourself with the medication, including its effects and side effects. Some medications, such as blood thinners, cause the client to be susceptible to bruising and may be a contraindication for some techniques.

QUICK QUIZ #1

1. The massage table height should be at your elbows when you stand next to the table with your arms at your sides.
   a. True
   b. False

2. The health survey includes: (Circle all that apply)
   a. Exercise habits
   b. Dietary habits
   c. Range of motion testing
   d. A treatment plan
   e. All of the above
   f. None of the above

3. The SOAP method is a style of record keeping that organizes information from the health survey, physical examination, assessment, and treatment plan.
   a. True
   b. False

4. Which of the following are important components of physical preparation for massage?
   a. Strengthening
   b. Flexibility
   c. Diet
   d. Rest
   e. All of the above
   f. a and b
   g. None of the above

5. The parasympathetic nervous system is associated with relaxation and can be stimulated by slowing the breath rate.
   a. True
   b. False

Physical Evaluation (Objective Information)

Postural Analysis

First observe the client. Note the posture, as well as the position of the joints in and around the pathology. If the position of a joint is distorted, this should give clues as to which areas are tense and will need therapy.

A simple method to help identify where the body is holding tension and how it is affecting the posture is to examine the balance of specific body landmarks. This allows you to compare both sides of the body with each other to see where the tension is being held. This process, called **postural analysis,** is a systematic way of observing the body from various angles to make these comparisons.

1. *Observe the client from the side.*   In a healthy posture, the following landmarks will be in a straight vertical line from head to toe (see Figure 1.4 ■):
   A. Ear—center of the *auditory meatus*
   B. Shoulder—tip of the *acromion*
   C. Pelvis—the greater trochanter
   D. Knee—center of the epichondile
   E. Ankle—the *lateral malleolus*

2. *Observe the client from the front.*   In a healthy posture, the following landmarks will be in a straight vertical line from head to toe (see Figure 1.5 ■):
   F. Nose—the center line
   G. Chest—center of the sternum
   H. Pelvis—center of the pubis
   I. Ankle—centered evenly between both feet
   J. Feet—the arches should be even and not flat or overarched.

3. *Observe the client from the front.*   In a healthy posture the following landmarks should be on the same plane in a horizontal line across the body (see Figure 1.6 ■):
   K. Ears—the opening of the external auditory meatus
   L. Shoulders—the clavicles and the tip of the acromium
   M. Arms—should hang freely at the same distance from midline.
   N. Pelvis—the crest of the *illium* and the *anterior superior iliac spine* (ASIS)
   O. Hands—the tips of the fingers
   P. Knees—the top of the patella
   Q. Ankles—malleolus

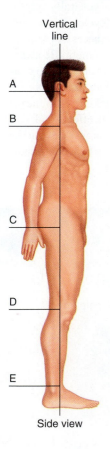

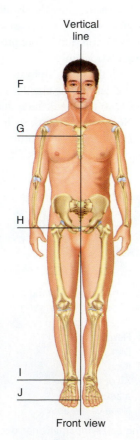

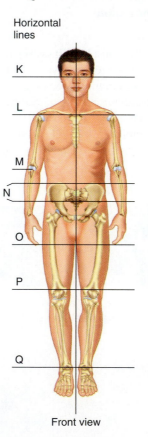

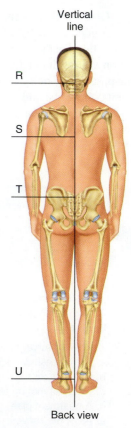

FIGURE 1.4

Landmarks on the Side of the Body Line Up Vertically in a Balanced Posture

FIGURE 1.5

Landmarks on the Front of the Body Line Up Vertically in a Balanced Posture

FIGURE 1.6

Landmarks on the Front of the Body Line Up Horizontally in a Balanced Posture

FIGURE 1.7

Landmarks on the Back of the Body Line Up Vertically in a Balanced Posture

4. ***Observe the client from the back.***   In a healthy posture the following landmarks will be in a straight vertical line from head to toe (see Figure 1.7 ■).

   R. Skull—the *nuchal line* of the occipital bone
   S. Vertebral column—entire center line (spinous processes)
   T. Pelvis—the center of the sacrum
   U. Ankle—should be centered evenly between both feet

This level of observation will give clues as to where the client is holding tension and where *compensation* has occurred. A client may have reported an injury to the right knee when you were taking the history. Your observation of posture could reveal that the right hip rests on a slightly higher plane than the left. This would indicate that compensation in the right lower back and hip has taken place. Table 1.1 ■ provides a list of muscles and how tension in them commonly affects posture.

It is important not only to observe your client while standing still, but to observe the client in motion as well. If possible, have the client attempt to perform any actions that are causing trouble so you can see the point at which the pain occurs. Have the client perform the motion on both sides of the body so you can compare the movement between the healthy side and the injured side.

Because most injuries affect many parts of the body at once, it is valuable to observe how the client walks. A healthy *gait* and *stride* should have the following characteristics:

- The head should rest evenly on the shoulders and remain steady with each stride.
- The torso should be vertical, and the shoulders should be level through the stride.
- The arms should swing freely along the sides of the body.
- The hips should move freely, rocking evenly on both sides with each stride.
- The knees should extend but not lock during the step.
- The stepping foot should clear the floor easily during the swing, then strike the floor heel first, rolling through the big toe to push off for the next step.

TABLE 1.1	**Common Effects of Muscle Tension on Posture and Movement**		
Muscle Group	**Name of Muscle**	**Effects on Posture**	**Effects on Movement**
Posterior shoulder	*Trapezius*	Elevated scapula (raised shoulders) Increased cervical curve Laterally flexed neck Head rotated to the side of tension Shoulders pulled back, "militaryshoulders"	Decreased lateral neck flexion and rotation to opposite side of tension Decreased neck flexion Shoulders held still during stride
	Levator scapulae	Elevated scapula (raised shoulders) Head rotated to the side opposite the tension	Decreased lateral neck flexion to same side of tension Decreased rotation to opposite side of tension Decreased neck flexion
	Latissimus dorsi	Medial rotation of arms (back of hand facing front) Rounded shoulders (pulled to the front)	Decreased arm abduction Decreased forward swing of arm during stride
Rotators of the shoulder	*Supraspinatus*	Arms abducted (arms hanging away from the body)	Arms swing away from body during stride
	Infraspinatus	Arms laterally rotated (palms facing front)	Decreased internal rotation of arm (palm facing forward during swing of arm)
	Subscapularis	Arms medially rotated (back of hands facing front)	Decreased lateral rotation of arm Back of hands face front during stride
Anterior shoulder	*Pectoralis major*	Medially rotated arms (back of hands face front) Rounded shoulders Thoracic *hyperkyphosis* (spine bent forward, "dowager's hump")	Decreased flexion and horizontal abduction of arm at the shoulder Arms swing across the front of the body during stride
	Pectoralis minor	Thoracic hyperkyphosis Scapular abduction (outward rotation of inferior angle) Lower border of scapula flares out, "scapular winging"	Decreased flexion of arm (at the shoulder), arms swing across the body during stride

(Continued)

TABLE 1.1 **Common Effects of Muscle Tension on Posture and Movement** *(Continued)*

Muscle Group	Name of Muscle	Effects on Posture	Effects on Movement
Anterior arm	*Biceps brachii*	Elbows chronically flexed (bent)	Decreased elbow extension
	Forearm flexors	Fingers, wrist chronically flexed	Decreased wrist and finger extension
Neck and Spine	*Sternocleidomastoid*	Craniocervical extension Cervical *hyperlordosis* Neck rotated to opposite side of tension	Decreased rotation of head to the side of tension Decreased cervical extension
	Scalenes	Shallow breathing Elevated first and second ribs	Increased shoulder elevation during inspiration Lateral neck flexion to the side of tension
	Erector spinae	"Forward head" posture Craniocervical extension Cervical hyperlordosis Lumbar hyperlordosis, "sway back" Anterior pelvic tilt	Decreased cervical flexion (difficulty bending neck forward) Decreased thoracic flexion (difficulty bending torso forward) Decreased lateral flexion of spine ("side bend") to the opposite side of tension
Lower torso	*Psoas*	Anterior pelvic tilt Lumbar hyperlordosis Lumbar rotation to the opposite side of tension	Decreased hip extension Decreased rotation of hip to side of tension Foot runs into floor during stride
	Quadratus lumborum	Ilium elevated on the side of tension Functionally shortened leg on side of tension	Decreased lateral flexion to the opposite side of tension
Hip	*Piriformis*	Lateral hip rotation to the side of tension Functional shortened leg	Decreased internal rotation of leg
	Tensor fascia lata	Medial hip rotation to the side of tension	Decreased posterior rotation of leg Difficulty sitting (esp. with legs crossed)
Thigh	*Hamstrings*	Posterior pelvic tilt Downward pull on ischium Locked knees when standing	Decreased hip flexion (difficulty bending forward) Decreased pelvic motion during stride Feet slap the ground during stride
	Adductors	Unlevel pubic bone (tilted down on the side of tension) "Bow-legged" stance	Decreased hip abduction (difficulty lifting leg to the side)
	Rectus femorus	Anterior pelvic tilt Raised patella Functionally shortened leg	Decreased lumbar and hip extension Foot runs into floor during forward stride
Posterior lower leg	*Gastrocnemius*	Plantar flexion when lying in supine position Locked knees when standing	Decreased dorsiflexion (difficulty pulling toes toward shins) Knees lock when stepping out Walking on toes with little heel strike
	Soleus	Plantar flexion when lying in supine position Locked knees when standing	Decreased dorsiflexion Walking on toes with little heel strike

(Lowe, 1997)

When any of these criteria are compromised, one can assume there is some form of tension affecting the client's ability to move. Table 1.1 provides a list of how tension and/or pathology in specific muscles commonly affects the body's posture and movement patterns. While this list is not exhaustive, it provides a good foundation for understanding the connections between posture, movement, and the muscles.

Palpation

The next step in the physical evaluation is palpating the tissues. Feel for tension, ropiness, *trigger points*, etc. Note the temperature of the tissues as well. Heat may indicate inflammation. Tissues with tension and lack of blood flow will feel colder than surrounding areas.

The evaluation should also include passive, active, and resisted *range of motion tests* on the affected and nonaffected sides of the client's body. Testing the side of the body that is healthy first will give a baseline as to how this client generally moves. Have the client relax, then move joints through a passive range of motion. If there is local pain during this movement, it suggests that the pathology is in the structures of the joint (i.e., the ligaments and joint capsule). The muscles are ruled out because the client's muscles are not active during this test. Only the joint and its related structures are involved.

Next, assist the client into a *static (isometric) contraction* for each of the directions the joint can be moved. Note the feeling of the muscles and related structures in each contraction. This will give insight into which muscles are involved.

It is important for the assessment to be thorough. You will be palpating all areas of possible pathology or compensation and be performing numerous range of motion tests. It is important to make note and remember all different areas of pathology. You may choose to begin palpating and testing in the primary area of complaint, then move outward from there. Or you may find a system for moving through the assessment that helps you to keep track of the various body parts and pathologies. Taking notes is an important part of the assessment and your records will help you to manage the details of your evaluation.

Assessment   This is where you combine all the information gathered through the subjective and objective processes and see how it all fits together. For example, a client complains of numbness in the fingers of the right hand (subjective information). You observe that the right shoulder is elevated. The muscles of the scalenes and trapezius are in a hypertonic state and have many trigger points (objective information). The subjective information suggests the nerve is being compressed (numbness), and the objective information suggests the muscles of the shoulder are very tense from the presence of the trigger points. Since the nerves that feed the hand pass through these affected muscles, you should assess that the nerve is possibly entrapped by the hypertonic muscles. From here you can formulate your plan on how to address the pathology found.

Treatment Plan   Once you have gathered the necessary information, it is time to develop a **treatment plan.** Sketch out the order in which the muscles will be treated. Then plan the specific techniques you will use and in what fashion you will use them. With a well thought out plan, the sessions will be more effective and efficient.

Occasionally, when executing the treatment plan formulated in your SOAP notes, you may discover that you need to change the course of the treatment and deviate from your original plan. This may be because you uncovered new information or new pathology while working on the client. It is important to make note of this new information in your notes as well as any other techniques you performed. Record this type of information in a separate "Session Comments" or "Session Notes" area of the record. You will then be able to refer back to this information when you see the client again. The newly discovered information (and any change in the treatment plan) from the previous session will be added to the objective section of the new SOAP note. The information from the previous session helps you formulate the new plan.

Any reports from the client of changes that occurred during or after the last session will go into the subjective section of the new SOAP note. An important concept to understand is that a new assessment and a new plan should be made for each treatment session. (See Appendix 1 for examples of SOAP note forms).

Preparing Your Client

Since bodywork is a powerful modality, it is especially important to prepare the client for the therapy session and for any side effects (i.e., releases and soreness) that may occur. Before the client gets on the table, sit down and explain the client's role in the process. Empower the client with control of the massage session. The client needs to know that it is important to communicate if the pressure is too much or too little. It is not uncommon for clients to resist telling the therapist that he or she is being too aggressive. This may be out of embarrassment for possibly being too sensitive, or because the thinking is that the therapist knows what he or she is doing, and if it hurts, well then, it is supposed to be that way.

Discuss with clients the different kinds of release that may occur during the therapy (the types of release are covered later in this chapter). Explain how the release of physical stress often allows an equal mental release. Make sure they are prepared to work through both levels.

 DID YOU KNOW

Tell the client to use a scale of 1 to 10 to describe the discomfort caused by your pressure. One means no discomfort; ten means too much. The scale can be used throughout the therapy to help facilitate communication and get the right pressure needed for the technique.

Explain the possibility of physical reactions to the bodywork such as nausea, vomiting, and headaches. The exact mechanism behind these types of physical reactions is unclear. There is some suggestion that a process known as rhabdomyolysis may be partly to blame. *Rhabdomyolysis* is the rapid breakdown of muscle tissue due to injury, immobility, or prolonged inflammation. Most cases of rhabdomyolysis develop as a result of muscle injury or strain, or other causes such as medications or drugs. Deep forms of bodywork may also damage the muscle causing rhabdomyolysis. The breakdown of muscle tissue leads to the release of substances including proteins (especially myoglobin), enzymes, and histamines into the bloodstream (Lai et al., 2006). Massage increases circulation of blood and lymph, essentially flushing these products through the bloodstream. Their increased presence in the bloodstream may directly stimulate the *emetic center* of the brain, located in the medulla, causing nausea and vomiting (Marieb, 2004). When discussing physical reactions with the client, it is not desirable to provoke anxiety; but explaining the possibilities ahead of time can save the client confusion if they do occur.

It is also important to explain the difference between therapeutic massage and relaxation massage. Therapeutic bodywork is not always comfortable. The client may become sore and stiff later on that evening and the next day. Delayed soreness may be the result of rhabdmyolysis and the toxins released from its process.

It is important that your client be instructed to drink twice the normal intake of water, both on the day of the massage and the day after. This will help to dilute the blood as well as increase kidney function to help eliminate these products from the blood and lymph. This will help minimize soreness after the therapy.

Finally, recommend that clients take it easy on therapy days. Their bodies need the energy to recover from the treatment. It is during the recovery time that the real healing takes place. Suggest a postmassage bath including a cup of Epsom salts (magnesium sulfate). This will help further relax and detoxify the client.

DID YOU KNOW

We store memories as neural input (such as sight, smell, and sound) from our sensory organs. Emotions and ideas associated with this neural input are connected in memory. For example, the smell of peanut butter cookies may remind you of grandma and make you feel happy.

Pain is also neural input, and can trigger a memory or a feeling the same way a smell or sound will.

During massage, we may recreate the memory of pain in an injured area. The client will often remember the feelings surrounding the injury and when it happened.

Tuning In to Your Client

During treatment, it is important to be present at all times for the client. Tune in to how the client's body is reacting to the therapy. Continuously focus on feeling the tissues, always looking for subtle levels of resistance. It is often difficult to feel tensions and other muscular pathology in the deeper tissues. The tension may not be as conspicuous, so look for subtle gradients of tension. Constantly compare the tissues being massaged with the surrounding tissues. This will increase success in identifying exactly where the therapy is most needed.

Watch the client's face, body, and hands for cues as to the level of tolerance of the treatment. If wincing or clenching of fists occurs, it may be a response to using too much pressure. You must stay in constant communication with the client, asking about the level of pressure. Also, look for changes in the client's breath rate. If the client is holding his or her breath, it means the client is resisting the pressure. React by backing off and/or instructing the client to "breathe through the tension." Breathing through the tension requires that the client breathe out during the down pressure. The client's body resists less when breathing out on the down stroke. In this way the body can accept the pressure and release the tension.

Tuning in to the client involves being aware and allowing the client to release mentally as well as physically. Often, when releasing physical tension, a client must also release the mental tension that contributed to the physical tension. As clients relax into the therapy, it is not uncommon for them to begin to talk about the causes of the stress. This is a way of unloading the mental stress as the massage releases the physical stress. This release of tension also manifests in other ways. The following is a short list of common forms of **release.**

- *Sighing* is probably the most common mental and physical release. When clients begin to relax they will sometimes spontaneously take deep breaths and sigh.
- *Moving* around during therapy, such as shifting or giving in to the pressure, is also common. As long as the movement isn't a *guarding* response, it is confirmation that the techniques are working.
- *Yawning* is a way to expel built up carbon dioxide, which often accumulates in patterns of shallow, stressed breathing. As the clients relax, they may yawn to cleanse the lungs. This may also be a release of tension in the face and neck.
- *Crying and yelling* are probably the most severe types of release. These strong forms of release are sometimes seen in clinic. They occur because the emotions tied to the stressful holding pattern may be so strong that when the body physically lets go, the related emotions are also released.

The body can release stress in as many ways as the tension was created. Responses can be as subtle as slight changes in breathing patterns or more obvious vocal releases, such as moaning. They can also be very strong reactions, like shivering.

HOLISTIC CONNECTION

Before and during the application of traditional Chinese therapies such as acupressure, it is very important for the therapist and client to focus their Qi, or "energy." Working with energy, intention, and focus is a common thread in holistic healing practices. To learn more about Qi see Chapters 14–16.

Be prepared to assist a client if an especially strong release occurs. If a client does experience a particularly strong reaction, be aware that the client is very vulnerable in this condition. The best response is just to be there for the client. Avoid offering any advice unless you are a qualified counselor. Sit quietly or hold the client's hand and let the client work through it. You may need to suspend the treatment for a few moments or the entire day. This will give the client time to reconcile emotions.

INITIATING BODYWORK

There are many different ways to begin massage. You may choose to begin a massage in a variety of areas of the body and with the client in any of several common positions. In the **prone position,** the client is lying face down, and in the **supine position** the client lies face up. You may choose to have the client in a **side-lying position** or even in a seated position at a massage chair. It is important to take into consideration a few key concepts when choosing the first area to treat and the initial position for the client. Ask yourself important questions such as these:

- What is the most comfortable position for the client?
- Does the client have experience receiving massage? (If so, where and what type?)
- Where is the client comfortable receiving massage?
- Where is the focal area of therapy?
- Where is the client storing most of the tension?
- How do you plan to work through your treatment plan? (Arrange to maximize time for target areas, minimize redraping, repositioning, etc.)
- Do you want to apply heat to any areas while working another area?

Remember that lying on the massage table may cause some clients to feel vulnerable. Clients receiving massage for the first time may be more comfortable receiving massage on particular areas of the body (e.g., neck, shoulders, feet). Each body position has its own set of benefits and challenges. Keep these ideas in mind as you consider your starting position.

QUICK QUIZ #2

1. Sighing, moving, and yawning are common forms of release.
   a. True
   b. False

2. Which of the following are important ways to prepare clients for massage? (Circle all that apply)
   a. Inform the client about possible physical and emotional releases.
   b. Instruct the client to drink plenty of water following massage.
   c. Explain to the client that feedback on the massage therapy and pressure is important.
   d. All of the above
   e. None of the above

3. Which of the following are indicators of compromised posture? (Circle all that apply)
   a. When viewed from the side, the ear is in a straight vertical line with the shoulder.
   b. When viewed from the side, the ear sits in a plane forward of the shoulder.
   c. When viewed from the front, the tips of the left fingers rest higher than the tips of the right fingers.
   d. When walking, the knees are extended.
   e. When walking, the head bounces with each stride.

4. When deciding how to initiate a massage session, it is important to consider: (Circle all that apply)
   a. the comfort level of the client.
   b. the primary complaint of the client.
   c. the overall treatment plan.
   d. All of the above
   e. None of the above

SUMMARY

Preparation is extremely important to the effective application of bodywork. A massage space should be set up for the comfort of the client and for the ease of movement of the therapist.

Massage is quite physically demanding of the therapist. It requires an understanding of the correct application of techniques, as well as physical and mental focus on the task at hand.

Before beginning treatment with massage it is important to gather a comprehensive history and assessment, and to work out a treatment plan. It is best to use a SOAP note format to properly document the assessment and massage session.

Postural assessment is a significant component of gathering information about the client's condition. It is important to become familiar with a variety of symptoms of posture, gait, and stride and how they are related to muscle tension and pathology.

Bodywork requires good communication between therapist and client. Ask clients to assign a number to the level of discomfort they are feeling using the scale of 1 to 10. Be sure to tell them that they are in control of the session and that their feedback is important to the session. They can request more or less pressure, or stop the treatment at any time. Be sure that clients are as mentally present as possible.

Bodywork and massage is a dance that takes two people. Learning to adjust the work to the client's needs and tolerance will make for very effective therapy. Learn to turn personal thoughts off and listen to the client's words and body. Ask for feedback as to how the client is doing and what the client is experiencing, as things change from minute to minute.

Massage is applied intensively on the client's body. Remember that release can come about in many ways including shaking, yawning, sighing, crying, and more. Be prepared to work with the client and possibly interrupt a session if serious releases occur.

How and where to start a massage depends on many factors and is an important consideration in the application of the treatment plan. The most important component to consider is the comfort of the client.

DISCUSSION QUESTIONS

1. Why is it important to prepare mentally and physically for massage therapy?
2. Why is it important to make a new assessment and treatment plan for each session with a client?
3. Explain the differences between the parasympathetic and sympathetic nervous systems.
4. In what ways might tension and pathology in the posterior shoulder affect a client's posture and movement?

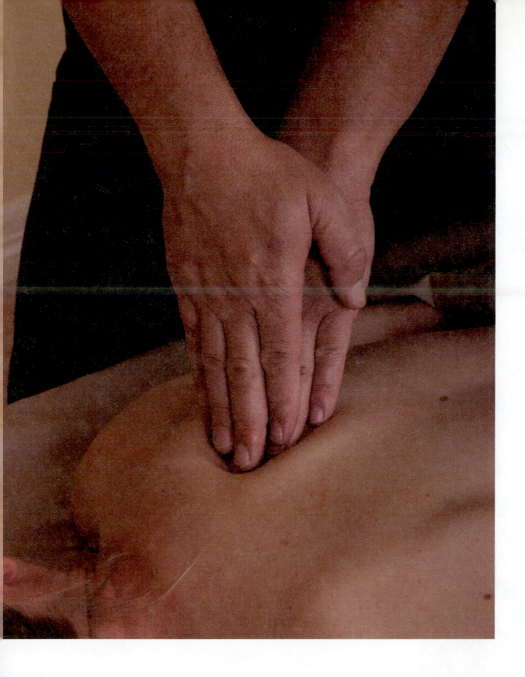

PART

2

The Deep Tissue Approach

2 A Study of Tissues

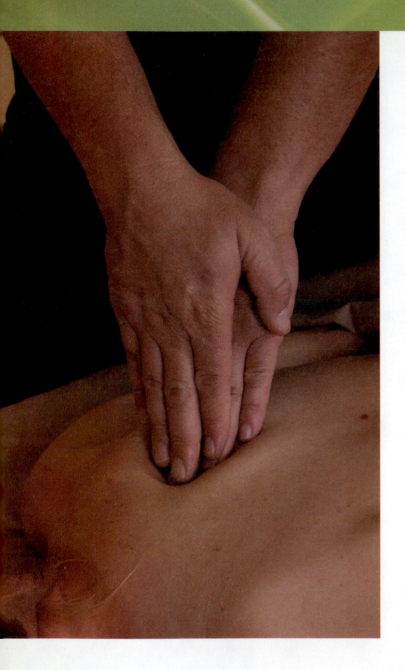

CHAPTER HIGHLIGHTS

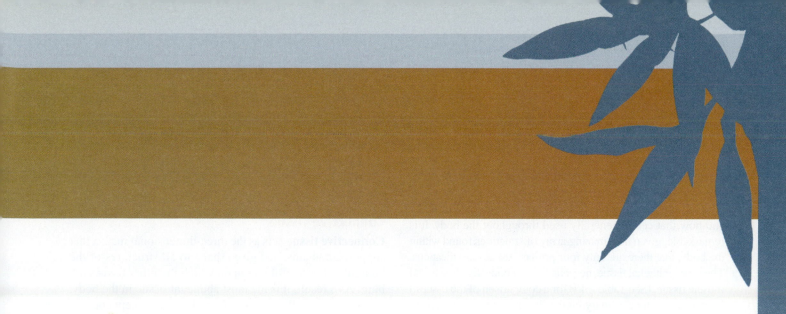

CHAPTER OBJECTIVES

- Classify and recognize different tissue types
- Understand the concept of deep tissue
- Explore the injury process and its effect on the body

KEY TERMS

CLASSIFYING TISSUES

Massage therapists are specialists in working with the soft tissues of the body. Therefore, it is important to have a strong foundation of knowledge about the physiology of tissues. In the field of **histology,** the study of tissues, "deep tissue" is not a common classification of tissues. In fact, the tissues of the body are classified according to each tissue's individual structure and function. Classification depends on what type of cell the tissue is made of and how that cell is generally used throughout the body. It is remarkable, given the amazing array of structures found within the body, that there are only four primary tissue classifications. They are: epithelial tissue, nervous tissue, connective tissue, and muscle tissue. (See Table 2.1 ■ for a comparison of the tissues.) Each of these four primary classes has numerous sub-classes. This discussion will focus on the four primary classifications and will elaborate upon those most relevant to massage.

Epithelial Tissue

Epithelial tissue acts as the covering for the body's structures. It functions to protect underlying tissues and provide the surface for absorption and secretion. This tissue makes up the outer surface of the skin (including the eye) and lines the interior of the respiratory and digestive tracts. It also lines the interior of blood vessels and organs and provides the interior surface for all body cavities.

Nervous Tissue

Nervous tissue provides the electrical control and communication system for the body. It is composed of the nerve fibers called *neurons*, which branch from the brain and spinal cord along the spinal column and reach into all structures of the body. They provide the pathway for the exchange of information between organs, other nervous tissues, the brain, and the spinal cord. The spinal cord is a fast moving information interchange system between the nerves and brain. The brain is the master controller, taking in information, analyzing it, and then sending out a proper response.

Connective Tissue

Connective tissue acts as the three-dimensional matrix that supports, contains, and gives shape to all structures of the body. It is the scaffolding upon which the other tissues are built. As a result, it is the most abundant tissue in the body. If one removed all the tissues from the body except connective tissue, all of the individual structures such as muscles, organs, etc., would still be discernable because connective tissue makes up most of their structure. The amount of connective tissue, however, is not evenly distributed. It is most abundant in structures needed for support, and is found in its most profound quantities in bone, *tendons*, *ligaments*, cartilage, and the skin. The brain, by contrast, contains very little connective tissue (Turchaninov, 2006).

Connective tissue is composed of a matrix of three major substances:

- **Collagen fibers** are white fibers that are often visible in tendons and *fascia*. Collagen fibers are strong and unyielding. These fibers add stability to connective tissue due to their relative inflexibility and great tensile strength.

TABLE 2.1	Comparison of the Various Tissues of the Body	
	Primary Location	Function
Epithelial Tissue	• Outer surface of the skin (including the eye) • Interior of the respiratory and digestive tracts • Interior of blood vessels, organs • Interior surface for all body cavities	• Cover and protect the body's structures; function to protect underlying tissues • Provide location for absorption and secretion of nutrients and waste
Nervous Tissue	• Brain • Spinal cord • Reaches into all structures of the body	• Provides electrical control and communication system • Pathway for the exchange of information between organs, the brain, spinal cord, and other nervous tissues
Connective Tissue	• All structures of the body • Most abundant in bone, tendons, ligaments, cartilage, and the skin	• Supports, contains, and gives shape to all structures of the body
Skeletal Muscle Tissue	• All over the body, both superficially and deep within the core • Attached to bone and other structures	• Responsible for all of the movements of the body • Limb movement and locomotion
Cardiac Muscle Tissue	• Only found within the walls of the heart	• Propels the blood throughout the body
Smooth Muscle Tissue	• In the walls of hollow organs such as the intestines and blood vessels • Hollow canals of various organs	• Contractions propel material through vessels and the hollow canals of organs

- **Reticular fibers** are very fine fibers containing a slightly altered form of collagen protein. They branch throughout the matrix forming a type of spider web of support and stability.
- **Elastic fibers** are yellow fibers that have some ability to stretch and recoil. They contain the protein elastin and add flexibility to the connective tissue matrix.
- **Ground substance** is a semigelatinous material that fills in the space between the cells and fibers. This material varies in *viscosity* depending on warmth and hydration. The warmer the ground substance, the more fluid it is. The colder the ground substance, the thicker it becomes.

These four substances make up all connective tissue. However, the ratio of each varies depending on the tissue's individual function. For example, tendons and ligaments are classified as "dense, regular connective tissue." They have a higher ratio of aligned collagen fibers and less elastin and ground substance. Tendons connect muscles to bone, and ligaments connect bone to bone. Therefore, they need a high ratio of strong collagen fibers to give them the ability to withstand external forces on the joints and muscles (Turchaninov, 2006).

Fascia, on the other hand, is classified as "loose, irregular connective tissue," which has a higher ratio of elastin and reticular fibers and more ground substance. Fascia is a flexible netting that provides form and stability to the body's organs, muscles, and vessels. Since fascia wraps and provides structure to all of the body's organs and tissues, it needs flexibility. The irregularity of the fiber arrangement helps it withstand forces in all directions (Turchaninov, 2006).

It is important to understand the form and function of fascia, because it plays an important role in the structure of muscles. All muscle fibers are wrapped in fascia (*endomysium*). All groups (*fascicles*) of muscle fibers are also wrapped in fascia (*perimysium*). Then the whole muscle is wrapped in fascia (*epimysium*). All of the fascia continues out of the muscle, thickens, and becomes the tendon (see Figure 2.1 ■).

Fascia performs the role of both separating and joining different parts of the muscle to and from other muscle groups as well as the bones. Figure 2.2 ■ shows a cross section of a lower leg. The figure shows the bones wrapped in fascia and the fascial seams that separate and surround the muscles.

Fascia not only provides structure for the muscle, it is also involved in healing and managing pathology or injury to the muscle. When muscle fibers are torn, the surrounding connective tissue grows a matrix in the form of a scar across the tear. The scar matrix contains a high ratio of collagen fibers. Therefore, it is not very flexible. Because of this rigidity, it can be a source of chronic pain (Werner, 2005).

Muscle Tissue

Muscle tissue is responsible for all of the movements of the body. All muscle tissue is made up of thousands of elongated cells called *muscle fibers*, which contain myofilaments made of the proteins *actin* and *myosin*. These myofilaments have the ability to slide across each other in a ratchetlike action.

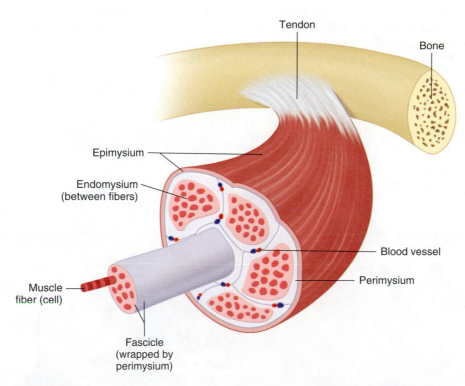

FIGURE 2.1

The Components of the Muscle Are Individually Wrapped in Fascia.

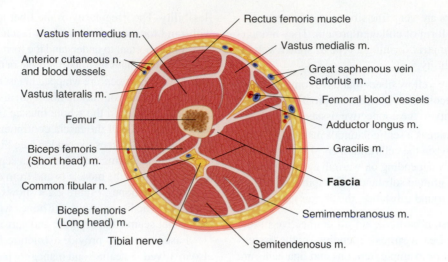

Vastus intermedius m.

Rectus femoris muscle

Anterior cutaneous n. and blood vessels

Vastus medialis m.

Vastus lateralis m.

Great saphenous vein
Sartorius m.

Femur

Femoral blood vessels

Biceps femoris (Short head) m.

Adductor longus m.

Common fibular n.

Gracilis m.

Biceps femoris (Long head) m.

Fascia

Tibial nerve

Semimembranosus m.

Semitendenosus m.

FIGURE 2.2

A Cross Section of the Lower Leg Shows How the Individual Muscles, Bones, Vessels and Nerves Are Divided by Fascia

This is what makes the muscle fiber contract (see Figure 2.3 ■). There are three kinds of muscle in the body:

- **Skeletal muscle** is made from striated muscle fibers wrapped within fascia into bundles. Muscles are attached to bone and other structures by projections of the fascia called *tendons*. As skeletal muscles contract they pull on those bones and other structures via the tendon, creating movement and locomotion. Skeletal muscles are found all over the body, both superficially and deep within the core. Skeletal muscles are often grouped into **myotatic units.** A myotatic unit includes all the muscles that act on a specific joint. The components of a myotatic unit include:

- Agonist or "prime mover"–creates an action at a joint
- Antagonist–opposes an action at a joint
- Synergist–assists an action at a joint
- Stabilizer–helps to stabilize an action
- Fixator–holds a bone or muscle still during action

- **Cardiac muscle** is only found within the walls of the heart and is responsible for the contractions that propel the blood throughout the body.

- **Smooth muscle** occurs in the walls of hollow organs such as the intestines and blood vessels. Its contractions act to squeeze material through the hollow canals of those organs.

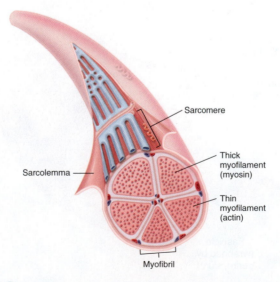

Sarcomere

Thick myofilament (myosin)

Sarcolemma

Thin myofilament (actin)

Myofibril

FIGURE 2.3

The Basic Arrangement of the Contractile Structures (Actin and Myosin Filaments) Within a Muscle Fiber

Generally speaking, all of the various organs, muscles, vessels, etc., are made from two, three, or all four tissue types. Each tissue works in concert with the others to perform that organ's particular functions. The structures we commonly refer to as "muscles" use three tissue types. They have muscle tissue to provide the contractile function. They also contain connective tissue to attach to bones and to provide structure and support. In addition, muscles have nervous tissue that permeates them to send and receive information about when to contract or relax. Skin, on the other hand, includes all four tissue types. Epithelial tissue provides a barrier to the environment. Nervous tissue senses pressure, pain, and temperature. Connective tissue provides structure to the skin. There are even tiny muscles located in the skin, called *arrector pili muscles*, that contract and raise the hairs.

WHAT IS DEEP TISSUE?

So, if deep tissue is not a common histological classification of tissues, what does it mean? The term *deep tissue* comes from the field of massage therapy. It is a compound phrase consisting of two parts: deep + tissue.

- **Deep** is an anatomical location referring to the opposite of superficial. It means "closer to the bone or to the center of the body."
- **Tissue,** in this context, refers to the **myofascial** and the **neuromuscular tissues** located in those deeper regions.

The terms *myofascial* and *neuromuscular* are medical terms that encompass three of the four tissue classes. These words can be simplified by looking at their meanings and origins (see Figure 2.4 ■).

These terms (*myofascial* and *neuromuscular*) are the clinical terms that refer to skeletal muscles and their respective nerves and connective tissues. In general conversation, we typically use the word *muscle* as a collective term to refer to skeletal muscle and the related connective and nervous tissues (i.e., myofascial and neuromuscular structures). For clarity and simplicity in this book, we will use the word *muscle* in this way. The proper medical terminology will be used when a concept warrants more detail.

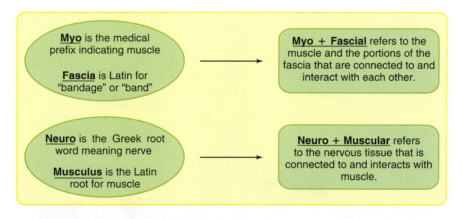

FIGURE 2.4

The Meaning of the Terms Myofascial and Neuromuscular

QUICK QUIZ #3

1. Connective tissue is comprised of: (Circle all that apply)
   a. Elastin fibers
   b. Muscle fibers
   c. Ground substance
   d. Collagen fibers
   e. All of the above
   f. None of the above

2. Smooth muscle is found only within the heart.
   a. True
   b. False

3. Fascia is composed of: (Circle all that apply)
   a. Loose connective tissue
   b. Ground substance
   c. Tendons
   d. All of the above
   e. None of the above

4. Ground substance is more fluid at warmer temperatures.
   a. True
   b. False

THE LAYERING OF MUSCLES

The muscles of the body are arranged in layers. Deep tissues are essentially those muscles found in the deeper layers of the body. For example, the back has two large superficial muscles (see Figure 2.5 ■). These are the trapezius (a diamond-shaped muscle that covers the posterior neck and shoulders) and the latissimus dorsi (a large, flat muscle that covers the entire lower back). Layered beneath those muscles is an intricate muscular network forming a middle layer. This layer is comprised of muscles such as the rhomboids, which retract and stabilize the shoulder blades. Deeper still is a layer of muscles called the erector spinae, which extend and support the spinal column (see Figure 2.6 ■). This type of arrangement of muscle layers occurs throughout the entire body. The limbs, hands, feet, torso, neck, and head all have layers of muscles that are set up in crossing patterns or reinforcing patterns.

Each muscle layer has its own purpose and varies depending upon the needs of the structure. Some muscle layers reinforce the action of other muscles, while others act only as support and stabilization. Since the deep tissues are close to the bone, they often provide a greater proportion of the stabilizing function.

The erector spinae muscles are a good example of how the deep muscles function as a stabilizing force. They lie along either side of the posterior spinal column and are deeper than most other major back muscles (see Figure 2.6). This group of muscles performs extension of the back. The muscles also assist in holding each individual vertebra in position during lateral flexion, anterior flexion, extension, and rotation of the torso. The rotator cuff muscles also provide an example of muscles with a deep stabilizing function (see Figure 2.7 ■). These deep-shoulder muscles function not only to rotate the arm as prime movers, but also help to hold the end of the humerus into the joint cavity. Therefore, the rotator cuff is responsible for a large portion of the stability of the shoulder during all arm movements.

The Process of Injury

The layering of muscles over muscles provides a series of checks and balances wherein the muscles work to support each other. However, the layering also contributes to the process of managing injury and dysfunction. This concept is

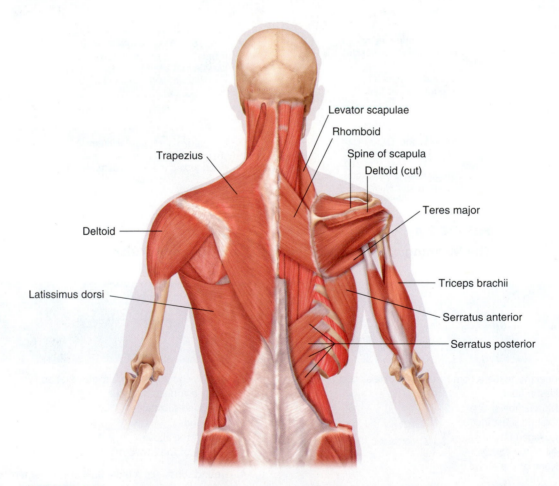

Levator scapulae
Rhomboid
Spine of scapula
Deltoid (cut)
Trapezius
Teres major
Deltoid
Triceps brachii
Latissimus dorsi
Serratus anterior
Serratus posterior

FIGURE 2.5

The Superficial Layer (Left Side) and the Middle Layer (Right Side) of Muscles on the Posterior Torso

HOLISTIC CONNECTION

The myofasia are so intimately connected that the layering of muscles and the layering of fascia are one and the same. Deep tissue massage treats fascia as well as muscle. Holistic therapies address multiple structures and multiple issues because the goal is to treat the body as a whole. For more about the layers of myofascia, see Chapters 10–13.

very important to massage therapy. Knowing how the process of injury develops in the layers assists in knowing how to relax them and encourage healing. The muscles, bones, and joints are constantly being subjected to stress from

- injury and/or repetitive strain
- gravity
- tension
- poor posture

- poor (work and hobby) ergonomics
- living habits.

The buildup of these events causes wear on the joints, ligaments, fascia, muscles, and tendons. When an area becomes overwhelmed, the body reacts by trying to **splint** the area. It does this by tightening the muscles around the affected site to hold the body secure so it can rest and heal. This splinting strategy works for the short-term, but when

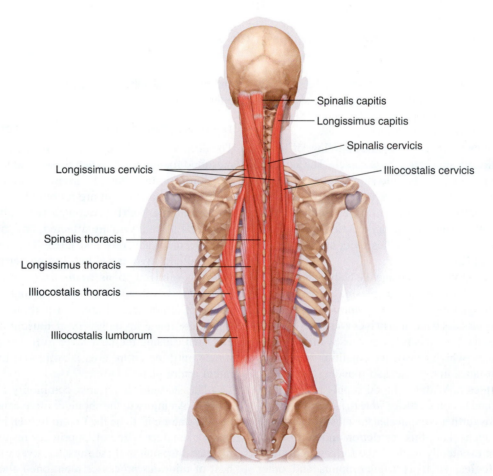

FIGURE 2.6

Depicts the Deep Layer of Muscles on the Posterior Torso

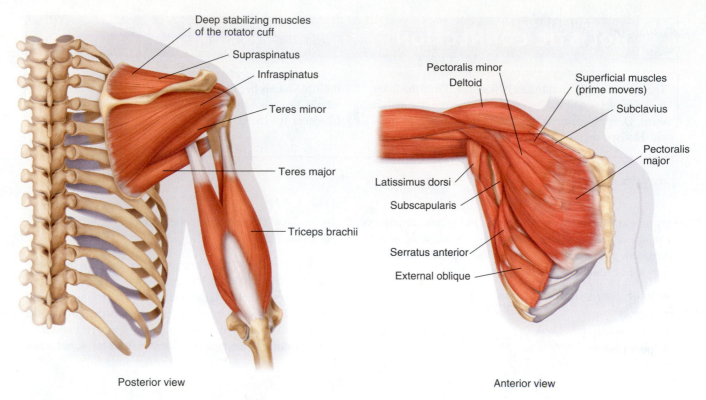

Posterior view

Anterior view

FIGURE 2.7

The Arrangement of the Rotator Cuff Muscles of the Shoulder

an injury or dysfunction is *chronic* (long-term), the splinting can have a deleterious effect on the surrounding structures and muscles. Chronic splinting can, itself, become the cause of serious injury (Turchaninov, 2006).

When muscles tighten they restrict the flow of blood and lymph by directly squeezing those vessels. The action is similar to crimping a garden hose to stop the flow of water. Without the flow of blood and lymph to the muscle cells, the muscles will lose nutrition, hydration, and the ability to expel metabolic waste. Poorly nourished, dry muscle fibers become brittle and inflexible, which makes them susceptible to damage or inflammation.

In the presence of tissue damage the body releases substances such as *bradykinin* (a plasma protein) and *prostaglandin* (a signaling molecule, or *hormone*) that stimulate the healing process but can also increase pain (Marieb, 2004). Typically, the body reacts to this pain by further tightening the muscles, which causes the condition to worsen. The ground substance in the fascia surrounding the muscle is especially affected. With the blood supply restricted, it tends to harden and become "sticky" due to lack of hydration and warmth. This further complicates the muscle's ability to function. Left unchecked, this restriction and build up of metabolic waste eventually leads to the formation of more serious **pathologies,** such as trigger points and other *myofascial adhesion* (Turchaninov, 2006). (Trigger points

and myofascial adhesions will be covered in more detail in later chapters.)

THE DEVELOPMENT OF MYOFASCIAL HOLDING PATTERNS

The deep muscles, being the stabilizers, are often the first recruited for splinting. When these deep muscles begin to develop pathology due to chronic tension, other muscles within the myotatic unit are recruited to help them. This cycle continues until it encompasses multiple layers. As more and more layers are affected, any movement at the joint becomes severely restricted. This process is clinically called a **myofascial holding pattern.** In the field, it is often referred to as **armoring,** or *armor plating*, because it is as though the body is laying down a series of plates of armor around areas of pathology. These armor plates are made up of layers of muscle clamping down and then causing the next layer to follow suit. This continues until the entire area is solid and immovable, like metal armor plates.

The shoulder is an area commonly affected by this process. An injury to the shoulder often causes the muscles of the rotator cuff to be the first to tighten because stabilizing the shoulder is one of its primary responsibilities. The increased tension in these muscles, over time, leads to the host of injurious processes mentioned above (e.g., metabolic waste build-up, brittleness, and adhesions, etc.). The

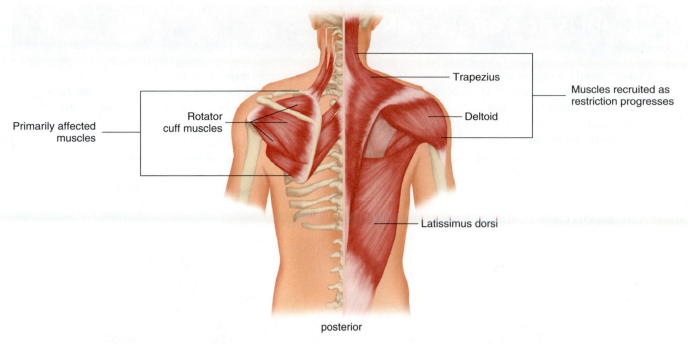

Primarily affected muscles

Rotator cuff muscles

Trapezius

Deltoid

Muscles recruited as restriction progresses

Latissimus dorsi

posterior

FIGURE 2.8

The Major Muscles of the Shoulder

restriction and developing pathology in a rotator cuff will then cause the pectoralis major, teres major, and deltoid muscles to be recruited into the action to protect it (see Figure 2.8 ■). These muscles will eventually become over-worked and chronically tense and will develop their own pathology. The resulting pain and restriction continues until all of the muscles of the shoulder (the myotatic unit) are recruited into the pathology.

The cycle may not end there. It may continue on to affect muscles outside the originally affected myotatic unit. As the first group of muscles stiffen and become less usable, other muscles and joints must do a larger portion of the work. This is called **compensation.** The body must compensate for the restriction of some muscles by using other muscles or mus-cle groups. The area doing the compensating may in turn be adversely affected since it is likely not used to this new action and may not even be built for it. Therefore, the new muscles may begin to splint up, creating new holding patterns, which lead to new compensations, and so on. This process can result in a **systemic postural dysfunction.** A systemic postural dysfunction occurs when the whole system (body) becomes affected by the original injury due to this process of com-pensation.

In other words, a local injury or holding pattern can spread from one area to another until the whole body is affected (see Figure 2.9 ■). For example, if a client injures his ankle, the muscles of the lower leg tighten to support it (1).

The restriction of movement in the tight muscles of the lower leg causes the knee to become overworked because it has to compensate (2). As the knee becomes more and more affected, the client may begin to compensate for that injury by lifting his hip on the injured side in order to take a step for-ward (3). This extra hip movement overworks the lower back muscles on that side (4). These lower back muscles become fatigued and fail to stabilize the lumbar vertebrae. This allows the back muscles to move out of place and causes pain for the client. Now the muscles of the back begin to splint to man-age the pain and injury (5). The tension alters the lateral curve of the spine causing the shoulders to be off-center (6). As the client struggles to keep his head level, his neck muscles become strained due to the imbalance caused by the offset shoulders (7). The imbalance in the neck will cause tilting of the skull, which often translates into a tilting in the jaw bone causing pain in the joint (8). What began as an ankle injury became an injury to the entire body. This process can begin to occur at any joint and may affect many other muscle groups, depending on the client and their individual circum-stances.

The longer the body continues the chronic process of splinting and compensating, the harder it becomes to treat the deep tissues. The armor plating, and often the pain toler-ance of the client, prevents getting deep enough to treat the tissues, thus requiring a specialized approach appropriately called *deep tissue massage* (DTM).

HOLISTIC CONNECTION

A fundamental concept in applying bodywork from a holistic perspective is that all areas of the body are connected. The myofascial meridians of myofascial therapy and the traditional Chinese channels of acupressure further explain the idea of how pathology is experienced throughout the whole body. See Chapters 10–13 for more about myofascial meridians. Refer to Chapters 14–17 for more information about the acupressure channels.

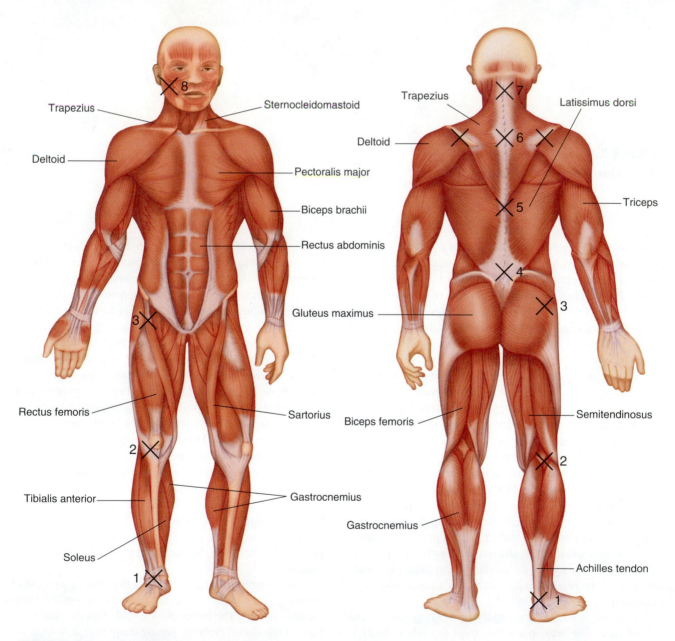

FIGURE 2.9

Beginning with an Ankle Injury, this Diagram Depicts the Sequence of Areas That May Become Affected Through the Process of Compensation.

QUICK QUIZ #4

1. Deep tissue is comprised of:
   a. Cardiac muscle
   b. Fascia and skeletal muscle in deeper anatomical regions
   c. Connective tissue in deeper anatomical regions
   d. Myofascial and neuromuscular structures in deeper anatomical regions
   e. All of the above
   f. None of the above

2. Muscles are arranged in layers only in the neck, shoulders, and back.
   a. True
   b. False

3. Deep muscle layers typically perform a greater proportion of _____.
   a. rotation
   b. anterior flexion
   c. stabilization
   d. extension

4. A systemic postural dysfunction occurs when:
   a. the entire body is affected by what was originally a local injury.
   b. the entire myotatic unit is recruited to help manage muscles affected by chronic tension.
   c. waste products such as prostaglandins and lactic acid build up in the fascia.

SUMMARY

Histology is the study of tissues. It classifies the tissues of the body into four general categories: nervous tissue, connective tissue, muscle tissue, and epithelial tissue. The structures of the body are made up of combinations of these four tissues. The muscular system of the body is constructed in layers, each having its own function. Deep tissue is a classification within the field of bodywork that refers to the muscles and connective tissues found in the deeper layers (i.e., closer to the bone).

When the body is subjected to injury, it undergoes a process called *splinting*. Splinting is essentially the tightening of the muscles and connective tissues around the injury site to secure the area so it may heal. If this splinting is present for a fair amount of time the body undergoes compensation in which new muscles and/or body parts take over for those affected. If the body parts doing the compensation become overworked, then they will begin their own splinting process. When this cycle repeats itself often enough, the whole body may become affected, causing a systemic postural dysfunction. The longer the body goes untreated, the more difficult it is to access the deeper layers of muscle which are often the first muscles recruited for splinting.

DISCUSSION QUESTIONS

1. What are the four types of tissues in the body, and what are their functions?
2. How are muscle, fascia, and tendons integrated?
3. How are the muscles of the body arranged, and how does this arrangement affect their function?
4. Describe how the layers of muscle and connective tissue respond to injury.
5. Explain how splinting causes further injury in the body.

3 Introduction to Deep Tissue Theory

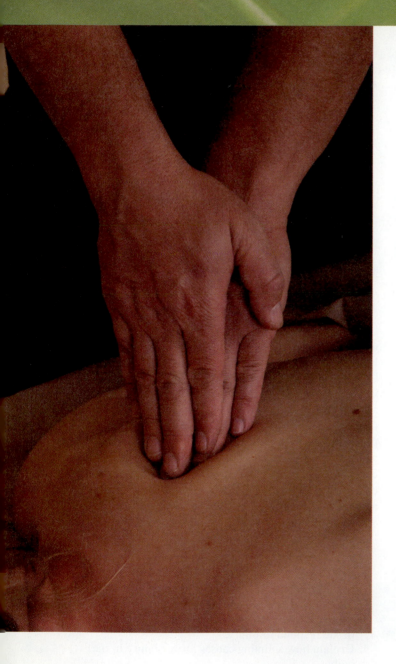

 CHAPTER HIGHLIGHTS

Chapter Objectives

Key Terms

Origins of Deep Tissue Massage

Basics of Deep Tissue Massage

Neurology and DTM

The Phases of Deep Tissue Massage

Summary

Discussion Questions

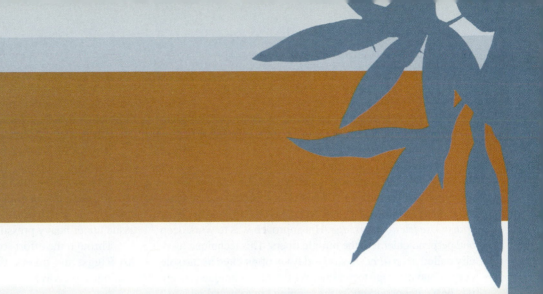

CHAPTER OBJECTIVES

- Survey the history of deep tissue massage
- Explore the connection between neurology and deep tissue massage

- Study the four phases of deep tissue massage

KEY TERMS

Proprioceptor *30*

Muscle spindle cells *31*

Golgi tendon organs *31*

Stretch reflex *31*

Guarding *31*

Reciprocal inhibition *32*

Golgi tendon reflex *33*

Passive stretch *34*

ORIGINS OF DEEP TISSUE MASSAGE

The roots of DTM reach as far back as Pehr Henrik Ling and his creation of the Swedish Movement Cure in 1814. In fact, almost all massage traditions employ some techniques aimed at working deeper into the tissues. One of the most well known deep techniques was developed by Dr. James Cyriax, a surgeon and the author of *The Textbook of Orthopedic Medicine*. In the 1940s and 1950s, he created the technique called *transverse friction massage*. His approach was to work deep and perpendicular into the muscle fibers. This technique (usually called *deep fiber friction* today) is often cited as the sole deep tissue massage technique. While this technique is deep, it is best categorized under the heading "myofascial release." This is because it focuses on the adhesions that develop in the fascial components of the muscle. (See information on deep fiber friction in the myofascial chapters of this book.)

Dr. Ben Benjamin was one of the first to design a specific system called *deep tissue massage*. He laid the groundwork for his system in the popular book, *Are You Tense*, in 1978. In this book he describes a systematic approach aimed specifically at working through the tissues to the deepest layers of muscles. He discusses the importance of using slow, even pressure to sink deeper into the fibers. To do this he developed the lean and drag technique. This technique generates pressure by leaning into the client using body weight instead of strength. The hands are then returned to the start of the stroke by firmly dragging back. Dr. Benjamin felt that staying in contact with the muscle facilitates relaxation and allows for deeper penetration of the stroke. Dr. Benjamin's ideas and his smooth, even approach laid the groundwork for modern deep tissue massage.

Today most therapists recognize the importance of treating the deep muscles, yet there is still no clear consensus about deep tissue theory and practice. There isn't even an industry-wide agreement as to its definition. To many therapists, deep tissue massage may simply mean using more pressure with regular massage strokes. While this is not entirely incorrect, there is a good argument for formalizing the theories and the best practices for working with the deep tissues of the body.

As early as the late 1980s, Art Riggs, a certified Rolfer, recognized the lack of a formal system of deep tissue massage. He developed a cohesive system of deep tissue massage and in 2002 wrote, *Deep Tissue Massage: A Visual Guide to Techniques*. In the preface to the book's second edition (2007), Riggs discusses the increasing need for certification in deep tissue massage and the industry's lack of a formalized system.

Riggs (2007) defines deep tissue massage as "The understanding of the layers of the body, and the ability to work with the tissue in these layers to relax, lengthen, and release holding patterns in the most effective and energy efficient way possible" (p. 3). Riggs' book offers one of the most cohesive systems of working from a DTM perspective. Like Ben Benjamin, Riggs discusses the importance of working efficiently by using body weight instead

of strength to apply pressure. He describes the need to work slowly. He also emphasizes the notion of getting the muscles to relax and "let go," instead of forcing the release through fast or forceful pressure.

Riggs (2007) also describes one very important element of deep tissue strokes. That is the use of oblique pressure that glides deeply through the skin's surface working the entire muscle origin to insertion. The idea is to "snowplow" through the entire muscle instead of just compressing the tissue under heavy pressure.

Through the efforts of practitioners like Ben Benjamin, Art Riggs, and others, the shape of deep tissue massage continues to evolve.

BASICS OF DEEP TISSUE MASSAGE

Deep tissue massage (DTM) is a therapeutic technique that helps reshape the client's body by treating the root of holding patterns in the deep myofascial structures. The end result is a more aligned and relaxed physique that is better able to handle the rigors of daily life. People often equate DTM with deep relaxation, when in fact DTM can be somewhat uncomfortable. There may even be a recovery time of a couple of days in which the client may experience some soreness. Deep relaxation is more likely found during a good Swedish relaxation massage.

Deep tissue massage is a modality designed to access the deeper stabilizing muscles, while simultaneously treating the more superficial ones. It is a unique system that breaks down the layers of armoring and stimulates deep neuromuscular receptors. This facilitates the release of myofascial holding patterns, allowing the body to return to normal function. When performed properly, DTM will release *systemic postural dysfunctions* (problems involving multiple joints) as well as local holding patterns (problems involving one or two joints) and adhesions. It can also assist in restoring proper breathing patterns and can even increase lung capacity when used in the thoracic region. DTM can actually treat myofascial pathology all over the body—from the hands to the feet and even the face.

Deep tissue massage affects muscles in two ways. First, it manipulates the muscle's neurological system causing it to relax and lengthen. Second, it uses a four-phased approach to systematically work through the superficial levels to disrupt then readjust the deeper layers. The four phases are elaborated upon later in the chapter. First, it is important to clarify how DTM manipulates neurological structures in order to facilitate lengthening and relaxation of muscles.

NEUROLOGY AND DTM

Within a muscle, one of the main neural structures responsible for sending and receiving information to and from the brain is the **proprioceptor.** Proprioceptors receive information from within the muscle and joint structure about the position of the body and the relative length of the muscle. They tell the brain and spinal cord when a muscle is stretching, contracting, or under stress. Through complex mechanisms, proprioceptors respond to the muscle's position and facilitate everything from contraction to relaxation. In short, proprioceptors allow for the smooth flow of all movements of the body. Different types of proprioceptors have different responsibilities and respond to different stimuli. **Muscle spindle cells** and **Golgi tendon organs** are important proprioceptors which are affected by DTM.

Muscle Spindle Cells

These proprioceptors are found in the belly of skeletal muscles (see Figure 3.1 ■). They detect when a muscle is stretched and initiate a reflex that resists that stretch. This is called a **stretch reflex.** The stretch reflex is an important safety measure. When a muscle is stretched fast and/or forcefully, the

muscle spindle initiates a contraction to protect the muscle and the joint from injury. During a physical examination, doctors test the stretch reflex of the quadriceps when they tap on the patellar ligament with a rubber mallet.

Massage therapists often experience the effects of muscle spindle cell stimulation. In the field it is called **"guarding."** A common lay term for this action is "flinching." This is a quick protective contraction of a muscle that occurs when a muscle is too tender to the touch or when the technique is applied too deeply and/or too quickly.

Muscle spindles also function to maintain muscle tone. Muscle tone (also called *tonus*) is the partial contraction of muscles. Muscle tone is important to many functions such as the ability to stand upright. Standing up requires the partial contraction of muscles of the whole upper torso as well as the legs so it can maintain an upright position.

If the posture is unbalanced, it can cause the spindle cell to become overstimulated. This will cause a muscle to be excessively or chronically contracted. A muscle in this state

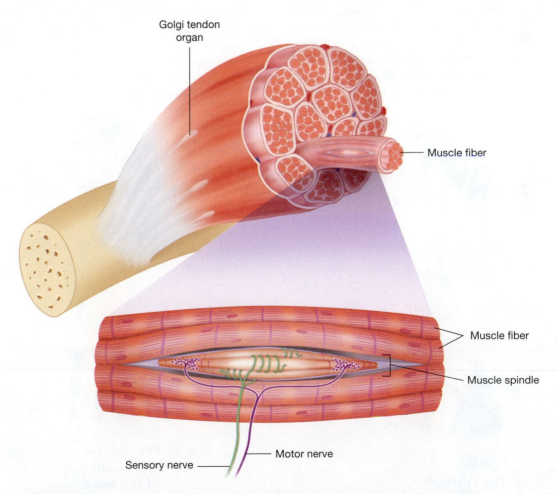

FIGURE 3.1

The Location of Muscle Spindle Cells and Golgi Tendon Receptors Within the Muscle

is called *hypertonic*. The neck commonly develops hypertonicity due to a condition called *head forward posture*, in which the torso is slumped slightly forward and the head hangs down in front (see Figure 3.2 ■). In a healthy posture, the head rests on top of, and is supported by, the spinal column (see Figure 3.3 ■). The unhealthy condition forces the muscles of the posterior neck to support more of the weight of the head. With every step taken, the head is slightly jarred. The spindle cells in the muscles of the posterior neck are repeatedly stimulated, causing the muscles to be chronically contracted. As this happens over and over, the muscles eventually become chronically tense.

THE STIMULATION OF MUSCLE SPINDLE CELLS

Spindle cells are active during three processes, and each has a special significance to massage therapy.

1. *When the entire muscle is stretched quickly through external force* When a heavy weight is applied to a limb causing the muscle to stretch quickly, the muscle spindles will cause a contraction to resist the movement. This is commonly experienced when grasping something that turns out to be heavier than expected. The arm must quickly increase its contraction to compensate for the heavier weight. The client's body will react the same way if a therapist moves the muscle into a stretch too quickly. This will stimulate the muscle spindle and cause contraction of the muscle that the therapist is trying to stretch. This is undesirable because now the muscle is

resisting the therapeutic action. It is best to stretch the muscle slowly to prevent this type of stimulation.

2. *During the contraction of muscles* When a muscle is contracting, its muscle spindles are actively sending signals to proprioceptors in the opposite muscle called the *antagonist*. The signals tell the antagonist to relax so the contracting muscle can move the body part. This allows for the smooth movement of the body. For example, when lifting an object, as soon as the biceps (the agonist) contract to move the arms, the triceps (the antagonist) are prevented from contracting so they don't counteract the action of the biceps (see Figure 3.4 ■). This process is called **reciprocal inhibition.**

   Reciprocal inhibition can be used as a tool to help relax a hypertonic muscle. Reciprocal inhibition is a popular facilitated stretching technique and is covered in detail in Chapter 7.

3. *When stretching a muscle at its midpoint* Since the spindles are concentrated in the belly of the muscle it makes sense that the muscle would be especially sensitive to a stretch here. This is important to massage therapy because direct stimulation of the muscle belly is a foundation of all types of massage, especially DTM. When a therapist moves into the muscle belly too quickly or with too much pressure, it can stimulate the spindles and cause guarding.

   Correct application of deep tissue massage prevents most guarding when it is performed methodically and

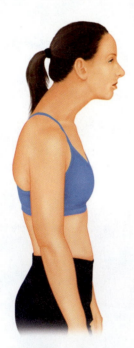

FIGURE 3.2

The Position of the Head and Shoulders in a "Head Forward" Posture

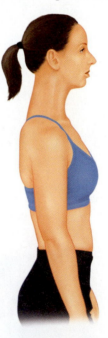

FIGURE 3.3

The Position of the Head and Shoulders in a Healthy, Balanced Posture

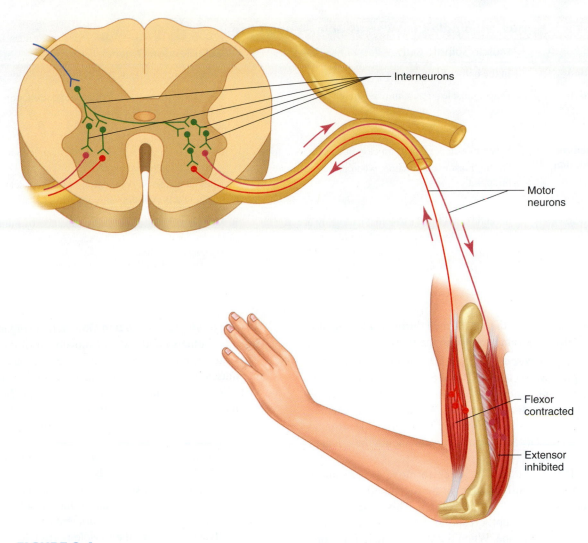

Interneurons

Motor neurons

Flexor contracted

Extensor inhibited

FIGURE 3.4

Bending the Elbow Demonstrates the Process of Reciprocal Inhibition. The Flexor (Biceps) Receives a Signal (in Red), Causing It to Contract. As This Occurs, the Extensor (Triceps) Receives a Signal (in Purple), Which Inhibits Its Contraction.

the techniques are applied very slowly. This tends to inhibit the stimulation of muscle spindle cells. By gently working into the tissues and slowly applying the strokes, you are less likely to stretch the muscle too quickly and cause the spindle to stimulate contraction. This allows for deeper and more effective work, without resistance on the part of the muscle. While DTM inhibits the action of muscle spindles, it actually encourages the action of Golgi tendon organs.

Golgi Tendon Organs

Golgi tendon organs are receptors found on the tendon where it blends into the muscle (Figure 3.1). They inhibit the contraction of muscles, causing them to relax. This inhibition is called the *Golgi tendon reflex.* This reflex causes the exact opposite of the stretch reflex. Where the stretch reflex causes the muscle to contract in response to a stretch, the Golgi tendon reflex causes the muscle to

lengthen and relax in response to a stretch. This is also a protective mechanism. In her popular text, *Human Anatomy and Physiology* (2004), Elaine Marieb highlights the protective nature of this mechanism. She states, "Golgi tendon organs protect muscles and tendons subjected to possible damaging stretching force from tearing" (p. 525). If a muscle is stretched too far and risks damage, the Golgi tendon reflex allows it to stretch a little further to prevent injury.

THE STIMULATION OF GOLGI TENDON ORGANS

Golgi tendon organs are active during three processes; each is significant to massage therapy.

1. *During muscle overload* When the muscle is overloaded, the Golgi tendon organ may be stimulated to cause the muscle to relax in order to prevent damage. This happens when an exhausted muscle gives way— as when lifting too heavy a weight. Slow, sustained

TABLE 3.1	Muscle Spindle Cells Versus Golgi Tendon Organs	
	Muscle Spindle Cells	Golgi Tendon Organs
Location	In the belly of muscles	On tendon as it blends into muscle
Function	Detect muscle stretch; initiate stretch reflex; causes muscle contraction.	Detect local muscle stretch; detect contraction in opposing muscle; initiate Golgi tendon reflex causing muscle relaxation.
Methods of Stimulation	When muscle lengthens quickly due to external force. During muscle contraction; when muscle is stretched at midpoint.	During prolonged stretch of local muscle; when local muscle is overloaded After an isometric contraction of local muscle; during contraction of opposing muscle
Significance to DTM	Should be inhibited to avoid guarding by use of cautious and slow application of pressure.	May be stimulated to induce relaxation by mimicking moderate stretch with massage or by performing passive stretch.

pressure such as that performed during DTM will also stimulate this same release in the muscle.

2. *During a stretch* Golgi tendon organs are active during **passive stretching.** Passive stretching occurs when the therapist moves the client into a stretch with no participation from the client. When passive stretching is applied slowly and gently, it increases the stimulation to the Golgi tendon organ enhancing the effect of the stretch.

It is a common practice to move slowly into a stretch and gently hold it for more than 30 seconds in order to get a full, proper stretch. This is because the Golgi tendon receptor responds to a stretch that is held for a length of time. When the stretch is held for a long duration, the Golgi tendon organ is stimulated, causing the muscle to relax and fully lengthen. In order to get the best results from therapy, hold the passive stretch long enough to engage the Golgi tendon organ.

Deep massage strokes can also take advantage of this proprioceptor by introducing pressure in a slow, deliberate way and keeping the pressure consistent. This gentle increase in tension and consistent pressure will help stimulate these important receptors to facilitate muscle relaxation and lengthening.

3. *During or after a contraction* Golgi tendon organs also function in the smooth flow of movement of the body. They are the proprioceptors that accept the signal from the muscle spindle of the contracting muscle (the agonist). When a muscle contracts, its muscle spindle sends a signal to the Golgi tendon organ in the antagonist. The Golgi tendon organ inhibits contraction of (i.e., relaxes) the antagonist, allowing the limb to move.

Interestingly, *isometric contractions* tend to activate the Golgi tendon organ as well. Just after an isometric contraction the Golgi tendon organ is activated, causing a temporary relaxation in the muscle. During some forms of bodywork this momentary relaxation is taken advantage of and the muscle is stretched to new longer lengths. (This is a technique of facilitated stretching that is discussed more fully in Chapters 6 and 7.) Table 3.1 ■ compares the significant features of Golgi tendon organs and muscle spindle cells. To sum up, the slow, deliberate, and systematic approach of DTM inhibits the function of muscle spindle cells, which are responsible for contracting a stretched muscle. On the other hand, it stimulates the Golgi tendon organ, which relaxes the muscle in response to a stretch, allowing the muscle to lengthen.

HOLISTIC CONNECTION

Treating the whole body means understanding and working with small and subtle components of the body as well as the larger, more obvious structures. When applying DTM it is important to understand neurological structures such as Golgi tendon receptors and muscle spindle cells. Using this type of structure to your advantage is the focus of neuromuscular therapy. For more about neurology and massage, see Chapters 6–9.

QUICK QUIZ #5

1. Muscle spindle cells are located where the tendon blends with the muscle.
   a. True
   b. False

2. Golgi tendon receptors are responsible for the stretch reflex.
   a. True
   b. False

3. Muscle spindle cells are stimulated by:
   a. slow passive stretching.
   b. isometric contraction.
   c. contraction of an antagonist muscle.

4. During deep tissue massage, it is beneficial for a therapist to use techniques that will:
   a. stimulate both muscle spindle cells and Golgi tendon receptors.
   b. inhibit muscle spindle cells and stimulate Golgi tendon receptors.
   c. stimulate muscle spindle cells and inhibit Golgi tendon receptors.
   d. inhibit both muscle spindle cells and Golgi tendon receptors.

THE PHASES OF DEEP TISSUE MASSAGE

With an understanding of how deep tissue massage works with the body's neuromuscular structures, a closer examination of the phases of DTM is warranted. Effective DTM is best achieved using four phases. It is a process that works from light pressure towards deep pressure, and then back to light pressure. In this way the body is gradually acclimated to deeper pressure. The work is finished gently to flush and relax the muscles. During DTM you must carefully approach the client's body and never rush into the deeper layers. This is accomplished by following the phases. Each phase includes specific techniques as well as a rate, rhythm, and direction of strokes designed to achieve the goals of that phase.

Warm-up Phase

This phase is made up of Swedish strokes such as effleurage and petrissage, rocking and jostling. It is light, soothing work designed to prepare the client mentally and physically for the deeper work to follow. The Swedish strokes increase circulation, and gently relax and warm the tissues, making them more pliable. During this phase, begin to assess the layers of muscle, looking for tension and other pathologies (such as trigger points, adhesions, etc.).

Separation Phase

This phase separates the fibers of muscle and fascia. It breaks down any adhesions or holding patterns. By separating the fibers of the muscle and fascia, they will be able to move more freely and independently, which balances function.

There are two steps to this phase. Both steps use the points of the fingers, knuckles, and elbows to dig in and separate fibers. The first step employs deep longitudinal strokes that work along the grain of the muscle. This separates the

fibers by working down between them. In the second step, the work travels across the grain of the muscle trying to pull apart the fibers one by one like strumming a guitar. This is the deepest phase of DTM and has the potential to meet with resistance or guarding by the client. While this work can be intense, if applied properly, the client should not experience discomfort. It is important to remind the client to exhale during the strokes to minimize resistance.

Realignment Phase

This phase gently works to encourage realignment of muscle tissue by engaging the muscle along its length. It uses deep pressure that compresses muscle fibers together, further encouraging them to reform and realign. The techniques in this phase use a broad application surface, such as the palm and forearm. They are used mostly along the length of the muscle. By using pressure that is evenly spread out across the broad surface of the muscle, the fibers are thoroughly compressed and realigned. These techniques also encourage relaxation and lengthening. They provide constant pressure on the muscle group to stimulate the Golgi tendon relaxation response.

Integrating and Closing Phase

The techniques of this phase are designed to integrate and re-educate muscles toward better functioning. Here, you will connect the body parts using general Swedish strokes. Kneading the tissues of an area together helps relax the body and allows the muscles to fall into their preferred patterns. Light passive stretching is employed in this phase as a way to re-educate or "teach" the muscle a new length.

This phase is also focused on encouraging the flow of blood and lymph to help remove metabolic wastes and other inflammatory substances from the tissues. The strokes increase circulation towards the liver and kidneys to speed up

TABLE 3.2	The Four Phases of Deep Tissue Massage	
Phase	**Goals**	**Techniques**
Warm-up	Prepare client for deeper work. Increase circulation. Relax and warm tissues to make them more pliable.	Swedish strokes including: rocking, jostling, effleurage, and petrissage.
Separation	Separate fibers of muscle and fascia. Break down adhesions and holding patterns.	Use of fingers, knuckles, and elbows. Longitudinal strokes with the grain of the muscle followed by strokes against the grain of the muscle.
Realignment	Encourage realignment of muscle tissue. Compress muscle fibers back together. Encourage relaxation and lengthening of muscles.	Use of broad surfaces such as forearms and palms of hands. Constant pressure on muscle group. Stimulation of Golgi tendon relaxation response.
Integration and Closing	Integrate and re-educate muscles. Encourage removal of waste products from muscles for elimination from the body.	Light passive stretching for re-education of muscles. Swedish strokes, especially kneading, to encourage movement of toxins into circulation toward heart and kidneys.

the removal process. Often, this is the portion of the massage that is the most enjoyable for the client.

Table 3-2 ■ compares the goals and techniques used in each of the four phases of DTM.

The time that is spent in each phase is dictated by the needs of the client. Some clients may require more warm-up than others. If it is cold outside, then all clients may need more warm-up. During the two middle phases, it is important to watch the client for clues as to when to move on and work another area. Usually you will know when to move on because the pathology in the tissues has diminished. If, however, the tissues are not responding or are becoming too inflamed, it may be prudent to work somewhere else and come back to that area later in the massage or to save it for another session. Some of this becomes intuitive with experience. However, it is important to remember to communicate with your client to see if they want you to continue in that area or to move on.

QUICK QUIZ #6

1. The warm-up phase uses light passive stretching to prepare the tissues for deeper work to follow.
   a. True
   b. False

2. Which of the following are goals of the realignment phase of deep tissue massage? (Circle all that apply)
   a. Encourage relaxation and lengthening of muscles
   b. Encourage realignment of muscle tissue
   c. Encourage removal of waste products
   d. Compress muscle fibers back together

3. Which of the following are techniques used in the separation phase of deep tissue massage?
   a. Use of broad surfaces such as forearms and palms
   b. Longitudinal strokes with the grain of the muscle
   c. Strokes against the grain of the muscle
   d. Effleurage and petrissage

4. The closing and integrating phase uses light passive stretching to re-educate the muscles for a new resting length.
   a. True
   b. False

SUMMARY

Deep tissue massage is a four-phased approach that systematically works into the deeper tissues. The focus is to break down pathology, such as postural holding patterns, and relax and realign the body's muscular system by stimulating neuromuscular structures. DTM stimulates Golgi tendon receptors and inhibits muscle spindle cells to relax and lengthen the muscle. Each phase has its own techniques and goals that are reflected in their titles. The four phases are (a) the warm-up phase, which prepares the body for deeper work using gentle techniques; (b) the separation phase, which breaks down myofascial adhesions and trigger points; (c) the realignment phase, which realigns the fibers previously disrupted; and (d) the integration and closing phase, which relaxes the worked tissue and helps to reintegrate the muscles with other surrounding myotatic units.

DISCUSSION QUESTIONS

1. Explain the importance of treating the deeper layers of muscles.
2. How are muscle spindle cells and Golgi tendon receptors important to DTM?
3. What are the goals of each of the four phases of DTM?
4. What are the two steps to the separation phase, and how do they differ?

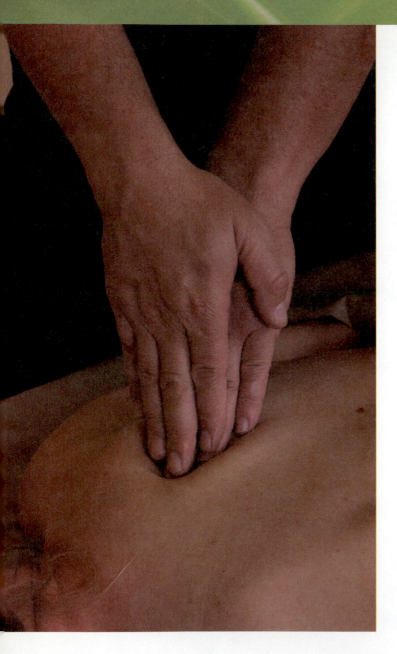

 CHAPTER HIGHLIGHTS

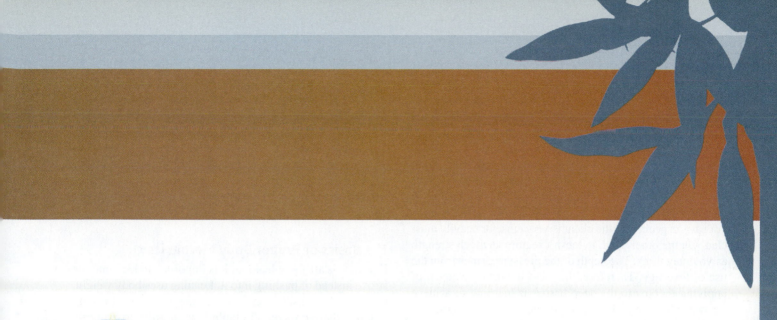

CHAPTER OBJECTIVES

- Understand proper body mechanics
- Establish general guidelines for applying deep tissue massage (DTM) techniques
- Analyze individual techniques of DTM
- Identify the contraindications for DTM

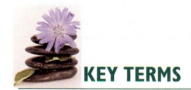

KEY TERMS

PROPER BODY MECHANICS

Before discussing the individual techniques of deep tissue massage, it is important to consider the proper body mechanics required to perform all of the movements. The use of proper body mechanics is important to the application of all forms of massage. However, in deep tissue massage (DTM) it is especially important because it requires that you reach the deepest levels of tension in the client's body. This is often not easy, especially if the client is very tense or heavily muscled. On the other hand, it doesn't require as much strength as you may think. The depth of the pressure comes from the use of **leverage.** Therefore, the most important element of applying therapy to the deep tissues is learning to achieve good depth through the use of proper body mechanics.

Proper body mechanics draws on the principles of using weight and leverage to apply pressure instead of using brute strength. With leverage, we can make use of a pivot point to multiply the mechanical force applied for massage. The principals of leverage allow a person to generate more power using a smaller force. Basically it allows people of differing size and strength to be able to generate the same level of deep pressure. The martial arts use leverage in this same way. People with petite bodies are able to generate enough power to break stacks of bricks using leverage and technique. Certainly the goal of massage is not to break things, but the principles are the same. Leverage is a much more efficient way to apply pressure and provides two important benefits:

1. *Saves physical wear and tear* When you are not using leverage to apply massage, the muscles are forced to do the majority of the work. This leads to tired muscles. Overworked, fatigued muscles will not properly support the joints, leaving them vulnerable to injury. Complicated joint structures, such as the carpals in the wrist, can take quite a beating if the surrounding muscles do not properly stabilize them. Using leverage places less demand on the muscles and keeps them from becoming fatigued.

   In addition, using muscle strength instead of leverage causes your muscles to be tense through the stroke. This tension will transfer to the client's body, increasing their level of tension. Furthermore, tension will accumulate in your body, which can, over time, develop into pathology such as inflammation and trigger points. Leverage allows you to stay relaxed throughout the treatment. This will minimize stress buildup and allow for a long and healthy career.

2. *Deeper pressure with less effort* By using leverage, your body is as fresh at the end of the massage as it is at the beginning. This ensures that the treatment is effective throughout the entire procedure. It is important to treat all the tissues with the same intensity. Overworking your muscles and becoming fatigued during the massage will at best cheat the client out of therapy, and at worst injure the client due to lack of focus. Fatigue also affects sensitivity and will diminish your ability to feel

the deeper layers of muscle. Constant changes that are occurring in the deep tissues can be very subtle, so it is important to be relaxed and focused to feel them.

One of the most important benefits of working with less effort is that it allows the performance of multiple massages in a single day, all with the same intensity and focus. The clients with late appointments deserve the same quality of therapy as those at the beginning of the day.

The Basics of Proper Body Mechanics

Leverage is all about leaning. It is important to lean into the stroke instead of pushing into it. Leaning uses body weight, where pushing uses more muscle than necessary. Leaning requires that you keep the table low. In order to properly perform the lean, some pointers on body position should be discussed.

PROPER STANCE

Placement of the feet is extremely important to proper body mechanics. DTM employs the **"archer stance"** (see Figure 4.1 ■). You stand as if you were trying to shoot a bow and arrow. It's the same position you might use to push a heavy object like a car. One leg is set back and the other is in front (in a type of lunge). The hips should face the same direction as the legs. The toes of the front leg should be pointing forward and the toes of the back leg are at a 45-degree angle.

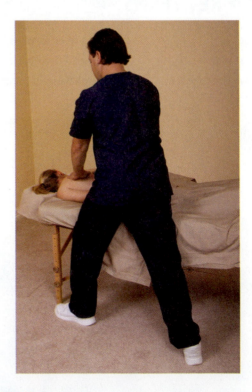

FIGURE 4.1

Correct Position of the Feet and Hips for the Proper Application of Deep Tissue Massage

Your shoulders and hands are relaxed. Your arms are extended to meet the client, and the elbows are firm but not locked (see Figure 4.2 ■). Your body weight should be balanced between the legs with a slight emphasis on the back leg.

Stay in the archer stance during all bodywork. When you need to sink lower into the client, just widen your stance by dropping your back leg farther back. This way your body will sink closer to the table. You never want to bend over at the waist to get closer to the client, as this puts your lower back at risk of strain (see Figure 4.3 ■).

When you want to move up or down the table length while still engaging the client, you will need to stay in the deep lunge. To maintain contact, shuffle your feet by first moving the back leg forward and then stepping forward with the front leg. For example, you may work on a tall client and will need to perform a stroke that travels the length of her back. Slide your back leg forward to meet the front leg, and then step forward with your front leg while keeping your body weight leaning into the client (see Figure 4.4 ■). If you need to take another step, perform the same procedure each time. Shuffle this way until you complete the movement and then settle back into the posture to finish your specific work.

When simply moving from one side of the client to the other (i.e., to begin a new move, or to redrape), keep a light touch with one of your hands on the client and walk naturally to the other side. Some prefer to break contact when moving to a different part of the body. This may give the client's body a brief relief from stimulation to integrate the effects of the

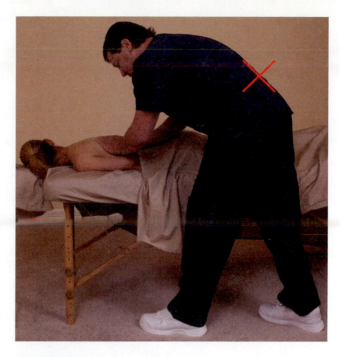

FIGURE 4.3

Incorrect Posture for Application of Deep Tissue Massage. The Therapist Is Bent Over Too Far at the Waist.

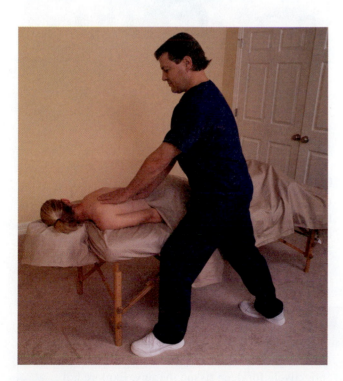

FIGURE 4.2

Correct Position of the Shoulders and Arms for the Proper Application of Deep Tissue Massage

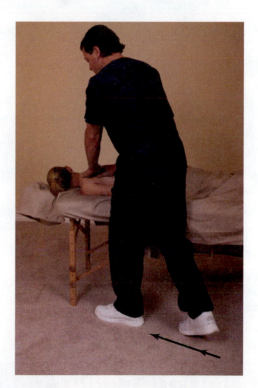

FIGURE 4.4

Maintain Contact and Good Posture While Moving Forward During a Massage by Sliding the Back Leg Forward to Meet the Front Leg. Then Step Out with the Front Leg. The Arrows Show the Forward Motion of the Back Leg.

work. The only time you need to shuffle in the lunge position is when you are moving while engaging the client during a deep stroke.

PROPER BALANCE

The point of contact with the client is called the *balance point*. When you lean forward you are slightly off balance, and the contact with the client provides the support to keep from falling forward. Your center of gravity should be focused around your hips, and they should direct all movements. The hips should always be turned in the direction of the stroke. When you lean forward, take some weight off of your back leg, and then use the contact with the client to counterbalance.

You should not position your body directly over the client (see Figure 4.5 ■). Ideally, you should be slightly behind and leaning into the client. Always keep your back straight and head slightly up during the stroke. This encourages leaning rather than muscling or pushing. Stay behind the stroke (see Figure 4.6 ■).

GENERAL CONSIDERATIONS FOR DEEP TISSUE MASSAGE

Proper Stroke

To begin a stroke, lean forward and sink into the client's tissues, to a depth in the middle range of the client's tolerance level (6–8 on a scale of 1–10). Then, move through the stroke, attempting to maintain the same level of pressure throughout the whole stroke. (Think of plowing through the tissues rather than gliding over the top.) You must be careful during this process and constantly monitor the client's reaction to the pressure. Make adjustments as warranted.

It is important to keep firm contact with the client at all times during a stroke as this helps prevent stimulation of the muscle spindle and encourages stimulation of the Golgi tendon receptor. You may recall that stimulation of the Golgi tendon receptor encourages relaxation in the muscles, and

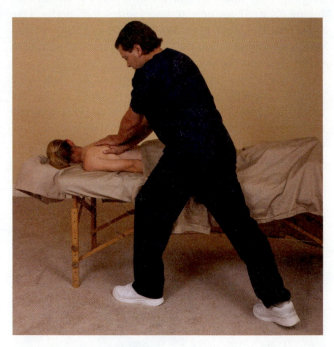

FIGURE 4.6
Correct Posture for Applying Deep Tissue Massage. The Therapist Is Slightly Behind the Client, with a Straight Back and His Head Facing Forward.

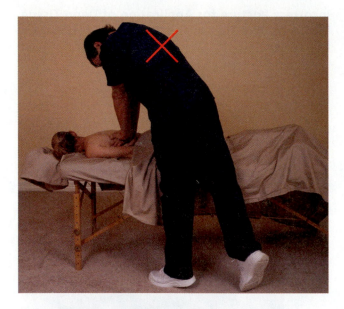

FIGURE 4.5
Incorrect Posture for Application of Deep Tissue Massage. The Therapist Is Leaning Too Far over the Client.

HOLISTIC CONNECTION

One way to increase access to the deeper layers is the use of additional tools. Hot stones provide deep, penetrating heat and glide across the skin very effectively for deep tissue therapy. Explore hot stone massage to expand the effectiveness of your holistic treatments.

stimulation of the muscle spindle creates contraction (guarding) in the muscle.

The contact should also be maintained by adding a firm "drag-back" at the end of the forward portion of the stroke. When working down into the tissues lean into the movement. When moving back to reset at the starting point of the stroke, keep contact and firmly drag your hands back across the tissues.

Rate and Rhythm

The rate of each stroke is as slow and deliberate as possible. By moving slowly there is more time to feel how the tissues are responding to the pressure. Furthermore, the client will have more time to adjust to and accept the pressure. When you move too quickly, the client's body will resist the movement by *guarding*. Guarding is caused by stimulation of the muscle spindle, which will stimulate a contraction of the muscle to resist the pressure.

The slow deliberate approach is used for all phases of massage. However, you may increase the speed slightly during the warm-up phase and the integration and closing phase. These phases use a softer touch. They also give priority to increasing circulation of blood and lymph, rather than working depth. During the deeper phases, it is very important to move as slowly as possible, as these phases are much more invasive.

Much as it is important to be slow during each stroke, it is important that the rhythm between movements should flow slowly from point to point in a constant tempo. When the rhythm is constant and even, the client's body will synchronize with the strokes. Their breathing patterns will be much more consistent with each downstroke, and they will be able to anticipate each stroke, allowing them to relax into it. If the rhythm is inconsistent, it keeps the client guessing and increases the possibility of a guarding response.

Lubrication

Many deep tissue specialists recommend using only balms or cocoa butter for lubrication. While those mediums are certainly appropriate, the type of lubrication used is not as important as the amount that is used. DTM requires very little lubrication.

In order to sink into the deeper tissues it is important to have a fair amount of friction. If there is too much lubricant (lotion, oils, balms, etc.), you will slip off of the contact point and be unable to grip the muscle sufficiently. Use only a small amount of lubricant, just enough to allow for free movement across the skin but not enough to make it slippery.

It is not practical to prescribe a measured amount of lubricant, because conditions and clients can be so variable. For example, in dry climates or during dry times of the year you may need to use a little more. The client's level of hydration will affect how much the skin will absorb. A good technique to follow is to place a small amount of lubrication in your hand, warm it up, and then apply it to the client. If this amount is sufficient, then work with it. If it is not, apply another small amount and try again. Using small amounts at a time minimizes the chances of getting too much. It is a good idea to keep a small hand towel close by to wipe off the excess if too much lubricant is present.

THE TECHNIQUES OF DEEP TISSUE MASSAGE

The Warm-up Phase

The warm-up phase consists of the basic Swedish massage movements: effleurage, petrissage, and jostling. To perform DTM, it is best that you have prior knowledge and practice using Swedish massage or some form of general relaxation massage. This text will not describe these basic massage movements. Therefore, it is advised that you review your basic massage techniques and apply them to this phase. However, some general rules apply to the application of the strokes in this phase.

This phase should be kept relatively short, and the strokes should be applied with a moderate tempo. The strokes are used to warm up the tissues and are not the main treating modality. The main goal here is to relax the client and increase circulation. Therefore, it is advised that you arrange your techniques to facilitate this objective.

In addition to preparing the tissues, you must assess the layers of muscle. During the performance of the Swedish strokes, it is important to feel for which tissues are tense and knotted. Make note of the depth and direction of the fibers that are holding the tension. This will help you to focus your work during the separation and realignment phases.

The Separation Phase

This phase is the deepest phase of DTM. The techniques used here employ points (i.e., fingertips, elbows, and knuckles) to work deeply between the muscle fibers, creating space between them. This phase is broken into two steps which use two different types of strokes.

1. The first step works along the grain of the muscle using **lengthwise strokes** (aka *linear strokes*). Working with the grain allows your contact point to slip between the fibers of the muscle, gently separating them (see Figure 4.7a ■).
2. The second step works across the grain of the muscle as if strumming the strings of a guitar. Using **cross-fiber strokes** (aka *transverse strokes*) further separates the adhered fibers (see Figure 4.7b ■).

During this phase it is very important to work the entire muscle, from attachment to attachment (along the grain) and side to side across the width. The best way to ensure that you completely treat the muscle is to

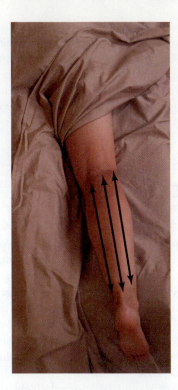

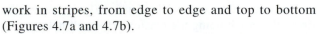

FIGURE 4.7a

The Arrows Show the Direction of the Lengthwise Strokes Performed on the Calf During the First Step of the Separation Phase of DTM.

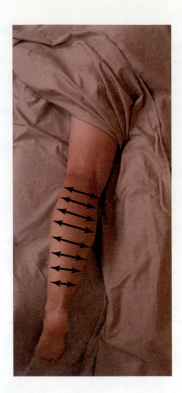

FIGURE 4.7b

The Arrows Show the Direction of the Cross-fiber Strokes Performed on the Calf During the Second Step of the Separation Phase of DTM.

work in stripes, from edge to edge and top to bottom (Figures 4.7a and 4.7b).

Each of the movements chosen for this phase is applied using the **lean and drag-back** technique. To apply the lean and drag-back technique, begin each stroke by engaging the client with the desired hand position. Next, sink your body weight into the client until you reach a depth that is well into the muscle, without being overwhelming to the client. Maintain this depth while leaning forward, and push through the muscle in a straight line. Use this method during both lengthwise and cross-fiber strokes. When you get to the end of the stroke, maintain pressure and position, and then firmly drag back to the starting position. Begin the next stroke without breaking contact with the client.

Try to maintain the initial depth throughout the stroke, easing up slightly if you feel the client start to guard or resist. If the client does begin to resist, slow down the movement or maintain pressure and pause for a moment. This allows the client time to adjust and accept the pressure. Often just by slowing down the stroke, you can maintain a deeper pressure without the need to ease off. Since each technique uses the lean and drag-back, the difference between each stroke is the method used to make contact with the client.

The following are descriptions of the various ways in which you can make contact with the client during this phase. Depth is always the primary concern. Therefore, the hand positions are presented in order, starting with the lightest technique and progressing to the deepest techniques. Lighter techniques should be used when you are first engaging the muscle. They should also be used on sensitive areas, or places where there is less muscle mass. However, all of the techniques may be appropriate on any body part if applied with care and focus on the client's tolerance. Be patient and creative, and use the client's feedback to help guide your choice of technique.

THE TECHNIQUES OF THE SEPARATION PHASE

FOUR FINGERS TECHNIQUE

- **Direction of stroke:** Lengthwise and cross-fiber
- **Contact point:** Pads of fingers and the fingertips
- **Physical description:** The four fingers of one hand are supported by the four fingers of the other hand by placing one hand on top of the other (see Figure 4.8a ■). This adds stability to the treating hand and decreases fatigue. It is important that the bones of the fingers are relatively straight (the finger

bones are stacked on top of each other) and the wrist is in a relatively straight line with the fingers. The elbows should be slightly bent but not too flexible. It is important that the arms stay rigid enough to transfer the weight of your body into the client (see Figure 4.8b ■).

- **Common areas of use:** Broad surfaces (e.g., back and legs). Sensitive areas where you need to work gradually into the depth of the muscle.
- **Special considerations:** In less muscular areas, a single hand can be used. However, use the single hand method sparingly to avoid fatigue.

SUPPORTED FINGERS TECHNIQUE

- **Direction of stroke:** Lengthwise or cross-fiber
- **Contact point:** Pads/tips of fingers
- **Physical description:** This is a single-handed technique in which the fingers of one hand are stacked or bunched together (see Figure 4.9a ■). The finger bones are stacked on top of each other and the wrist is in a straight line with the fingers (see Figure 4.9b ■).
- **Common areas of use:** Smaller or more delicate muscles, like the neck muscles. Also good for areas which are difficult to access, such as the deep pectoral region.
- **Special considerations:** This technique will allow for deeper work than the four fingers technique because

of the focused point of contact. However, it should be used sparingly due to the relative weakness of the fingers. Although the fingers are supported, they do not provide as much strength as the thumbs or knuckles. Therefore, this technique is best when applied on small or tender muscles that don't require a lot of pressure or depth.

SUPPORTED THUMB TECHNIQUE

- **Direction of stroke:** Lengthwise or cross-fiber
- **Contact point:** Pad and tip of thumb
- **Physical description:** Make a fist and press the thumb against the closed fist. Extend the tip of the thumb past the knuckles of the index finger (see Figure 4.10a ■). Be sure the hand and wrist are in a straight line, so that the bones of the thumb are also aligned. The hand should be aligned with the wrist. The wrist and forearm are aligned with the upper arm and the shoulders are relaxed (see Figure 4.10b ■).
- **Common areas of use:** This technique is strong enough for sections of large, tense muscles, such as back muscles. It is also well suited for smaller muscles in areas like the arms, hands, and feet.

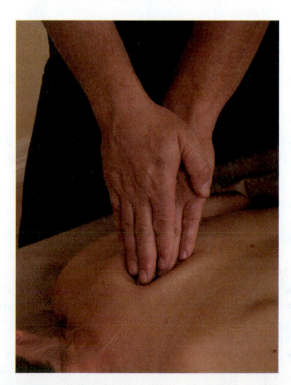

FIGURE 4.8a

The Hand Position for Applying the Four Fingers Technique

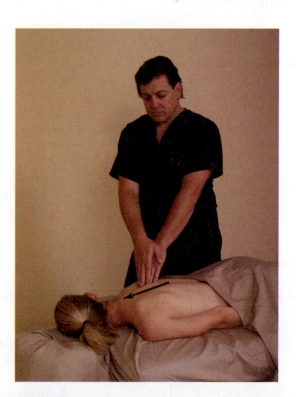

FIGURE 4.8b

The Correct Position for Applying the Four Fingers Technique. The Stroke Should Always Be Applied in a Forward Direction as Indicated by the Arrows. To Change the Direction of the Stroke, You Must Reposition Your Body.

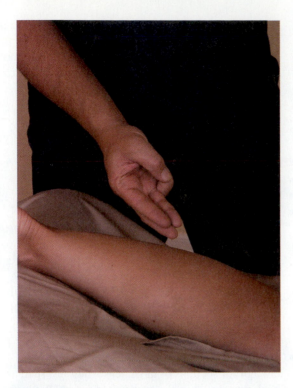

FIGURE 4.9a

The Hand Position for Applying the Supported Fingers Technique

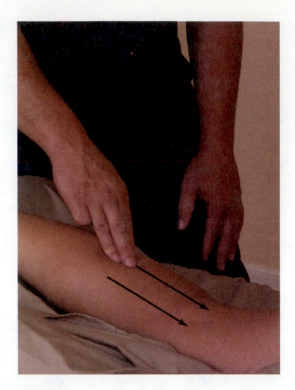

FIGURE 4.9b

The Correct Position for Applying the Supported Fingers Technique. The Stroke Should Always Be Applied in a Forward Direction, as Indicated by the Arrows. To Change the Direction of the Stroke, You Must Reposition Your Body.

- **Special considerations:** Thumb strokes have the capacity to work very deeply because of the focused point of contact. They can also be adjusted for thin or sensitive areas. When first beginning to use the thumb stroke, make sure the thumb is held tightly to the fist for support. When you begin to get the feel, you may slightly move the thumb away from the fist. However when doing so, always make sure to push down longitudinally through the thumb and not at right angles to the thumb joint (see Figure 4.11 ■).

KNUCKLE STROKE TECHNIQUE

- **Direction of stroke:** Lengthwise or cross-fiber
- **Contact point:** Knuckles, also called **interphalangeal joints**
- **Physical description:** Begin by making a fist. Then, push out the knuckle of the index finger while using the thumb to support it (see Figure 4.12a ■). Make contact using the first interphalangeal joint, and begin the stroke (see Figure 4.12b ■). Be sure to ease the pressure on the drag-back since this is a deeper method.
- **Common areas of use:** This technique is best for thicker and more muscular areas, such as the legs and larger shoulder muscles. Since the knuckle is a "boney" contact point, it is likely to be too firm for thin sensitive areas such as over the client's ribs.

- **Special considerations:** A variation on this technique is to use two or more knuckles to engage the client. Multiple knuckles may be best in broader areas requiring fairly deep pressure. Using more than one knuckle will be a little less invasive than a single knuckle, but it will still be important to ease pressure on the drag-back. Because knuckle strokes can be quite invasive, it is important that the tissues are thoroughly warmed up.

ELBOW STROKE TECHNIQUE

- **Direction of stroke:** Lengthwise, cross-fiber
- **Contact point: Olecranon process** (tip of the elbow) and the *proximal* third of the ulnar side of forearm (see Figure 4.13a ■).
- **Physical description:** When using elbow strokes you will need to be able to get in a little closer to the client. Therefore, begin by adjusting to a wider stance. A wider stance will lower your body while keeping your back straight. Initially the point of contact should primarily be the proximal third of

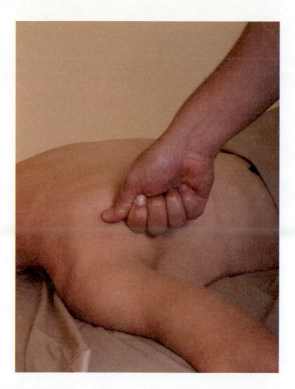

FIGURE 4.10a

The Hand Position for Applying the Supported Thumb Technique

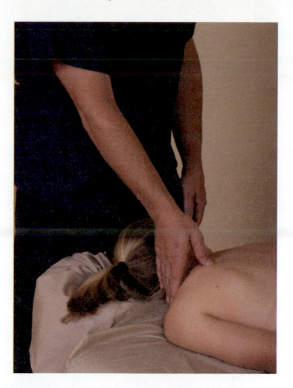

FIGURE 4.11

The Position of the Hand, Wrist, and Elbow for Applying Nonsupported Thumb Pressure

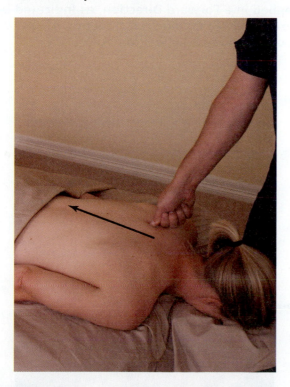

FIGURE 4.10b

The Correct Position for Applying the Supported Thumb Technique. The Stroke Should Always Be Applied in a Forward Direction as Indicated by the Arrows. To Change the Direction of the Stroke, You Must Reposition Your Body.

the forearm (see Figure 4.13b ■). The proximal forearm is less invasive than the tip of the elbow, so beginning the pressure there will allow the client to adjust and help prevent guarding. Then, as the client's tissues begin to soften to the initial pressure, gradually transfer the point of contact to the tip of the elbow (see Figure 4.13c ■).

- **Common areas of use:** Thicker more muscular areas (e.g., thighs, muscular backs, and shoulders).
- **Special considerations:** Elbow strokes have the capacity to work very deep into the tissues. They are excellent to use in thick or heavily muscled areas because they save wear and tear on your wrists and hands. They will allow you to work deeper with less effort.

MUSCLE ROLLING TECHNIQUE

- **Direction of stroke:** Cross-fiber
- **Contact point:** Tips of fingers and thumbs
- **Physical description:** Squeeze the muscle between the thumb and fingers (see Figure 4.14a ■). Work the tissues by rolling the muscle between the thumb and fingertips, slowly grinding the tissues back and forth. Grind down the fibers until the desired level of softness is reached. A variation on this technique is to grasp the

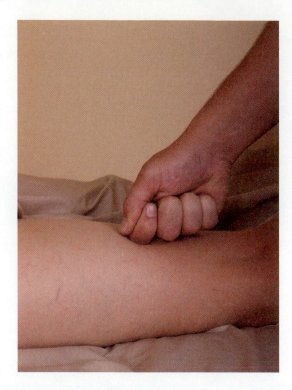

FIGURE 4.12a

The Hand Position for Applying the Knuckle Stroke Technique

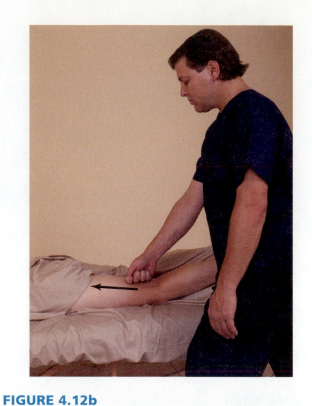

FIGURE 4.12b

The Correct Position for Applying the Knuckle Stroke Technique. The Stroke Should Always Be Applied in a Forward Direction, as Indicated by the Arrows. To Change the Direction of the Stroke, You Must Reposition Your Body.

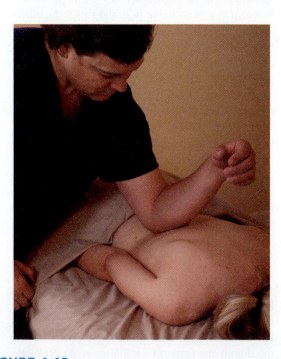

FIGURE 4.13a

The Arm Position for Applying the Elbow Stroke Technique

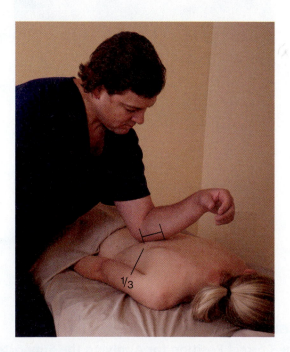

FIGURE 4.13b

Begin the Stroke with the Proximal 1/3 of the Forearm

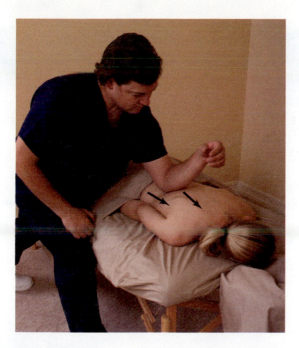

FIGURE 4.13c

The Correct Position for Applying the Elbow Stroke Technique. The Stroke Should Always Be Applied in a Forward Direction, as Indicated by the Arrows. To Change the Direction of the Stroke, You Must Reposition Your Body.

muscle by clamping the thumb onto the side of the index finger, and then roll the muscle between them (see Figure 4.14b ■).

- **Common areas of use:** Muscle rolling is commonly used across joints where you can grab a section of the muscle. The most common muscles treated with this technique are the pectoralis major, sternocleidiomastiod, trapezius, and the lower calf.
- **Special considerations:** This technique is excellent to use in areas where it is difficult to use weight to apply pressure, and where the muscle can be grasped easily. To prevent guarding, be sure to stay in the appropriate comfort range of the client.

The Realignment Phase

This phase is carried out with as much pressure as the separation phase. However, the contact with the client is much less invasive. Instead of the techniques being focused on separating fibers, this phase uses broad contact surfaces to help realign the fibers. In addition, the techniques are applied along the grain of the fibers to facilitate cohesiveness in the muscle. These techniques are performed slowly and smoothly to relax and realign. Like the separation phase, the lean and drag-back method is used, except, in

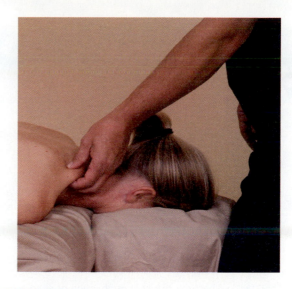

FIGURE 4.14a

The Position of the Hand when Performing Muscle Rolling with the Tips of the Fingers

this phase the broad contact point with the client is very soothing. The following is a selection of movements that can be employed during this phase. This is by no means an exhaustive list of the ways to work in this phase. However, it presents a strong foundation of techniques that employ a flat, broad contact point to move slowly and deeply along the grain of the muscles. The key is to use even pressure during these movement, and not to dig into or between the muscle fibers.

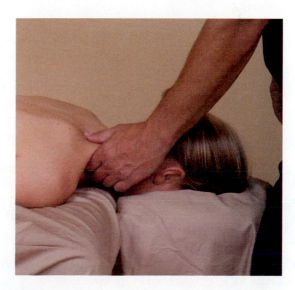

FIGURE 4.14b

The Position of the Hand When Performing Muscle Rolling Between the Thumb and the Index Finger

QUICK QUIZ #7

1. Proper body mechanics: (Circle all that apply)
   a. allow for the use of leverage to provide more power with less force.
   b. allow the therapist's muscles and joints to become fatigued quickly.
   c. take advantage of low table height, allowing the therapist to bend over the client to achieve greater pressure.
   d. allow the therapist to maintain contact through a long stroke by shuffling the feet while in the lunge position.
   e. All of the above
   f. None of the above

2. For DTM, it is best to use just enough lotion or oil to allow for free movement across the skin, but not enough to make it slippery.
   a. True
   b. False

3. Because it is used in less muscular areas, the single hand method of the four fingers technique can be used often, without worry of fatigue to the therapist.
   a. True
   b. False

4. Thumbs, elbows, and knuckles are generally more invasive and will achieve greater depth than the fingertips.
   a. True
   b. False

THE TECHNIQUES OF THE REALIGNMENT PHASE
STRAIGHT-LINE FOREARM TECHNIQUE

- **Direction of stroke:** Lengthwise
- **Contact point:** Unlike the elbow strokes of the separation phase, the point of contact is the flat, ulnar surface of the entire forearm (see Figure 4.15a ■). On smaller body parts, use the area proximal to the elbow without engaging the olecranon process (tip of the elbow).
- **Physical description:** Bend the elbow to about 45 degrees. Keep the shoulders relaxed and the back straight. Before engaging the client, you will need to get closer. Drop your back leg farther back to lower your entire torso toward the client. Begin the stroke by making contact with the entire forearm. Then sink to the desired depth in the tissue. Glide along the length of the muscle, maintaining the same depth throughout the stroke (see Figure 4.15b ■). At the end of the stroke, ease the pressure slightly and drag the forearm back to the starting position.
- **Common areas of use:** This technique can be used in any area large enough to accommodate the forearm. The back, thighs, and calves are common areas for this technique.
- **Special considerations:** This technique is particularly useful for large clients and very tense muscles, because it affords deep pressure with little effort. When performing the stroke, keep your hand relaxed. There is a natural tendency to tense the hand while applying this stroke, so concentrate on relaxing the

hand to avoid undue stress to your forearm. Be sure the shoulders are firm but not tense. Any tension in your body is counterproductive and may be felt by the client. Let the weight of your body do the work, rather than your arm muscles.

STRAIGHT-LINE FLAT-FIST TECHNIQUE

- **Direction of stroke:** Lengthwise
- **Contact point:** Contact is made using the flat surfaces of the finger bones, between the first proximal knuckles and the second proximal knuckles (see Figure 4.16a ■). Let the flat part of the fist do most of the work.
- **Physical description:** Make contact with the flat surface of the fist as described above. The hand should be in line with the wrist. The elbow should be in line with the wrist but not locked. Keep the entire arm and hand firm but not tense. Lean into the movement, using body weight rather than muscle, and glide along the length of the muscle (see Figure 4.16b ■). At the end of the stroke, ease the pressure slightly and drag the fist back to the starting position.
- **Common areas of use:** This technique is commonly used on the back, thighs, calf, forearms, and feet.
- **Special considerations:** This technique is good for areas of heavy muscle or *adipose*. It is deeper than most techniques in the Realignment Phase because it involves the knuckles. The key is to spread the pressure over the flat surface of all the finger bones to minimize the impact of the individual knuckles.

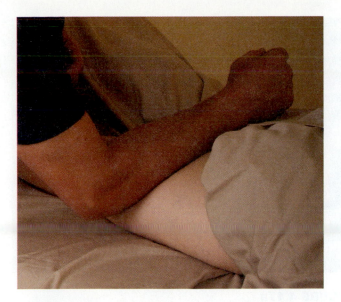

FIGURE 4.15a

The Arm Position for Applying the Straight Line Forearm Technique

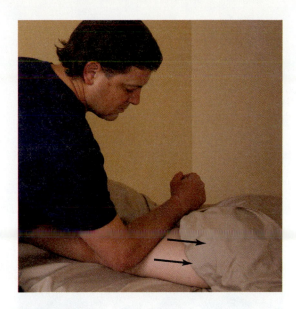

FIGURE 4.15b

The Correct Position for Applying the Straight Line Forearm Technique. The Stroke Should Always Be Applied in a Forward Direction, as Indicated by the Arrows. To Change the Direction of the Stroke, You Must Reposition Your Body.

PALM PRESS TECHNIQUE

- **Direction of stroke:** Lengthwise
- **Contact:** Contact is made with the palm of the hand, keeping the pressure spread evenly throughout the palm (see Figure 4.17a ■)
- **Physical description:** The wrist is bent but not hyperextended. The elbow is slightly bent but remains firm. Begin the move by leaning into the client, pressing with the palm (see Figure 4.17b ■). Glide along the length of the muscle, and, at the end, ease up and drag the palm back to the starting position.
- **Common areas of use:** This technique is easy to use on almost all areas of the body. It is ideal for heavily muscled areas.
- **Special considerations:** Be sure to keep the fingers relaxed in order to minimize fatigue to the forearm and to keep the pressure centered in the middle of the hand. It is very important to resist the urge to dig in with the heel of the palm to achieve depth or pressure. This will tend to hyperextend the wrist and place stress on the carpals. Excessive pressure on the carpals can irritate the meridian nerve, creating injury to the carpal tunnel. When the need to back off the pressure arises, there is a tendency to soften the pressure of this stroke by bending the elbows. Rather than bending the elbows to adjust the depth, use your legs to adjust by increasing or decreasing the width of your stance. When your elbows become bent, your arm muscles must do more work to apply pressure.

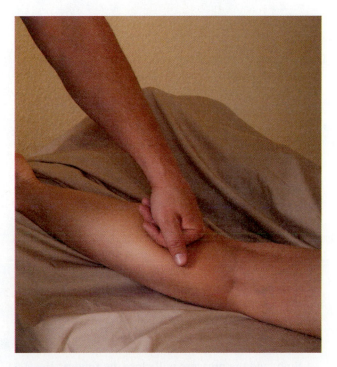

FIGURE 4.16a

The Hand Position for Applying the Straight Line Flat-Fist Technique

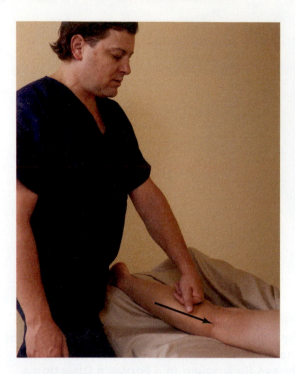

FIGURE 4.16b

The Correct Position for Applying the Straight-Line Flat-Fist Technique. The Stroke Should Always Be Applied in a Forward Direction, as Indicated by the Arrows. To Change the Direction of the Stroke, You Must Reposition Your Body.

LIMB STROKE TECHNIQUE

- **Direction of stroke:** Lengthwise
- **Contact point:** The surface of the entire palm, including the hand and fingers; essentially, the thumb and fingers are used to grasp the limb being treated (see Figure 4.18a ■)
- **Physical description:** Begin by holding the distal end of the limb elevated with one hand. Grasp the area to be worked between the thumb and fingers of the other hand. Keep the elbow relatively straight (but not locked) and the shoulders relaxed. While facing the area to be worked, lean into the limb and let your hand slide down the limb (see Figure 4.18b ■). At the end of the stroke, drag back to the starting position.
- **Common areas of use:** This stroke is mostly used on the shin, calf, and forearm muscles.
- **Special considerations:** Avoid squeezing your hand together during this movement to avoid fatigue of the hand muscles. Instead, press the hand into the limb, and the pressure will close the fingers. Be careful not to hunch your shoulders, and remember to keep them relaxed.

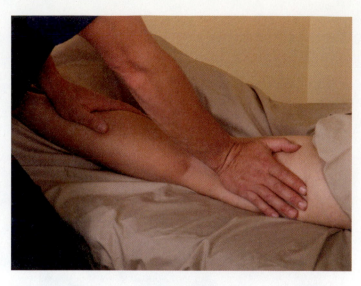

FIGURE 4.17a

The Hand Position for Applying the Palm Press Technique

SUPPORTED PALMS TECHNIQUE

- **Direction of stroke:** Lengthwise
- **Contact point:** The palm of one hand makes contact with the client, while the second hand is stacked on top for support (see Figure 4.19a ■); emphasize pressure at the center of the palm, to ensure that pressure is dispersed evenly.

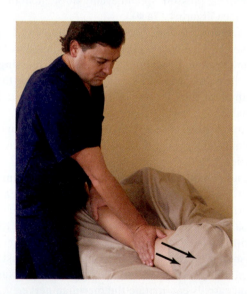

FIGURE 4.17b

The Correct Position for Applying the Palm Press Technique. The Stroke Should Always Be Applied in a Forward Direction, as Indicated by the Arrows. To Change the Direction of the Stroke, You Must Reposition Your Body.

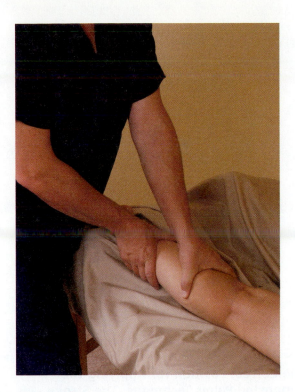

FIGURE 4.18a

The Hand Position for Applying the Limb Stroke Technique

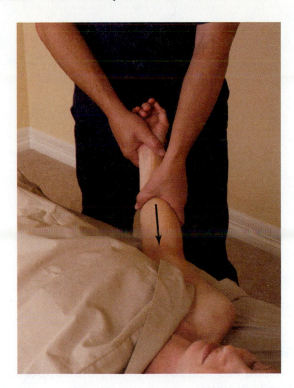

FIGURE 4.18b

The Correct Position for Applying the Limb Stroke Technique. The Stroke Should Always Be Applied in a Forward Direction, as Indicated by the Arrows. To Change the Direction of the Stroke, You Must Reposition Your Body.

- **Physical description:** Begin by facing the direction in which the stroke will be performed. Make contact by placing down first the hand that is closest to the client. Then place the second hand on top, perpendicular to the first. Keep your hands slightly in front of you to prevent leaning directly over the hands and hyperextending the wrists. The elbows should be kept firm but not locked. Keep the shoulders, hands, and especially the fingers relaxed. Begin the stroke by leaning into the palms. Move in a straight line, up the muscle, being sure to treat its entire length (see Figure 4.19b ■). The greatest depth is applied with the initial lean; however, the drag-back should be slow and quite deep as well.
- **Common areas of use:** This technique can be used anywhere the area is large enough to receive the pressure of both hands. The back and the thighs are common areas to use the supported palms technique.
- **Special considerations:** With all the weight driving through the hands, it is easy to hyperextend the wrist of the bottom hand. Also, there is a tendency to tense the elbows, shoulders, hands, or fingers in order to place more weight on the client. Avoid

both of these tendencies. Remember to keep your hands in front of you, and use your body weight to increase pressure.

ONE-TWO TECHNIQUE
- **Direction of stroke:** Lengthwise
- **Contact point:** The hand position and contact point can vary for this technique; there will be different needs in different situations; the palms and "flat-fists" are the most common contact points (see Figure 4.20a ■)
- **Physical description:** Begin the technique by leaning into one hand which initiates the move. Then, at the end of the stroke, the body weight shifts to the second hand as it begins at the same starting point and follows the same path as the first (see Figure 4.20b ■). Once the second hand reaches the end of the stroke, the first hand picks up again and the process is repeated. The result of this technique is a smooth, fluid transition from one hand to the next.

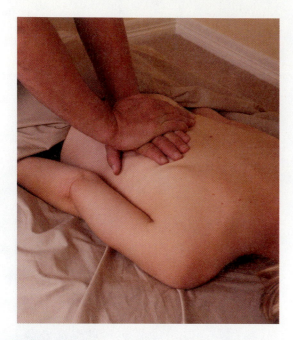

FIGURE 4.19a

The Hand Position for Applying the Supported Palms Technique

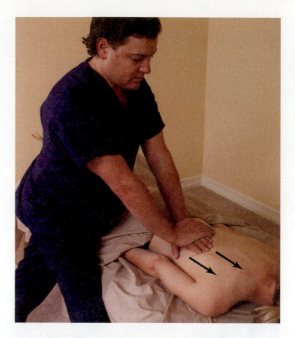

FIGURE 4.19b

The Correct Position for Applying the Supported Palms Technique. The Stroke Should Always Be Applied in a Forward Direction, as Indicated by the Arrows. To Change the Direction of the Stroke, You Must Reposition Your Body.

- **Common areas of use:** This technique can be used on legs, arms, and back.
- **Special considerations:** The one-two technique thoroughly relaxes the muscles, and the rhythm of the stroke works in addition to the depth. Because this is a "timing" move, the hand position is not the most important part: it is most important that the movement be deep and fluid.

The Integration and Closing Phase

This phase consists primarily of Swedish massage movements with the addition of stretching. The strokes during this phase should be gentle and primarily in the direction of the core of the torso. This assists in metabolic waste removal by moving lymph and blood towards the eliminatory organs. Often this phase is referred to as the "make nice" phase because of the gentle nature of the strokes.

Stretching is also an important element in this phase. It is often called "re-education" because it teaches the muscle a new, longer resting length. It should be applied at the end of the massage to ensure that the muscle is relaxed and receptive to the new length.

A passive stretch should be applied to all the muscles treated. Allow the client to relax and gently move the body part through its range of motion. Finish by taking the muscles into a full stretch and hold for 30 seconds. In order to properly stretch the client you must have sound knowledge of the range of motion and actions of the

muscles and joints you wish to stretch. Please review this before including stretching in the integration and closing phase. Refer to Chapter 7 for more information on proper stretching techniques.

CONTRAINDICATIONS FOR DEEP TISSUE MASSAGE

Deep Tissue Massage, like any massage modality has its **contraindications.** That is to say, there are times when DTM should not be applied. The following is a list of contraindications for DTM. Keep in mind that no list, including this one, can take into account all of the circumstances that might suggest a contraindication. So it is highly important to employ clinical experience and common sense to decide whether it is appropriate to use DTM. When in doubt, contact the client's physician for consultation.

- **Acute inflammation.** Inflamed conditions such as *neuritis, tendonitis, epichondolitis,* and *tenosynovitis* may be aggravated by DTM. Putting deep pressure on the muscles may cause excessive movement and strain on inflamed tissues, making the condition worse. However, if applied appropriately, DTM can be used in therapy for these conditions.

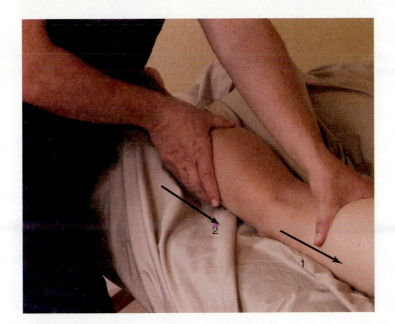

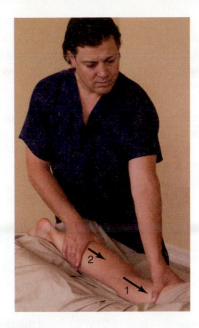

FIGURE 4.20a

The Hand Position for Applying the One-Two Technique

FIGURE 4.20b

The Correct Position for Applying the One-Two Technique. The Numbers Represent the Order in Which the Strokes Are to Be Performed. The Stroke Should Always Be Applied in a Forward Direction, as Indicated by the Arrows. To Change the Direction of the Stroke, You Must Reposition Your Body.

- **Acute injuries.** Torn ligaments, tendons, muscles, unhealed fractures, and postsurgical sites should be given the proper healing time before DTM is applied. To determine the proper healing time, consult with the client's physician. If DTM is used too soon, it may further tear the damaged tissue.
- **New scar tissue.** If a scar is not completely healed/formed, DTM may reinjure the site by pulling the unhealed fibers apart. It is best to make sure the scar is fully stitched together before using DTM. As a general rule wait 6 to 8 weeks or get clearance from the client's physician before you begin DTM. At this point, the techniques may be used to make the scar more functional by increasing its flexibility and decreasing adhesions.
- **Gross swelling.** This is typically the result of an acute injury. The pressure from DTM can aggravate the injury by placing stress on the healing myofascial structures.
- **During flair-ups of osteoarthritis and rheumatoid arthritis.** The pressure from DTM causes movement in the joints. If those joints are inflamed by arthritis, the increase in movement and pressure caused by DTM may exacerbate the condition.
- **Excess fatigue.** If clients are extremely tired, it is best that they rest before undergoing the rigors of DTM. A body that is exhausted from jet-lag or a marathon may not respond as well to a rigorous deep tissue massage.
- **Infection.** DTM can tax the body, taking energy away from the body's efforts at healing an infection. There is also the risk of cross-infection from the

client, meaning the therapist and other clients are at risk of exposure.
- **Just after a meal.** One should wait 40 minutes to an hour after eating before receiving DTM. This will help prevent reactions such as nausea and vomiting.
- **Atrophied muscles.** Very weak muscles often cannot tolerate the pressure of DTM. These muscles are often dehydrated and brittle, making them even more fragile and unable to withstand DTM.
- **Flaccid paralysis.** This indicates nerve damage. The proper application of DTM involves paying close attention to how the client's body is responding, so as not to push too far. Muscles lacking nervous sensation will be unable to provide that feedback, making it very hard to discern whether you are working at a safe level.
- **High blood pressure or other heart conditions aggravated by an increase in blood pressure.** The pressure from deep tissue massage may increase internal pressure, especially if the client has a tendency to hold his breath. This internal pressure aggravates high blood pressure conditions.
- **Hyperesthesia.** This is an increased sensitivity to pain and/or touch. There are many reasons why a client may have hyperesthesia. Most involve injury to nerves. DTM may provide too much stimulation for these clients.

- **Marked or pitted edema.** This occurs when there is a systemic problem such as congestive heart failure or renal failure. DTM moves body fluids (i.e., blood and lymph). This may further tax a system already overwhelmed due to poor function of the heart and kidneys.
- **Plaque filled arteries or history of stroke.** These are commonly found in geriatric clients, but are not limited to geriatrics. The plaque can be destabilized and sent back into the bloodstream to become lodged in a smaller vessel. This can cause serious problems for the client. The carotid arteries in the neck are a common site for plaque buildup.
- **Venous stasis.** Pathology such as varicose veins should be avoided during DTM. This modality may break up the clotted blood stagnated in the vessel and allow it to flow to sensitive areas such as the brain or heart. If clots find their way to these structures, it may cause a stroke or heart attack.

QUICK QUIZ #8

1. The realignment phase of DTM:(Circle all that apply)
   a. is less invasive than the separation phase.
   b. uses similar depth of pressure as the separation phase.
   c. uses broad contact surfaces.
   d. focuses on realignment of the fibers.
   e. All of the above
   f. None of the above

2. The straight-line forearm technique is most commonly used
   a. on the shin, calves, and forearms.
   b. on the back, thighs, and calves.
   c. All of the above
   d. None of the above

3. The integration and closing phase includes which elements? (Circle all that apply)
   a. Lengthwise supported palms strokes
   b. Swedish massage strokes
   c. Straight-line flat-fist strokes
   d. Re-education and stretching
   e. All of the above
   f. None of the above

4. Acute injuries such as unhealed fractures or torn ligaments are a contraindication for deep tissue work.
   a. True
   b. False

5. Deep tissue massage is very effective for breaking down myofascial adhesions and for the treatment of varicose veins.
   a. True
   b. False

SUMMARY

The use of proper body mechanics in bodywork is important to save wear and tear on the therapist's body. Proper body mechanics also facilitate working deeper with less effort, which benefits the client because the therapist does not become fatigued and loose focus.

To perform proper body mechanics, use an "archer stance" and lean into the client. The feet are positioned one in front and one in back. Balance is centered between both legs with an emphasis on the back leg. When leaning, the weight is counterbalanced by the point of contact with the client. After leaning into the stroke, the hands are dragged back to the starting position for the next move.

The rate and rhythm of techniques is slow and deliberate to facilitate relaxation. Use minimal lubrication in order to grip the muscle and work deeper. The warm-up phase consists of light relaxation techniques designed to get the tissues ready for the deeper work to follow. The separation phase is the most invasive as it is designed to separate the fibers of the muscle. It consists of specialized techniques using small points of contact to penetrate deeper. The realignment phase consists of broad deep pressure moves designed to compress and bring the tissues back together. This phase contains techniques that use the forearm and hand. The integration and closing phase relaxes and renews the tissues. It uses techniques that encourage circulation and relaxation. This phase also contains stretching techniques.

Finally, there are a number of contraindications for performing DTM, and they range from mild illness to certain forms of heart disease.

DISCUSSION QUESTIONS

1. Why is the use of leverage important during the application of DTM?
2. What is the best rate and rhythm for applying DTM techniques? Why is this important?

3. How are the techniques in the warm-up and integration and closing phases similar, and how are they different?
4. Why is stretching included in the integration and closing phase?

5 Sample Protocols for Deep Tissue Massage

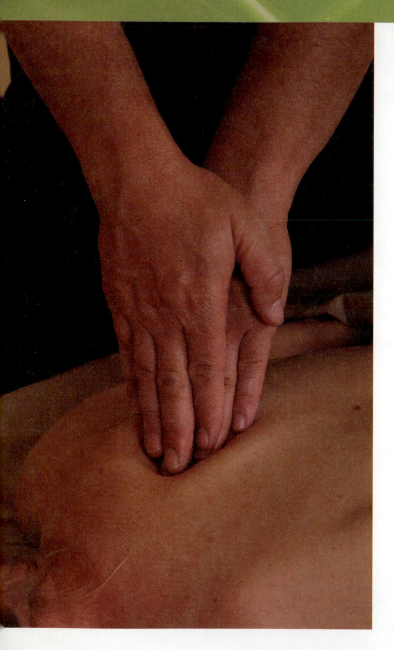

 CHAPTER HIGHLIGHTS

Chapter Objectives

Key Terms

Application of the Techniques

Sample Protocols

Summary

Discussion Questions

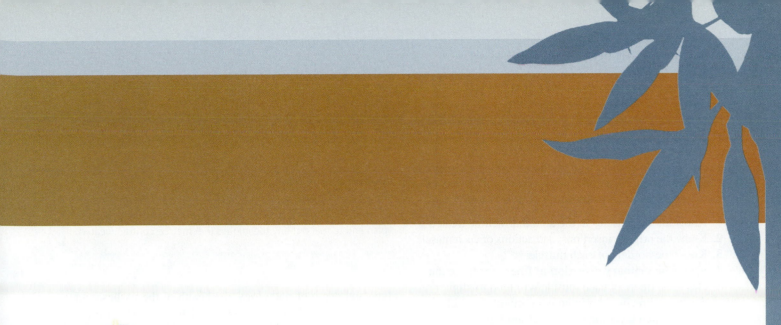

CHAPTER OBJECTIVES

- Understand how to combine the techniques of deep tissue massage
- Explore sample deep tissue massage protocols for various body parts
- Rehearse assessment skills and practice deep tissue massage techniques

KEY TERMS

APPLICATION OF THE TECHNIQUES

The techniques of deep tissue massage can be combined in a variety of ways, limited only by the area being treated and the creativity of the therapist. The four phases of DTM are set up to provide a systematic method for working through the layers and addressing pathology. Here are a few key concepts to consider when formulating your DTM protocols.

1. Know all the muscles in the area that will be treated
2. Know the origins, insertions, and actions of each muscle
3. Know the borders of each muscle
4. Know the **primary direction of fibers** for those muscles (The fibers of each muscle will tend to align in the same direction throughout a particular muscle.)
5. Know which layer the muscle is found in

A suitable protocols will be easy to prepare if you match your understanding of the muscles being treated with the relative benefits of the various techniques. Keep in mind that some deep tissue techniques and contact points are inherently more invasive than others. Use those techniques and contact points later in the sequence. Lead into the more invasive techniques by first using less invasive techniques. The

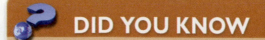

DID YOU KNOW

Before Every Massage

Remember to obtain a proper client history and perform a thorough assessment. This is important in order to develop a good plan and to rule out any techniques that may be contraindicated.

type and depth of pathology, the health of the tissues, and the comfort level of the client will determine which technique is chosen. In addition, as discussed in Chapter 4, certain massage strokes are better suited for each particular phase of treatment. Use Table 5.1 ■ as a quick reference to the appropriate strokes for each phase.

Also, as discussed in Chapter 4, some techniques are better suited for certain areas and types of pathology. Table 5.2 ■ provides a quick reference to the common uses for each of the deep tissue massage techniques.

TABLE 5.1	Strokes for the Phases of DTM		
Warm-up Phase	Separation Phase	Realignment Phase	Integration and Closing Phase
Rocking, effleurage, light petrissage, light compression	Lengthwise and cross-fiber strokes using various contact points	Lengthwise strokes using various contact points	Effleurage, light petrissage, jostling, stretching

TABLE 5.2	Common Uses of Deep Tissue Techniques		
	Description	Common Uses	Direction of Stroke
Separation Phase			
Four Fingers Technique	Moderate depth of pressure. Easy to adjust pressure. Fairly durable contact point for frequent use	Good for broad surfaces and sensitive areas. Back and legs	Lengthwise or cross-fiber
Supported Fingers Technique	Moderate to strong depth of pressure. Easy to adjust pressure. Less durable contact point. Use sparingly	Good for small and sensitive areas. Neck, inner arm, inner thigh, forearm, face, hands, and feet	Lengthwise or cross-fiber
Supported Thumb Technique	Strong depth of pressure. Easy to adjust pressure. Durable contact point for frequent use	Good for robust muscles. Shoulders, arms, legs, gluteals, and chest	Lengthwise or cross-fiber
Knuckle Stroke Technique	Moderate to strong depth of pressure. Easy to adjust pressure. Durable contact point for frequent use	Good for robust muscles. Shoulders, arms, legs, gluteals, and chest	Lengthwise or cross-fiber
Elbow Stroke Technique	Very strong depth of pressure. Not as easy to adjust pressure. Very durable contact point for frequent use	Good for large, robust muscles. Back, shoulders, legs, and gluteals	Lengthwise or cross-fiber
Muscle Rolling Technique	Moderate depth of pressure. Easy to adjust pressure. Less durable contact point. Use sparingly	Used in only a few areas. Neck, pectoral muscles, calves, and axillary area	Cross-fiber

TABLE 5.2	**(Continued)**		
	Description	Common Uses	Direction of Stroke
Realignment Phase			
Straight-Line Forearm Technique	Moderate to strong depth of pressure. Not as easy to adjust pressure. Very durable contact point for frequent use	Good for large areas. Back, legs, arms, and shoulders	Lengthwise
Straight-Line Flat-Fist Technique	Moderate to strong depth of pressure. Fairly easy to adjust pressure. Durable contact point for frequent use	Good for smaller areas. Arms, neck, shoulders, sacrum, and feet	Lengthwise
Palm Press Technique	Moderate depth of pressure. Easy to adjust pressure. Durable contact point but use sparingly due to pressure on wrists. Relatively gentle technique	Good for use anywhere on body	Lengthwise
Limb Stroke Technique	Moderate depth of pressure. Easy to adjust pressure. Used in limited areas	Arms and legs	Lengthwise
Supported Palms Technique	Strong depth of pressure. Not as easy to adjust pressure. Durable contact point. Can be used more frequently because palm is supported, but be aware of pressure it puts on your wrists	Good for large areas. Legs, shoulders, chest, and back	Lengthwise
One-Two Technique	Variable moderate depth of pressure. Easy to adjust pressure. Durability depends on hand position	Can be used anywhere on body	Lengthwise

SAMPLE PROTOCOLS

The Posterior Neck

☑ Review the muscles of the posterior neck (see Figure 5.1 ■).

☑ Review the primary direction of the fibers in the muscles of the posterior neck (see Table 5.3 ■).

☑ Review the deep tissue techniques and contact points to help choose those that are best suited for use on the posterior neck, and for the particular pathology and the specific client: Table 5.2.

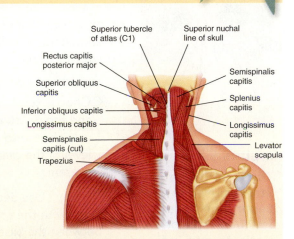

FIGURE 5.1

The Major Muscles of the Posterior Neck

TABLE 5.3   Direction of Fibers in the Muscles of the Posterior Neck

Muscle Group (from superficial to deep)	Name of Muscle	Direction of Fibers (from origin to insertion)
Attaching to vertebra, scapula, and clavicle	*Trapezius*	medial to lateral
Cervical vertebral	*Splenius capitus* *Splenius cervicis*	inferior to superior
Erector spinae	*Iliocostalis cervicis* *Longissimus capitis* *Longissimus cervicis* *Spinalis capitis* *Spinalis cervicis*	inferior to superior
Transversospinalis	*Semispinalis capitis* *Semispinalis cervicis*	inferior to superior
Suboccipital neck muscles	*Rectus capitis posterior major* *Rectus capitis posterior minor* *Obliquus capitis inferior* *Obliquus capitis superior*	inferior to superior
Vertebral muscles	*Multifidi* *Rotatores* *Interspinalis*	inferior to superior
Intertransversarii	*Intertransversarii posteriores*	inferior to superior

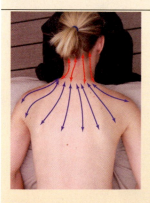

FIGURE 5.2

The Lengthwise Strokes Used in the Separation Phase for the Posterior Neck. Arrows Indicate Direction of Stroke and Colors Correspond to the Steps of Treatment.

WARM UP

Using a selection of appropriate warm-up techniques, begin to warm and encourage circulation to the neck. Make sure to work the entire area, including the shoulders as well as the upper back. This is because the neck muscles extend well into these areas.

SEPARATION PHASE (LENGTHWISE) FIGURE 5.2 ■

☑ Choose techniques and contact points suitable to the area being worked and the **depth of treatment** you want to achieve (see Table 5.4 ■). You may choose to use deeper or lighter pressure based on the tolerance level of the client as well as the specific location and type of pathology present.

Step 1: (red)   Use deep, short, **lengthwise strokes** (strokes which are applied along with the grain of the majority of muscle fibers) to work the neck between the base of the neck and the base of the skull.

Step 2: (blue)   Use deep, short, lengthwise strokes to work the superior shoulder between the base of the neck and the lateral shoulder.

SEPARATION PHASE (CROSS-FIBER) FIGURE 5.3 ■

☑ Choose techniques and contact points suitable to the area being worked and the depth of treatment you want to achieve (Table 5.4).

Step 1: (red) Use deep, short, **cross-fiber strokes** (strokes which are applied across the grain of the majority of muscle fibers) to work the neck between its base and the base of the skull.

Step 2: (blue) Use deep, short, cross-fiber strokes to work the upper back at the base of the neck.

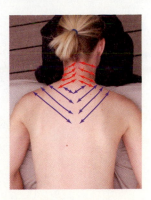

FIGURE 5.3

The Cross-Fiber Strokes Used in the Separation Phase for the Posterior Neck. Arrows Indicate Direction of Stroke and Colors Correspond to the Steps of Treatment.

REALIGNMENT PHASE FIGURE 5.4 ■

☑ Choose techniques and contact points suitable to the area being worked and the depth of treatment you want to achieve (Table 5.4).

Step 1: (red) Use long, continuous, lengthwise strokes to work the neck and superior shoulder between the base of the skull and the lateral shoulder.

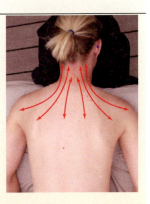

FIGURE 5.4

The Lengthwise Strokes to Be Applied to the Posterior Neck in the Realignment Phase. Arrows Indicate Direction of Stroke and Colors Correspond to the Steps of Treatment.

INTEGRATION AND CLOSING PHASE

Use a selection of appropriate closing techniques to encourage circulation to the posterior neck (Table 5.1). During this phase, it is important to include some long strokes to integrate the neck with the shoulders and upper back. Use effleurage strokes towards the core to encourage movement of blood and lymph through the area. Finish by applying range of motion movements or passive stretches to help re-educate the muscles being treated.

The Upper Back, Posterior Shoulder, and Upper Arm

☑ Review the muscles of the upper back, posterior shoulder, and upper arm (see Figure 5.5 ■).

☑ Review the primary direction of the fibers in the muscles of the upper back, posterior shoulder, and upper arm: Table 5.4.

☑ Review the deep tissue techniques and contact points to help choose those that are best suited for use on the upper back, posterior shoulder, and upper arm, and for the particular pathology and the specific client: Table 5.2.

FIGURE 5.5

The Major Muscles of the Upper Back, Posterior Shoulder, and Upper Arm

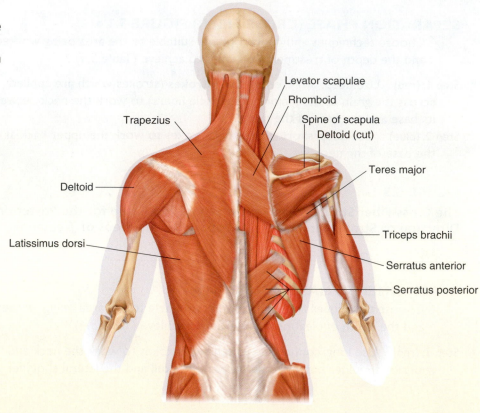

Levator scapulae
Rhomboid
Spine of scapula
Deltoid (cut)
Trapezius
Teres major
Deltoid
Triceps brachii
Latissimus dorsi
Serratus anterior
Serratus posterior

TABLE 5.4	Direction of Fibers in the Muscles of the Upper Back, Posterior Shoulder, and Upper Arm	
Muscle Group	Name of Muscle	Direction of Fibers (from origin to insertion)
Attaching to trunk and arm	*Trapezius*	medial to lateral & 45° inferior
	Latissimus dorsi	inferior to superior & 45° lateral
Attaching to scapula and arm	*Teres major*	medial to lateral & 45° superior
	Deltoid	superior to inferior
Attaching to scapula and trunk	*Levator scapulae*	superior to inferior
	Rhomboid major	medial to lateral & 45° inferior
	Rhomboid minor	
	Serratus anterior	lateral to medial
Rotators of the shoulder	*Supraspinatus*	medial to lateral
	Teres minor	
	Infraspinatus	
	Subscapularis	
Upper arm	*Triceps brachii*	proximal to distal
	Anconeus	superior to inferior

WARM UP

Using a selection of appropriate warm-up techniques, begin to warm and encourage circulation to the upper back, posterior shoulder, and upper arm (Table 5.1). Make sure to work the entire area including the neck and middle back. This is because the shoulder muscles extend well into these areas.

SEPARATION PHASE (LENGTHWISE) FIGURE 5.6 ■

☑ Choose techniques and contact points suitable to the area being worked and the depth of treatment you want to reach (Table 5.2).

Step 1: (red)   Work from medial to lateral and use deep, short, lengthwise strokes to work the superior shoulder between the base of the neck and the lateral shoulder.

Step 2: (blue)   Work from lateral to medial. Apply deep, short, lengthwise strokes from the lateral edge of the scapula to the vertebral column.

Step 3: (green)   Work from proximal to distal, and use deep, short, lengthwise strokes to work the upper arm between the shoulder and the elbow.

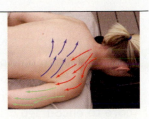

FIGURE 5.6

The Lengthwise Strokes Used in the Separation Phase for the Upper Back, Posterior Shoulder, and Upper Arm. Arrows Indicate Direction of Stroke and Colors Correspond to the Steps of Treatment.

SEPARATION PHASE (CROSS-FIBER) FIGURE 5.7 ■

☑ Choose techniques and contact points suitable to the area being worked and the depth of treatment you want to reach (Table 5.2).

Step 1: (red)   Use deep, short, cross-fiber strokes to work the superior shoulder between the base of the neck and the lateral shoulder cap.

Step 2: (blue)   Working from superior to inferior, apply deep, short, cross-fiber strokes over the entire scapula.

Step 3: (green)   Use deep, short, cross-fiber strokes to work just below the scapula. Begin at the posterior axilla and work medially, toward the vertebral column.

Step 4: (purple)   Use deep, short, cross-fiber strokes to work the upper arm between the shoulder and the elbow.

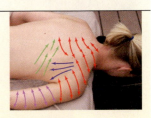

FIGURE 5.7

The Cross-Fiber Strokes Used in the Separation Phase for the Upper Back, Posterior Shoulder, and Upper Arm. Arrows Indicate Direction of Stroke and Colors Correspond to the Steps of Treatment.

REALIGNMENT PHASE FIGURE 5.8 ■

☑ Choose techniques and contact points suitable to the area being worked and the depth of treatment you want to reach (Table 5.2).

Step 1: (red)   Use long, continuous, lengthwise strokes to work the superior shoulder between the base of the neck over the lateral shoulder cap down to the elbow.

Step 2: (blue)   Work from lateral to medial. Apply long, lengthwise strokes from the lateral edge of the scapula to the vertebral column.

FIGURE 5.8

The Lengthwise Strokes to Be Used in the Realignment Phase Applied to the Posterior Upper Back, Shoulder, and Upper Arm. Arrows Indicate Direction of Stroke and Colors Correspond to the Steps of Treatment.

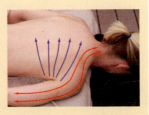

INTEGRATION AND CLOSING PHASE

Use a selection of appropriate closing techniques to encourage circulation to the upper back, posterior shoulder, and upper arm (Table 5.1). During this phase, it is important to include some long strokes to integrate these areas with the neck and middle back. Use effleurage strokes towards the core to encourage movement of blood and lymph through the area. Finish by applying range of motion movements or passive stretches to help re-educate the muscles being treated.

The Posterior Forearm and Hand

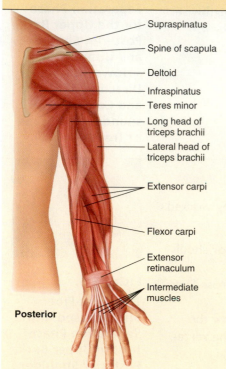

- Supraspinatus
- Spine of scapula
- Deltoid
- Infraspinatus
- Teres minor
- Long head of triceps brachii
- Lateral head of triceps brachii
- Extensor carpi
- Flexor carpi
- Extensor retinaculum
- Intermediate muscles

Posterior

THE POSTERIOR FOREARM

☑ Review the muscles of the posterior forearm and hand (see Figure 5.9 ■).

☑ Review the primary direction of fibers in the posterior forearm muscles: see Table 5.5 ■.

☑ Review the deep tissue techniques and contact points to help choose those that are best suited for use on the posterior forearm, and for the particular pathology and the specific client: Table 5.2.

FIGURE 5.9

The Major Muscles of the Posterior Forearm and Hand

TABLE 5.5	**Direction of Fibers in the Muscles of the Posterior and Lateral Forearm and Hand**	
Muscle Group	Name of Muscle	Direction of Fibers (from origin to insertion)
Muscles of forearm	*Brachioradialis*	
	Anconeus	proximal to distal
	Supinator	
Muscles that move the wrist	*Extensor carpi radialis longus*	
	Extensor carpi radialis brevis	proximal to distal
	Extensor carpi ulnaris	
Muscles that move the fingers	*Extensor digitorum communis*	
	Extensor digiti minimi	
	Abductor pollicis longus	
	Extensor pollicis brevis	proximal to distal
	Extensor pollicis longus	
	Extensor indicis	
Hand	*Dorsal interossei*	proximal to distal

WARM UP

Using a selection of appropriate warm-up techniques, begin to warm and encourage circulation to the posterior forearm. Make sure to work the entire area including the upper arm and hand. This is because the forearm muscles extend well into these areas.

SEPARATION PHASE (LENGTHWISE) FIGURE 5.10 ■

☑ Choose techniques and contact points suitable to the area being worked and the depth of treatment you want to achieve (Table 5.2).

Step 1: (red)   Use deep, short, lengthwise strokes to work the forearm between the elbow and wrist.

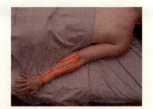

FIGURE 5.10

The Lengthwise Strokes Used in the Separation Phase for the Posterior Forearm. Arrows Indicate Direction of Stroke and Colors Correspond to the Steps of Treatment.

SEPARATION PHASE (CROSS-FIBER) FIGURE 5.11 ■

☑ Choose techniques and contact points suitable to the area being worked and the depth of treatment you want to achieve (Table 5.2).

Step 1: (red)   Use deep, short, cross-fiber strokes to work the forearm between the lateral and medial edges. Make sure to work the whole forearm between the elbow and hand.

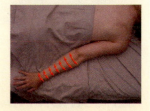

FIGURE 5.11

The Cross-Fiber Strokes Used in the Separation Phase for the Posterior Forearm. Arrows Indicate Direction of Stroke and Colors Correspond to the Steps of Treatment.

REALIGNMENT PHASE FIGURE 5.12 ■

☑ Choose techniques and contact points suitable to the area being worked and the depth of treatment you want to achieve (Table 5.2).

Step 1: (red)   Use long, continuous, lengthwise strokes to work the forearm between the elbow and hand.

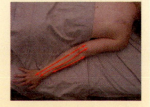

FIGURE 5.12

The Lengthwise Strokes to Be Applied to the Posterior Forearm in the Realignment Phase. Arrows Indicate Direction of Stroke and Colors Correspond to the Steps of Treatment.

INTEGRATION AND CLOSING PHASE

Use a selection of appropriate closing techniques to encourage circulation to the posterior forearm (Table 5.1). During this phase, it is important to include some long strokes to integrate the forearm with the upper arm and hand. Use effleurage strokes towards the core to encourage movement of blood and lymph through the area. Finish by applying range of motion movements or passive stretches to help re-educate the muscles being treated.

THE POSTERIOR HAND

☑ Review the muscles of the posterior forearm and hand (Figure 5.9).

☑ Review the primary direction of fibers in the muscles of the posterior hand: Table 5.5.

☑ Review the deep tissue techniques and contact points to help choose those that are best suited for use on the posterior hand, and for the particular pathology and the specific client: Table 5.2.

WARM UP

Using a selection of appropriate warm-up techniques, begin to warm and encourage circulation to the posterior hand. Make sure to work the entire hand as well as the forearm. This is because the hand muscles extend well into the forearm.

SEPARATION PHASE (LENGTHWISE) FIGURE 5.13 ■

☑ Choose techniques and contact points suitable to the area being worked and the depth of treatment you want to achieve (Table 5.2).

Step 1: (red)   Use deep, short, lengthwise strokes to work the posterior hand in either direction, including the wrist and fingers.

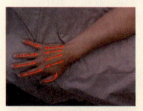

FIGURE 5.13

The Lengthwise Strokes Used in the Separation Phase for the Posterior Hand. Arrows Indicate Direction of Stroke and Colors Correspond to the Steps of Treatment.

SEPARATION PHASE (CROSS-FIBER) FIGURE 5.14 ■

☑ Choose techniques and contact points suitable to the area being worked and the depth of treatment you want to achieve (Table 5.2).

Step 1: (red)   Use deep, short, cross-fiber strokes to work the posterior hand between the lateral and medial edges. Make sure to work the entire posterior hand.

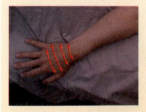

FIGURE 5.14

The Cross-Fiber Strokes Used in the Separation Phase for the Posterior Hand. Arrows Indicate Direction of Stroke and Colors Correspond to the Steps of Treatment.

REALIGNMENT PHASE FIGURE 5.15 ■

☑ Choose techniques and contact points suitable to the area being worked and the depth of treatment you want to achieve (see Table 5.2).

Step 1: (red)   Use long, continuous, lengthwise strokes to work the posterior hand, including the wrist and fingers.

FIGURE 5.15

The Lengthwise Strokes to Be Applied to the Posterior Hand in the Realignment Phase. Arrows Indicate Direction of Stroke and Colors Correspond to the Steps of Treatment.

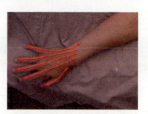

INTEGRATION AND CLOSING PHASE

Use a selection of appropriate closing techniques to encourage circulation to the posterior hand (Table 5.1). During this phase, it is important to include some long strokes to integrate the posterior hand with the forearm. Use effleurage strokes towards the core to encourage movement of blood and lymph through the area. Finish by applying range of motion movements or passive stretches to help re-educate the muscles being treated.

The Posterior Torso (Back and Sacrum)

☑ Review the muscles of the posterior torso (see Figure 5.16 ■).
☑ Review the primary direction of fibers in the muscles of the posterior torso: see Table 5.6 ■.
☑ Review the deep tissue techniques and contact points to help choose those that are best suited for use on the posterior torso, and for the particular pathology and the specific client: Table 5.2.

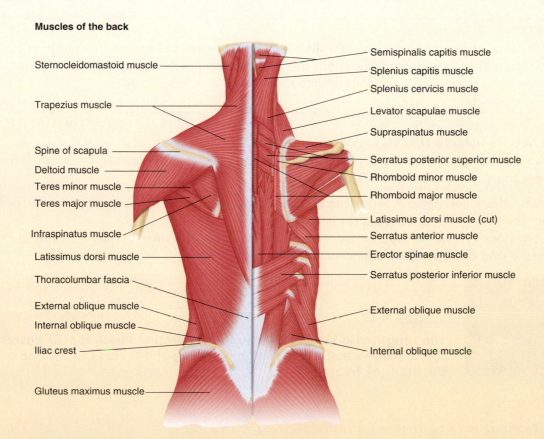

Muscles of the back

Sternocleidomastoid muscle

Trapezius muscle

Spine of scapula
Deltoid muscle
Teres minor muscle
Teres major muscle

Infraspinatus muscle

Latissimus dorsi muscle

Thoracolumbar fascia

External oblique muscle
Internal oblique muscle
Iliac crest

Gluteus maximus muscle

Semispinalis capitis muscle
Splenius capitis muscle
Splenius cervicis muscle
Levator scapulae muscle
Supraspinatus muscle

Serratus posterior superior muscle
Rhomboid minor muscle
Rhomboid major muscle

Latissimus dorsi muscle (cut)
Serratus anterior muscle
Erector spinae muscle
Serratus posterior inferior muscle

External oblique muscle

Internal oblique muscle

FIGURE 5.16

The Major Muscles of the Posterior Torso

TABLE 5.6   **Direction of Fibers in the Muscles of the Posterior Torso (Back and Sacrum)**

Muscle Group (from superficial to deep)	Name of Muscle	Direction of Fibers (from origin to insertion)
Attaching to trunk and arm	*Trapezius*	medial to lateral and 45° inferior
	Latissimus dorsi	inferior to superior and 45° lateral
Erector spinae	*Iliocostalis thoracis*	inferior to superior
	Iliocostalis lumborum	
	Longissimus thoracis	
	Spinalis thoracis	
Transversospinalis	*Semispinalis thoracis*	inferior to superior
Muscles of inspiration	*Serratus posterior inferior*	medial to lateral and 45° superior
	Serratus posterior superior	medial to lateral and 45° inferior
Vertebral muscles	*Multifidi*	inferior to superior
	Rotatores	
	Interspinalis	
Intertransversarii	*Intertransversarii posteriores*	inferior to superior
	Intertransversarii lateralis	
	Intertransversarii mediales	
Attaching trunk to ilium	*Quadratus lumborum*	inferior to superior and 45° medial

WARM UP

Using a selection of appropriate warm-up techniques, begin to warm and encourage circulation to the posterior torso. Make sure to work the entire area, including the middle back and gluteals. This is because the lower back muscles extend well into these areas.

SEPARATION PHASE (LENGTHWISE) FIGURE 5.17 ■

☑ Choose techniques and contact points suitable to the area being worked and the depth of treatment you want to achieve (see Table 5.2).

Step 1: (red)   Work inferior to superior and use deep, short, lengthwise (diagonal) strokes to work the lower back between the ilium and the vertebral column.

Step 2: (blue)   Work inferior to superior and use deep, short, lengthwise strokes to work the lower back along the sides of the vertebral column out the sides of the torso.

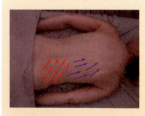

FIGURE 5.17

The Lengthwise Strokes Used in the Separation Phase for the Posterior Torso. Arrows Indicate Direction of Stroke and Colors Correspond to the Steps of Treatment.

SEPARATION PHASE (CROSS-FIBER) FIGURE 5.18 ■

☑ Choose techniques and contact points suitable to the area being worked and the depth of treatment you want to achieve (Table 5.2).

Step 1: (red)   Use deep, short, cross-fiber strokes to work the lower back between the lateral edge and the sacrum along the top of the ilium.

Step 2: (blue)   Use deep, short, cross-fiber strokes to work the entire lower back to the costal area.

Step 3: (green)   Working from the center of the sacrum out, apply deep, short, cross-fiber strokes over the entire sacrum.

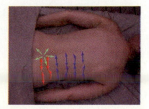

FIGURE 5.18

The Cross-Fiber Strokes Used in the Separation Phase for the Posterior Torso. Arrows Indicate Direction of Stroke and Colors Correspond to the Steps of Treatment.

REALIGNMENT PHASE FIGURE 5.19 ■

☑ Choose techniques and contact points suitable to the area being worked and the depth of treatment you want to achieve (Table 5.2).

Step 1: (red)   Use long, continuous, lengthwise strokes to work the lower back between the top of the ilium and the lower ribs.

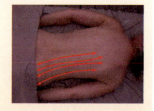

FIGURE 5.19

The Lengthwise Strokes to Be Applied to the Posterior Torso in the Realignment Phase. Arrows Indicate Direction of Stroke and Colors Correspond to the Steps of Treatment.

INTEGRATION AND CLOSING PHASE

Use a selection of appropriate closing techniques to encourage circulation to the posterior torso (Table 5.1). During this phase, it is important to include some long strokes to integrate the lower back with the buttocks and middle back. Use effleurage strokes towards the core to encourage movement of blood and lymph through the area. Finish by applying range of motion movements or passive stretches to help re-educate the muscles being treated.

The Posterior Hip and Thigh

THE POSTERIOR HIP

☑ Review the muscles of the posterior hip and thigh (see Figure 5.20 ■).
☑ Review the primary direction of fibers in the muscles of the posterior hip: see Table 5.7 ■.
☑ Review the deep tissue techniques and contact points to help choose those that are best suited for use on the posterior hip, and for the particular pathology and the specific client: Table 5.2.

FIGURE 5.20

The Major Muscles of the Posterior Hip and Thigh

Muscles of the posterior left hip and thigh

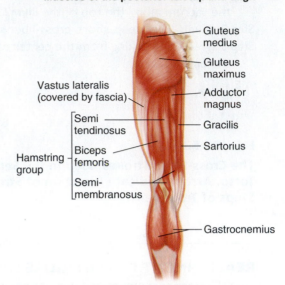

- Gluteus medius
- Gluteus maximus
- Adductor magnus
- Gracilis
- Sartorius
- Gastrocnemius

Vastus lateralis (covered by fascia)

Semi tendinosus

Biceps femoris

Semi-membranosus

Hamstring group

TABLE 5.7	Direction of Fibers in the Muscles of the Posterior Hip and Thigh	
Muscle Group (from superficial to deep)	Name of Muscle	Direction of Fibers (from origin to insertion)
Gluteal muscles	*Gluteus maximus*	
	Gluteus medius	medial to lateral and 45° superior
	Gluteus minimus	
Posterior thigh muscles	*Biceps femorus*	
	Semitendinosus	proximal to distal
	Semimembranosus	
Lateral rotators	*Piriformis*	
	Obturator internus	
	Gemellus superior	
	Gemellus inferior	medial to lateral
	Obturator externus	
	Quadratus femoris	

WARM UP

Using a selection of appropriate warm-up techniques, begin to warm and encourage circulation to the posterior hip. Make sure to work the entire area, including the lower back and posterior upper leg. This is because the posterior hip muscles have connections with these areas.

SEPARATION PHASE (LENGTHWISE) FIGURE 5.21 ■

☑ Choose techniques and contact points suitable to the area being worked and the depth of treatment you want to achieve (Table 5.2).

Step 1: (red)   Use deep, short, lengthwise strokes to work the gluteal muscles between the lateral edge of hip and sacrum.

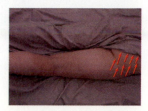

FIGURE 5.21

The Lengthwise Strokes Used in the Separation Phase for the Posterior Hip. Arrows Indicate Direction of Stroke and Colors Correspond to the Steps of Treatment.

SEPARATION PHASE (CROSS-FIBER) FIGURE 5.22 ■

☑ Choose techniques and contact points suitable to the area being worked and the depth of treatment you want to achieve (Table 5.2).

Step 1: (red)   Use deep, short, cross-fiber strokes to work the gluteal muscles between the gluteal fold and the top of the ilium.

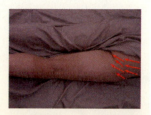

FIGURE 5.22

The Cross-Fiber Strokes Used in the Separation Phase for the Posterior Hip. Arrows Indicate Direction of Stroke and Colors Correspond to the Steps of Treatment.

REALIGNMENT PHASE FIGURE 5.23 ■

☑ Choose techniques and contact points suitable to the area being worked and the depth of treatment you want to achieve (Table 5.2).

Step 1: (red)   Use long, continuous, lengthwise strokes to work the gluteal muscles between the sacrum and lateral hip.

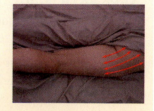

FIGURE 5.23

The Lengthwise Strokes to Be Applied to the Posterior Hip in the Realignment Phase. Arrows Indicate Direction of Stroke and Colors Correspond to the Steps of Treatment.

INTEGRATION AND CLOSING PHASE

Use a selection of appropriate closing techniques to encourage circulation to the posterior hip (Table 5.1). During this phase, it is important to include some long strokes to integrate the posterior hip with the lower back and upper thigh. Use effleurage strokes towards the core to encourage movement of blood and lymph through the area. Finish by applying range of motion movements or passive stretches to help re-educate the muscles being treated.

THE POSTERIOR THIGH

☑ Review the muscles of the posterior hip and thigh (Figure 5.20).
☑ Review the primary direction of fibers in the muscles of the posterior thigh: Table 5.7.
☑ Review the deep tissue techniques and contact points to help choose those that are best suited for use on the posterior thigh, and for the particular pathology and the specific client: Table 5.2.

WARM UP

Using a selection of appropriate warm-up techniques, begin to warm and encourage circulation to the posterior thigh. Make sure to work the entire area, including the gluteals and lower leg. This is because the upper leg muscles extend well into these areas.

SEPARATION PHASE (LENGTHWISE) FIGURE 5.24 ■

☑ Choose techniques and contact points suitable to the area being worked and the depth of treatment you want to achieve (Table 5.2).

Step 1: (red)   Use deep, short, lengthwise strokes to work the upper leg between the base of the buttocks and the knee.

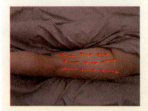

FIGURE 5.24

The Lengthwise Strokes Used in the Separation Phase for the Posterior Thigh Arrows Indicate Direction of Stroke and Colors Correspond to the Steps of Treatment.

SEPARATION PHASE (CROSS-FIBER) FIGURE 5.25 ■

☑ Choose techniques and contact points suitable to the area being worked and the depth of treatment you want to achieve (Table 5.2).

Step 1: (red)   Use deep, short, cross-fiber strokes to work the posterior upper leg between the lateral and medial edges. Make sure to work the whole upper leg between the hip and the knee.

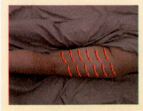

FIGURE 5.25

The Cross-Fiber Strokes Used in the Separation Phase for the Posterior Thigh. Arrows Indicate Direction of Stroke and Colors Correspond to the Steps of Treatment.

REALIGNMENT PHASE FIGURE 5.26 ■

☑ Choose techniques and contact points suitable to the area being worked and the depth of treatment you want to achieve (Table 5.2).

Step 1: (red)   Use long, continuous, lengthwise strokes to work the upper leg between the base of the buttocks and the knee.

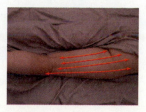

FIGURE 5.26

The Lengthwise Strokes to Be Applied to the Posterior Thigh in the Realignment Phase. Arrows Indicate Direction of Stroke and Colors Correspond to the Steps of Treatment.

INTEGRATION AND CLOSING PHASE

Use a selection of appropriate closing techniques to encourage circulation to the posterior thigh (Table 5.1). During this phase, it is important to include some long strokes to integrate the posterior thigh with the gluteals and lower leg. Use effleurage strokes towards the core to encourage movement of blood and lymph through the area. Finish by applying range of motion movements or passive stretches to help re-educate the muscles being treated.

The Posterior Lower Leg and Foot

THE POSTERIOR LOWER LEG

☑ Review the muscles of the posterior lower leg and foot (see Figure 5.27 ■).

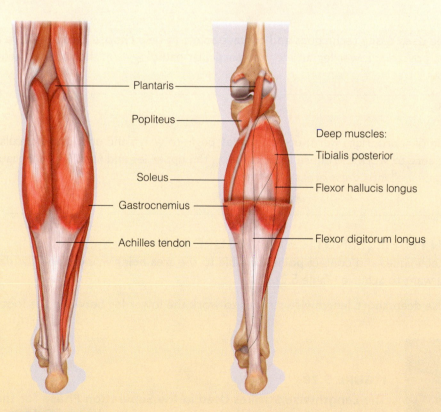

Plantaris
Popliteus
Soleus
Gastrocnemius
Achilles tendon

Deep muscles:
Tibialis posterior
Flexor hallucis longus
Flexor digitorum longus

FIGURE 5.27

The Major Muscles of the Posterior Lower Leg and Foot

☑ Review the primary direction of fibers in the muscles of the posterior lower leg: see Table 5.8 ■.

TABLE 5.8	**Direction of Fibers in the Muscles of the Posterior Lower Leg and Foot**	
Muscle Group (from superficial to deep)	Name of Muscle	Direction of Fibers (from origin to insertion)
Lower leg	*Gastrocnemius*	proximal to distal
	Soleus	
	Plantaris	
	Popliteus	
	Tibialis posterior	
Plantar surface of foot	*Abductor hallucis*	proximal to distal
	Flexor digitorum brevis	
	Abductor digiti minimi	
	Quadratus plantae	
	Lumbricales	
	Flexor hallucis brevis	
	Adductor hallucis	medial to lateral
	Flexor digiti minimi brevis	
	Dorsal interossei	proximal to distal
	Plantar interossei	
Lower leg/foot	*Flexor hallucis longus*	proximal to distal
	Flexor digitorum	

☑ Review the deep tissue techniques and contact points to help choose those that are best suited for use on the posterior lower leg, and for the particular pathology and the specific client: Table 5.2.

WARM UP
Using a selection of appropriate warm-up techniques, begin to warm and encourage circulation to the lower leg. Make sure to work the entire area, including the upper leg and foot. This is because the lower leg muscles extend well into these areas.

SEPARATION PHASE (LENGTHWISE) FIGURE 5.28 ■
☑ Choose techniques and contact points suitable to the area being worked and the depth of treatment you want to achieve (Table 5.2).

Step 1: (red)   Use deep, short, lengthwise strokes to work the lower leg between the foot and the knee.

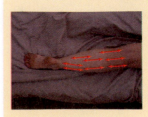

FIGURE 5.28 ■
The Lengthwise Strokes Used in the Separation Phase for the Posterior Lower Leg. Arrows Indicate Direction of Stroke and Colors Correspond to the Steps of Treatment.

SEPARATION PHASE (CROSS-FIBER) FIGURE 5.29 ■

☑ Choose techniques and contact points suitable to the area being worked and the depth of treatment you want to achieve (Table 5.2).

Step 1: (red)   Use deep, short, cross-fiber strokes to work the lower leg between the lateral and medial edges. Make sure to work the whole lower leg between the foot and the knee.

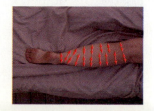

FIGURE 5.29

The Cross-Fiber Strokes Used in the Separation Phase for the Posterior Lower Leg. Arrows Indicate Direction of Stroke and Colors Correspond to the Steps of Treatment.

REALIGNMENT PHASE FIGURE 5.30 ■

☑ Choose techniques and contact points suitable to the area being worked and the depth of treatment you want to achieve (Table 5.2).

Step 1: (red)   Use long, continuous, lengthwise strokes to work the lower leg between the knee and the foot.

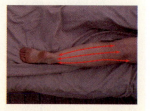

FIGURE 5.30

The Lengthwise Strokes to Be Applied to the Posterior Lower Leg in the Realignment Phase. Arrows Indicate Direction of Stroke and Colors Correspond to the Steps of Treatment.

INTEGRATION AND CLOSING PHASE

Use a selection of appropriate closing techniques to encourage circulation to the posterior lower leg (Table 5.1). During this phase, it is important to include some long strokes to integrate the lower leg with the upper leg. Use effleurage strokes towards the core to encourage movement of blood and lymph through the area. Finish by applying range of motion movements or passive stretches to help re-educate the muscles being treated.

THE POSTERIOR FOOT

☑ Review the muscles of the posterior lower leg and foot (Figure 5.27).
☑ Review the primary direction of fibers in the muscles of the foot: Table 5.8.
☑ Review the deep tissue techniques and contact points to help choose those that are best suited for use on the foot, and for the particular pathology and the specific client: Table 5.2.

WARM UP

Using a selection of appropriate warm-up techniques, begin to warm and encourage circulation to the foot. Make sure to work the entire area, including the lower leg. This is because the foot muscles extend well into that area.

SEPARATION PHASE (LENGTHWISE) FIGURE 5.31 ■

☑ Choose techniques and contact points suitable to the area being worked and the depth of treatment you want to achieve (Table 5.2).

Step 1: (red)   Use deep, short, lengthwise strokes to work the foot between the heel and the toes.

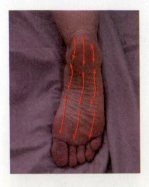

FIGURE 5.31

The Lengthwise Strokes Used in the Separation Phase for the Foot. Arrows Indicate Direction of Stroke and Colors Correspond to the Steps of Treatment.

SEPARATION PHASE (CROSS-FIBER) FIGURE 5.32 ■

☑ Choose techniques and contact points suitable to the area being worked and the depth of treatment you want to achieve (Table 5.2).

Step 1: (red)   Use deep, short, cross-fiber strokes to work the foot between the lateral and medial edges. Make sure to work the whole foot between the heel and the toes.

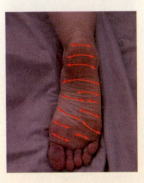

FIGURE 5.32

The Cross-Fiber Strokes Used in the Separation Phase for the Foot. Arrows Indicate Direction of Stroke and Colors Correspond to the Steps of Treatment.

REALIGNMENT PHASE FIGURE 5.33 ■

☑ Choose techniques and contact points suitable to the area being worked and the depth of treatment you want to achieve (Table 5.2).

Step 1: (red)   Use long, continuous, lengthwise strokes to work the foot between the heel and the toes.

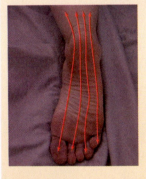

FIGURE 5.33

The Lengthwise Strokes to Be Applied to the Foot in the Realignment Phase. Arrows Indicate Direction of Stroke and Colors Correspond to the Steps of Treatment.

INTEGRATION AND CLOSING PHASE

Use a selection of appropriate closing techniques to encourage circulation to the foot (Table 5.1). During this phase, it is important to include some long strokes to integrate the foot with the lower leg. Use effleurage strokes towards the core to encourage movement of blood and lymph through the area. Finish by applying range of motion movements or passive stretches to help re-educate the muscles being treated.

QUICK QUIZ #9

1. Which of the following techniques are best suited for warming the tissues of the posterior neck? (Circle all that apply)
   a. Compression
   b. Effleurage
   c. Petrissage
   d. Muscle rolling
   e. All of the above
   f. None of the above

2. The elbow stroke technique is well suited for use on the large muscles of the back and shoulders during the realignment phase.
   a. True
   b. False

3. Which of the following techniques are well suited for use on the posterior forearm? (Circle all that apply)
   a. Supported thumb technique
   b. Knuckle stroke technique
   c. Straight-line forearm technique
   d. Limb stroke technique
   e. One-two technique
   f. All of the above
   g. None of the above

4. The primary direction of the muscle fibers in the Erector spinae muscles is from inferior to superior.
   a. True
   b. False

The Head and Face

☑ Review the muscles of the head and face (see Figure 5.34 ■).

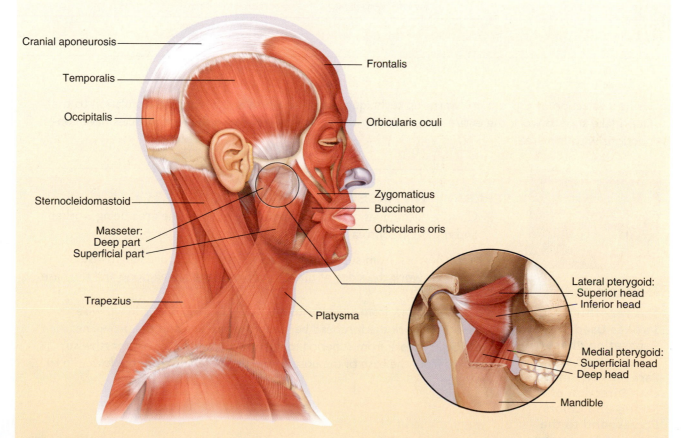

FIGURE 5.34

The Major Muscles of the Head and Face

☑ Review the primary direction of fibers in the muscles of the face: see Table 5.9 ■.

☑ Review the deep tissue techniques and contact points to help choose those that are best suited for use on the face, and for the particular pathology and the specific client: Table 5.2.

TABLE 5.9	Direction of Fibers in the Muscles of the Head and Face	
Muscle Group (from superficial to deep)	Name of Muscle	Direction of Fibers (from origin to insertion)
The muscles of the scalp	Epicranius—occipitalis	inferior to superior
	Epicranius—frontalis	superior to inferior
	Temporoparietalis	inferior to superior
The muscles of the ear	Auricularis anterior	anterior to posterior
	Auricularis posterior	posterior to anterior
	Auricularis superior	superior to inferior
The muscles of the eyelids	Orbicularis oculi	circular
	Levator palpebrae superioris	superior to inferior
	Corrugator supercilii	inferior to superior
The muscles of the nose	Procerus	inferior to superior
	Depressor septi	
	Nasalis	lateral to medial
The muscles of the jaw	Masseter	superior to inferior
	Temporalis	superior to inferior
	Lateral pterygoid	medial to lateral
	Medial pterygoid	superior to inferior

WARM UP

Using a selection of appropriate warm-up techniques, begin to warm and encourage circulation to the face. Make sure to work the entire area, including the neck. This is because the face muscles have connections with this area.

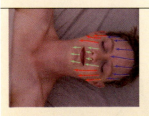

FIGURE 5.35

The Lengthwise Strokes Used in the Separation Phase for the Head and Face. Arrows Indicate Direction of Stroke and Colors Correspond to the Steps of Treatment.

SEPARATION PHASE (LENGTHWISE) FIGURE 5.35 ■

☑ Choose techniques and contact points suitable to the area being worked and the depth of treatment you want to achieve (Table 5.2).

Step 1: (red)   Work from superior to inferior. Use deep, short, lengthwise strokes to work the sides of the face between the cheek bone and the base of the jaw.

Step 2: (blue)   Work from superior to inferior. Use deep, short, lengthwise strokes to work the forehead between the hair line and the brow line.

Step 3: (green)   Work from superior to inferior. Apply deep, short, lengthwise strokes from the base of the nose to the upper lip, and from the lower lip to the chin.

SEPARATION PHASE (CROSS-FIBER) FIGURE 5.36 ■

☑ Choose techniques and contact points suitable to the area being worked and the depth of treatment you want to achieve (Table 5.2).

Step 1: (red)   Work from medial to lateral. Use deep, short, cross-fiber strokes to work the sides of the face between the cheek bone and the base of the jaw.

Step 2: (blue)   Work from medial to lateral. Use deep, short, cross-fiber strokes to work the forehead between the hair line and the brow line.

Step 3: (green)   Work from medial to lateral. Apply deep, short, cross-fiber strokes under the base of the nose to the upper lip and under the lower lip to the chin.

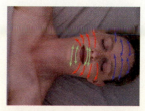

FIGURE 5.36

The Cross-Fiber Strokes Used in the Separation Phase for the Head and Face. Arrows Indicate Direction of Stroke and Colors Correspond to the Steps of Treatment.

REALIGNMENT PHASE FIGURE 5.37 ■

☑ Choose techniques and contact points suitable to the area being worked and the depth of treatment you want to achieve (Table 5.2).

Step 1: (red)   Work from superior to inferior. Use long, continuous, lengthwise strokes to work the sides of the face, between the temple and the base of the jaw.

Step 2: (blue)   Work from superior to inferior. Use long, continuous, lengthwise strokes to work the forehead, between the hair line and the brow line.

Step 3: (green)   Work from superior to inferior. Apply long, continuous, lengthwise strokes from the cheekbone to the upper lip and from the lower lip to the chin.

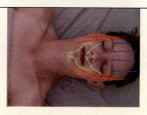

FIGURE 5.37

The Lengthwise Strokes to Be Applied to the Head and Face in the Realignment Phase. Arrows Indicate Direction of Stroke and Colors Correspond to the Steps of Treatment.

INTEGRATION AND CLOSING PHASE

Use a selection of appropriate closing techniques and contact points to encourage circulation to the face (Table 5.1). During this phase, it is important to include some long strokes to integrate the face with the neck. Use effleurage strokes towards the core to encourage movement of blood and lymph through the area. Finish by applying range of motion movements or passive stretches to help re-educate the muscles being treated.

The Anterior Neck

☑ Review the muscles of the anterior neck (see Figure 5.38 ■).
☑ Review the primary direction of fibers in the muscles of the anterior neck: see Table 5.10 ■.
☑ Review the deep tissue techniques and contact points to help choose those that are best suited for use on the anterior neck, and for the particular pathology and the specific client: Table 5.2.

FIGURE 5.38

The Major Muscles of the Anterior Neck

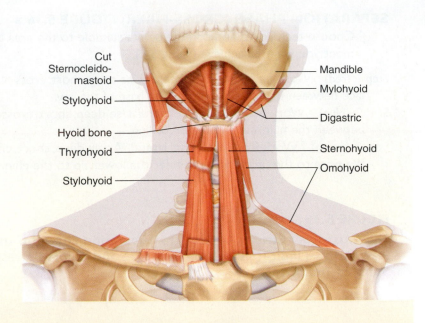

TABLE 5.10 | Direction of Fibers in the Muscles of the Anterior Neck

Muscle Group (from superficial to deep)	Name of Muscle	Direction of Fibers (from origin to insertion)
Superficial muscle	Platysma	inferior to superior
Suprahyoid muscles	Digastricus	lateral to medial and medial to lateral
	Stylohyoid	superior to inferior
	Mylohyoid	
	Geniohyoid	
Infrahyoid muscles	Sternohyoid	inferior to superior
	Sternothyroid	
	Thyrohyoid	
	Omohyoid	
Prime mover for head and neck	Sternocleidomastoid	inferior to superior
Vertebral muscles	Longus colli	inferior to superior
	Longus capitis	
	Rectus capitus anterior	
	Rectus capitus lateralis	
	Intertransversarii anteriores	
Lateral vertebral muscles	Scalenus anterior	superior to inferior
	Scalenus medius	
	Scalenus posterior	

WARM UP

Using a selection of appropriate warm-up techniques, begin to warm and encourage circulation to the anterior neck. Make sure to work the entire neck, including the chest. This is because the neck muscles extend well into the chest.

SEPARATION PHASE (LENGTHWISE) FIGURE 5.39 ■

☑ Choose techniques and contact points suitable to the area being worked and the depth of treatment you want to achieve (Table 5.2).

Step 1: (red) Working from superior to inferior, apply deep, short, lengthwise strokes over the anterior neck. Focus is on the sternocleidomastoid (SCM) muscle.

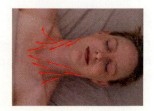

FIGURE 5.39

The Lengthwise Strokes Used in the Separation Phase for the Anterior Neck. Arrows Indicate Direction of Stroke and Colors Correspond to the Steps of Treatment.

SEPARATION PHASE (CROSS-FIBER) FIGURE 5.40 ■

☑ Choose techniques and contact points suitable to the area being worked and the depth of treatment you want to achieve (Table 5.2).

Step 1: (red) Working from medial to lateral, apply deep, short, cross-fiber strokes over the anterior neck. Focus is on the SCM muscle.

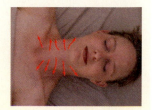

FIGURE 5.40

The Cross-Fiber Strokes Used in the Separation Phase for the Anterior Neck. Arrows Indicate Direction of Stroke and Colors Correspond to the Steps of Treatment.

REALIGNMENT PHASE FIGURE 5.41 ■

☑ Choose techniques and contact points suitable to the area being worked and the depth of treatment you want to achieve (Table 5.2).

Step 1: (red) Use long, continuous, lengthwise strokes to work the neck from superior to inferior, including the anterior chest.

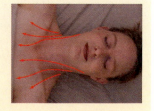

FIGURE 5.41

The Lengthwise Strokes to be Applied to the Anterior Neck in the Realignment Phase. Arrows Indicate Direction of Stroke and Colors Correspond to the Steps of Treatment.

INTEGRATION AND CLOSING PHASE

Use a selection of appropriate closing techniques to encourage circulation to the anterior neck (Table 5.1). During this phase, it is important to include some long strokes to integrate the neck with the chest and shoulder. Use effleurage strokes towards the core to encourage movement of blood and lymph through the area. Finish by applying range of motion movements or passive stretches to help re-educate the muscles being treated.

The Chest, Anterior Shoulder, and Upper Arm

THE CHEST AND ANTERIOR SHOULDER

☑ Review the muscles of the chest anterior shoulder and upper arm (see Figure 5.42 ■ and Figure 5.49).
☑ Review the primary direction of fibers in the muscles of the chest and anterior shoulder: see Table 5.11 ■.

☑ Review the deep tissue techniques and contact points to help choose those that are best suited for use on the chest and anterior shoulder, and for the particular pathology and the specific client: Table 5.2.

FIGURE 5.42

The Major Muscles of the Anterior Chest and Upper Arm

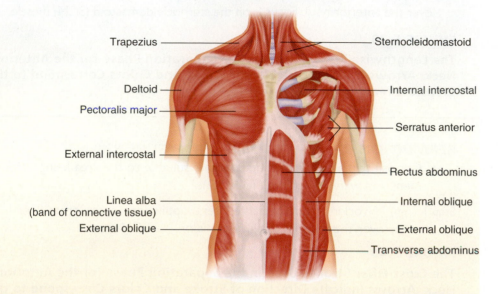

Trapezius

Sternocleidomastoid

Deltoid

Internal intercostal

Pectoralis major

Serratus anterior

External intercostal

Rectus abdominus

Linea alba
(band of connective tissue)

Internal oblique

External oblique

External oblique

Transverse abdominus

TABLE 5.11	Direction of Fibers in the Muscles of the Chest, Anterior Shoulder, and Upper Arm	
Muscle Group (from superficial to deep)	Name of Muscle	Direction of Fibers (from origin to insertion)
Attaching to trunk and arm	*Pectoralis major*	medial to lateral
Attaching clavicle to arm	*Deltoid*	superior to inferior
Attaching to arm and scapula	*Biceps brachii* *Coracobrachialis*	proximal to distal
Attaching to scapula and trunk	*Pectoralis minor* *Subclavius*	inferior to superior
Upper arm	*Brachialis*	proximal to distal

WARM UP

Using a selection of appropriate warm-up techniques, begin to warm and encourage circulation to the chest and anterior shoulder. Make sure to work the entire area, including the neck and lateral shoulder. This is because the chest and shoulder muscles extend well into these areas.

SEPARATION PHASE (LENGTHWISE) FIGURE 5.43 ■

☑ Choose techniques and contact points suitable to the area being worked and the depth of treatment you want to achieve (Table 5.2).

Step 1: (red)   Work from lateral to medial, and apply deep, short, lengthwise strokes from the lateral edge of the shoulder to the sternum.

Step 2: (blue)   Use deep, short, lengthwise strokes to work the anterior shoulder.

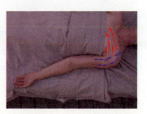

FIGURE 5.43

The Lengthwise Strokes Used in the Separation Phase for the Anterior Chest. Arrows Indicate Direction of Stroke and Colors Correspond to the Steps of Treatment.

SEPARATION PHASE (CROSS-FIBER) FIGURE 5.44 ■

Choose techniques and contact points suitable to the area being worked and the depth of treatment you want to achieve (Table 5.2).

Step 1: (red)   Working from superior to inferior, apply deep, short, cross-fiber strokes over the entire anterior chest.

Step 2: (blue)   Use deep, short, cross-fiber strokes to work the anterior shoulder.

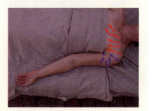

FIGURE 5.44

The Cross-Fiber Strokes Used in the Separation Phase for the Anterior Chest. Arrows Indicate Direction of Stroke and Colors Correspond to the Steps of Treatment.

REALIGNMENT PHASE FIGURE 5.45 ■

Choose techniques and contact points suitable to the area being worked and the depth of treatment you want to achieve (Table 5.2).

Step 1: (red)   Use long, continuous, lengthwise strokes to work the anterior shoulder and chest.

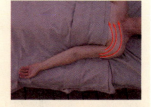

FIGURE 5.45

The Lengthwise Strokes to Be Applied to the Anterior Chest in the Realignment Phase. Arrows Indicate Direction of Stroke and Colors Correspond to the Steps of Treatment.

INTEGRATION AND CLOSING PHASE

Use a selection of appropriate closing techniques to encourage circulation to the chest and anterior shoulder (Table 5.1). During this phase, it is important to include some long strokes to integrate the chest and shoulder with the neck and upper arm. Use effleurage strokes towards the core to encourage movement of blood and lymph through the area. Finish by applying range of motion movements or passive stretches to help re-educate the muscles being treated.

THE UPPER ARM
- ☑ Review the muscles of the chest, shoulder, and upper arm (Figure 5.42).
- ☑ Review the primary direction of fibers in the muscles of the upper arm: Table 5.11.
- ☑ Review the deep tissue techniques and contact points to help choose those that are best suited for use on the upper arm, and for the particular pathology and the specific client: Table 5.2.

WARM UP

Using a selection of appropriate warm-up techniques, begin to warm and encourage circulation to the upper arm. Make sure to work the entire area, including the shoulder and forearm. This is because the upper arm muscles extend well into these areas.

SEPARATION PHASE (LENGTHWISE) FIGURE 5.46 ■

☑ Choose techniques and contact points suitable to the area being worked and the depth of treatment you want to achieve (Table 5.2).

Step 1: (red)   Use deep, short, lengthwise strokes to work the upper arm between the shoulder and elbow.

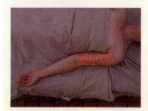

FIGURE 5.46

The Lengthwise Strokes Used in the Separation Phase for the Upper Arm. Arrows Indicate Direction of Stroke and Colors Correspond to the Steps of Treatment.

SEPARATION PHASE (CROSS-FIBER) FIGURE 5.47 ■

☑ Choose techniques and contact points suitable to the area being worked and the depth of treatment you want to achieve (Table 5.2).

Step 1: (red)   Use deep, short, cross-fiber strokes to work the upper arm between the lateral and medial edges. Make sure to work the whole arm between the shoulder and elbow.

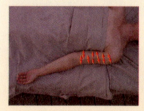

FIGURE 5.47

Cross-Fiber Strokes Used in the Separation Phase for the Upper Arm. Arrows Indicate Direction of Stroke and Colors Correspond to the Steps of Treatment.

REALIGNMENT PHASE FIGURE 5.48 ■

☑ Choose techniques and contact points suitable to the area being worked and the depth of treatment you want to achieve (Table 5.2).

Step 1: (red)   Use long, continuous, lengthwise strokes to work the upper arm between the shoulder and elbow.

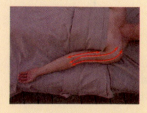

FIGURE 5.48

The Lengthwise Strokes to Be Applied to the Upper Arm in the Realignment Phase. Arrows Indicate Direction of Stroke and Colors Correspond to the Steps of Treatment.

INTEGRATION AND CLOSING PHASE

Use a selection of appropriate closing techniques to encourage circulation to the upper arm (Table 5.1). During this phase, it is important to include some long strokes to integrate the upper arm with the shoulder and forearm. Use effleurage strokes towards the core to encourage movement of blood and lymph through the area. Finish by applying range of motion movements or passive stretches to help re-educate the muscles being treated.

The Anterior Forearm and Hand

THE ANTERIOR FOREARM

☑ Review the muscles of the anterior forearm (see Figure 5.49 ■).

☑ Review the primary direction of fibers in the muscles of the anterior forearm: see Table 5.12 ■.

☑ Review the deep tissue techniques and contact points to help choose those that are best suited for use on the anterior forearm, and for the particular pathology and the specific client: Table 5.2.

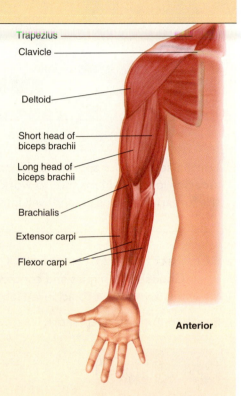

Trapezius
Clavicle
Deltoid
Short head of biceps brachii
Long head of biceps brachii
Brachialis
Extensor carpi
Flexor carpi

Anterior

FIGURE 5.49

The Major Muscles of the Anterior Forearm and Hand

TABLE 5.12	Direction of Fibers in the Muscles of the Anterior and Medial Forearm and Hand	
Muscle Group (from superficial to deep)	**Name of Muscle**	**Direction of Fibers (from origin to insertion)**
Forearm/hand muscles	*Pronator teres*	
	Flexor carpi radialis	
	Palmaris longus	
	Flexor carpi ulnaris	proximal to distal
	Flexor digitorum superficialis	
	Flexor digitorum profundus	
	Flexor pollicis longus	
	Pronator quadratus	medial to lateral

(Continued)

TABLE 5.12 *(Continued)*		
Muscle Group (from superficial to deep)	Name of Muscle	Direction of Fibers (from origin to insertion)
Hand	*Palmaris brevis*	
	Abductor pollicis	
	Flexor pollicis brevis	medial to lateral
	Opponens pollicis	
	Adductor pollicis	
	Abductor digiti minimi	proximal to distal
	Flexor digiti minimi brevis	
	Opponens digiti minimi	lateral to medial
	Palmar interossei	
	Lumbricales	proximal to distal

WARM UP

Using a selection of appropriate warm-up techniques, begin to warm and encourage circulation to the anterior forearm. Make sure to work the entire area, including the upper arm and hand. This is because the forearm muscles extend well into these areas.

SEPARATION PHASE (LENGTHWISE) FIGURE 5.50 ■

☑ Choose techniques and contact points suitable to the area being worked and the depth of treatment you want to achieve (Table 5.2).

Step 1: (red)   Use deep, short, lengthwise strokes to work the forearm between the elbow and wrist.

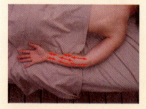

FIGURE 5.50

The Lengthwise Strokes Used in the Separation Phase for the Anterior Forearm. Arrows Indicate Direction of Stroke and Colors Correspond to the Steps of Treatment.

SEPARATION PHASE (CROSS-FIBER) FIGURE 5.51 ■

☑ Choose techniques and contact points suitable to the area being worked and the depth of treatment you want to achieve (Table 5.2).

Step 1: (red)   Use deep, short, cross-fiber strokes to work the forearm between the lateral and medial edges. Make sure to work the whole forearm between the elbow and hand.

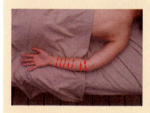

FIGURE 5.51

The Cross-Fiber Strokes Used in the Separation Phase for the Anterior Forearm. Arrows Indicate Direction of Stroke and Colors Correspond to the Steps of Treatment.

REALIGNMENT PHASE FIGURE 5.52 ■
☑ Choose techniques and contact points suitable to the area being worked and the depth of treatment you want to achieve (Table 5.2).

Step 1: (red)   Use long, continuous, lengthwise strokes to work the forearm between the elbow and hand.

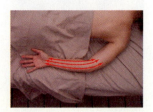

FIGURE 5.52

The Lengthwise Strokes to be Applied to the Anterior Forearm in the Realignment Phase. Arrows Indicate Direction of Stroke and Colors Correspond to the Steps of Treatment.

INTEGRATION AND CLOSING PHASE
Use a selection of appropriate closing techniques to encourage circulation to the anterior forearm (Table 5.1). During this phase, it is important to include some long strokes to integrate the forearm with the upper arm. Use effleurage strokes towards the core to encourage movement of blood and lymph through the area. Finish by applying range of motion movements or passive stretches to help re-educate the muscles being treated.

THE ANTERIOR HAND
☑ Review the muscles of the hand (Figure 5.49).
☑ Review the primary direction of fibers in the muscles of the anterior hand: Table 5.12.
☑ Review the deep tissue techniques and contact points to help choose those that are best suited for use on the anterior hand, and for the particular pathology and the specific client: Table 5.2.

WARM UP
Using a selection of appropriate warm-up techniques, begin to warm and encourage circulation to the anterior hand. Make sure to work the entire hand as well as the forearm. This is because the hand muscles extend well into the forearm.

SEPARATION PHASE (LENGTHWISE) FIGURE 5.53 ■
☑ Choose techniques and contact points suitable to the area being worked and the depth of treatment you want to achieve (Table 5.2).

Step 1: (red)   Use deep, short, lengthwise strokes to work the hand either direction, including the wrist and fingers.

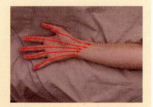

FIGURE 5.53

The Lengthwise Strokes Used in the Separation Phase for the Hand. Arrows Indicate Direction of Stroke and Colors Correspond to the Steps of Treatment.

SEPARATION PHASE (CROSS-FIBER) FIGURE 5.54 ■
☑ Choose techniques and contact points suitable to the area being worked and the depth of treatment you want to achieve (Table 5.2).

Step 1: (red) Use deep, short, cross-fiber strokes to work the hand between the lateral and medial edges. Make sure to work the entire hand.

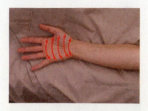

FIGURE 5.54

The Cross-Fiber Strokes Used in the Separation Phase for the Hand. Arrows Indicate Direction of Stroke and Colors Correspond to the Steps of Treatment.

REALIGNMENT PHASE FIGURE 5.55 ■

☑ Choose techniques and contact points suitable to the area being worked and the depth of treatment you want to achieve (Table 5.2).

Step 1: (red) Use long, continuous, lengthwise strokes to work the hand including the wrist and fingers.

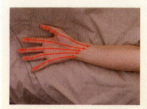

FIGURE 5.55

The Lengthwise Strokes to Be Applied to the Hand in the Realignment Phase. Arrows Indicate Direction of Stroke and Colors Correspond to the Steps of Treatment.

INTEGRATION AND CLOSING PHASE

Use a selection of appropriate closing techniques to encourage circulation to the anterior hand (Table 5.1). During this phase, it is important to include some long strokes to integrate the hand with the forearm. Use effleurage strokes towards the core to encourage movement of blood and lymph through the area. Finish by applying range of motion movements or passive stretches to help re-educate the muscles being treated.

The Anterior Torso (Abdomen)

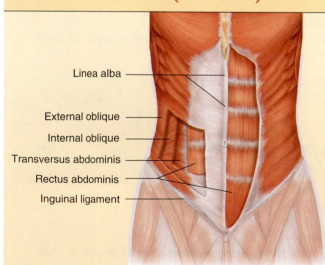

Linea alba

External oblique

Internal oblique

Transversus abdominis

Rectus abdominis

Inguinal ligament

☑ Review the muscles of the anterior torso (see Figure 5.56 ■).
☑ Review the primary direction of fibers in the muscles of the anterior torso: see Table 5.13 ■.
☑ Review the deep tissue techniques and contact points to help choose those that are best suited for use on the anterior torso, and for the particular pathology and the specific client: Table 5.2.

FIGURE 5.56

The Major Muscles of the Anterior Torso

TABLE 5.13	Direction of Fibers in the Muscles of the Anterior Torso (Abdomen)	
Muscle Group (from superficial to deep)	**Name of Muscle**	**Direction of Fibers (from origin to insertion)**
Abdominal muscles	*Obliquus externus abdominis*	lateral to medial and 45° inferior
	Rectus abdominis	inferior to superior
	Obliquus internus abdominis	lateral to medial and 45° inferior
	Transverses abdominis	lateral to medial
	Cremaster	superior to inferior
Thoracic muscles	*Intercostales externi*	
	Intercostales interni	superior to inferior
	Subcostales	
	Transverses thoracis	medial to lateral and 45° superior
	Levatores costarum	superior to inferior
	Diaphragm	lateral to medial

WARM UP

Using a selection of appropriate warm-up techniques, begin to warm and encourage circulation to the anterior torso. Make sure to work the entire area, including the costal area and hips. This is because the abdominal muscles extend well into these areas.

SEPARATION PHASE (LENGTHWISE) FIGURE 5.57 ■

☑ Choose techniques and contact points suitable to the area being worked and the depth of treatment you want to achieve (Table 5.2).

Step 1: (red) Use deep, short, lengthwise strokes to work the abdomen between the *xiphoid* and the *pubis*.
Step 2: (blue) Work from lateral to medial (at a slight angle) and apply deep, short, lengthwise strokes from the lateral edge of the torso to the center of the abdomen.

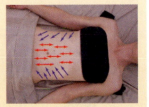

FIGURE 5.57

The Lengthwise Strokes Used in the Separation Phase for the Anterior Torso. Arrows Indicate Direction of Stroke and Colors Correspond to the Steps of Treatment.

SEPARATION PHASE (CROSS-FIBER) FIGURE 5.58 ■

☑ Choose techniques and contact points suitable to the area being worked and the depth of treatment you want to achieve (Table 5.2).

Step 1: (red)   Use deep, short, cross-fiber strokes to work the entire abdomen between the lateral and medial edges. Make sure to work the whole area between the ribs and the hips.

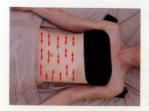

FIGURE 5.58

The Cross-Fiber Strokes Used in the Separation Phase for the Anterior Torso. Arrows Indicate Direction of Stroke and Colors Correspond to the Steps of Treatment.

REALIGNMENT PHASE FIGURE 5.59 ■

☑ Choose techniques and contact points suitable to the area being worked and the depth of treatment you want to achieve (Table 5.2).

Step 1: (red)   Work from superior to inferior and apply long, lengthwise strokes from the lower ribs to the hips.

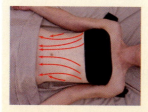

FIGURE 5.59

The Lengthwise Strokes to be Applied to the Anterior Torso in the Realignment Phase. Arrows Indicate Direction of Stroke and Colors Correspond to the Steps of Treatment.

INTEGRATION AND CLOSING PHASE

Use a selection of appropriate closing techniques to encourage circulation to the anterior torso (Table 5.1). During this phase, it is important to include some long strokes to integrate the area with the lower ribs and the hips. Use effleurage strokes towards the core to encourage movement of blood and lymph through the area. Finish by applying range of motion movements or passive stretches to help re-educate the muscles being treated.

The Anterior Hip and Thigh

☑ Review the muscles of the anterior hip and thigh (see Figure 5.60 ■).

☑ Review the primary direction of fibers in the muscles of the anterior hip and thigh: Table 5.14 ■.

☑ Review the deep tissue techniques and contact points to help choose those that are best suited for use on the anterior hip and thigh, and for the particular pathology and the specific client: Table 5.2.

FIGURE 5.60

The Major Muscles of the Anterior Hip and Thigh

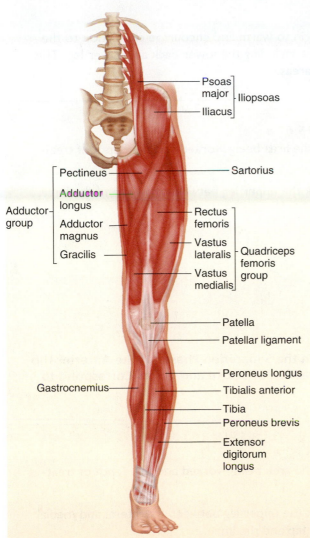

Psoas major ⎤
Iliacus ⎦ Iliopsoas

Pectineus

Adductor longus

Adductor group

Adductor magnus

Gracilis

Sartorius

Rectus femoris ⎤
Vastus lateralis ⎥ Quadriceps femoris group
Vastus medialis ⎦

Patella

Patellar ligament

Gastrocnemius

Peroneus longus

Tibialis anterior

Tibia

Peroneus brevis

Extensor digitorum longus

TABLE 5.14   Direction of Fibers in the Muscles of the Anterior and Medial Hip and Thigh

Muscle Group (from superficial to deep)	Name of Muscle	Direction of Fibers (from origin to insertion)
Anterior thigh muscles	*Tensor fascia latae*	proximal to distal
	Sartorius	
	Rectus femoris	
	Quadriceps vastus lateralis	
	Vastus medialis	
	Vastus intermedius	
Medial thigh muscles	*Gracilis*	proximal to distal
	Adductor longus	
	Adductor magnus	
	Adductor brevis	
	Pectineus	medial to lateral and 45° inferior
Hip muscles	*Psoas major*	superior to inferior
	Iliacus	

WARM UP

Using a selection of appropriate warm-up techniques, begin to warm and encourage circulation to the anterior hip and thigh. Make sure to work the entire area, including the lower back and lower leg. This is because the upper leg muscles extend well into these areas.

SEPARATION PHASE (LENGTHWISE) FIGURE 5.61 ■

☑ Choose techniques and contact points suitable to the area being worked and the depth of treatment you want to achieve (Table 5.2).

Step 1: (red)   Use deep, short, lengthwise strokes to work the upper leg between the hip and the knee.

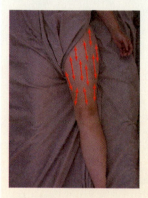

FIGURE 5.61
The Lengthwise Strokes Used in the Separation Phase for the Anterior Hip and Thigh. Arrows Indicate Direction of Stroke and Colors Correspond to the Steps of Treatment.

SEPARATION PHASE (CROSS-FIBER) FIGURE 5.62 ■

☑ Choose techniques and contact points suitable to the area being worked and the depth of treatment you want to achieve (Table 5.2).

Step 1: (red)   Use deep, short, cross-fiber strokes to work the upper leg between the lateral and medial edges. Make sure to work the upper leg between the hip and the knee.

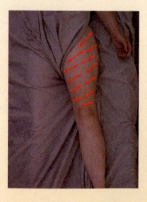

FIGURE 5.62
The Cross-Fiber Strokes Used in the Separation Phase for the Anterior Hip and Thigh. Arrows Indicate Direction of Stroke and Colors Correspond to the Steps of Treatment.

REALIGNMENT PHASE FIGURE 5.63 ■

☑ Choose techniques and contact points suitable to the area being worked and the depth of treatment you want to achieve (Table 5.2).

Step 1: (red)   Use long, continuous, lengthwise strokes to work the upper leg between the hip and the knee.

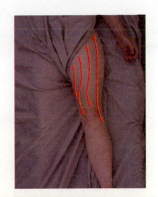

FIGURE 5.63

The Lengthwise Strokes to Be Applied to the Anterior Hip and Thigh in the Realignment Phase. Arrows Indicate Direction of Stroke and Colors Correspond to the Steps of Treatment.

INTEGRATION AND CLOSING PHASE

Use a selection of appropriate closing techniques to encourage circulation to the anterior hip and thigh (Table 5.1). During this phase, it is important to include some long strokes to integrate the anterior hip and thigh with the lower back and lower leg. Use effleurage strokes towards the core to encourage movement of blood and lymph through the area. Finish by applying range of motion movements or passive stretches to help re-educate the muscles being treated.

The Anterior Lower Leg and Foot

THE ANTERIOR LOWER LEG

- ☑ Review the muscles of the anterior lower leg and foot (see Figure 5.64 ■).

- ☑ Review the primary direction of fibers in the muscles of the anterior lower leg: see Table 5.15.

- ☑ Review the deep tissue techniques and contact points to help choose those that are best suited for use on the anterior lower leg, and for the particular pathology and the specific client: Table 5.2.

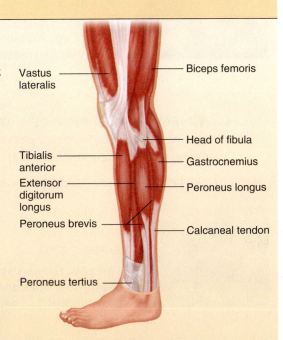

FIGURE 5.64

The Major Muscles of the Anterior Lower Leg and Foot

WARM UP

Using a selection of appropriate warm-up techniques, begin to warm and encourage circulation to the anterior lower leg. Make sure to work the entire area, including the upper leg and foot. This is because the lower leg muscles extend well into these areas.

SEPARATION PHASE (LENGTHWISE) FIGURE 5.65 ■

☑ Choose techniques and contact points suitable to the area being worked and the depth of treatment you want to achieve (Table 5.2).

Step 1: (red) Use deep, short, lengthwise strokes to work the lower leg between the knee and foot.

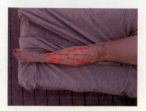

FIGURE 5.65

The Lengthwise Strokes Used in the Separation Phase for the Anterior Lower Leg. Arrows Indicate Direction of Stroke and Colors Correspond to the Steps of Treatment.

SEPARATION PHASE (CROSS-FIBER) FIGURE 5.66 ■

☑ Choose techniques and contact points suitable to the area being worked and the depth of treatment you want to achieve (Table 5.2).

Step 1: (red) Use deep, short, cross-fiber strokes to work the lower leg between the lateral and medial edges. Make sure to work the whole leg between the knee and the foot.

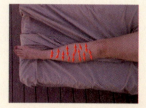

FIGURE 5.66

The Cross-Fiber Strokes Used in the Separation Phase for the Anterior Lower Leg. Arrows Indicate Direction of Stroke and Colors Correspond to the Steps of Treatment.

REALIGNMENT PHASE FIGURE 5.67 ■

☑ Choose techniques and contact points suitable to the area being worked and the depth of treatment you want to achieve (Table 5.2).

Step 1: (red) Use long, continuous, lengthwise strokes to work the lower leg between the knee and foot.

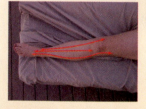

FIGURE 5.67

The Lengthwise Strokes to be Applied to the Anterior Lower Leg in the Realignment Phase. Arrows Indicate Direction of Stroke and Colors Correspond to the Steps of Treatment.

INTEGRATION AND CLOSING PHASE

Use a selection of appropriate closing techniques to encourage circulation to the anterior lower leg (Table 5.1). During this phase, it is important to include some long strokes to integrate the lower leg with the upper leg and foot. Use effleurage strokes towards the core to encourage movement of blood and lymph through the area. Finish by applying range of motion movements or passive stretches to help re-educate the muscles being treated.

THE ANTERIOR FOOT

☑ Review the muscles of the anterior foot (see Figure 5.64).

☑ Review the primary direction of fibers in the muscles of the anterior foot: Table 5.15.

☑ Review the deep tissue techniques and contact points to help choose those that are best suited for use on the anterior foot, and for the particular pathology and the specific client: Table 5.2.

WARM UP

Using a selection of appropriate warm-up techniques, begin to warm and encourage circulation to the anterior foot. Make sure to work the entire area, including the lower leg. This is because the foot muscles extend well into that area.

SEPARATION PHASE (LENGTHWISE) FIGURE 5.68 ■

☑ Choose techniques and contact points suitable to the area being worked and the depth of treatment you want to achieve (Table 5.2).

Step 1: (red)   Use deep, short, lengthwise strokes to work the anterior foot between the ankle and the toes.

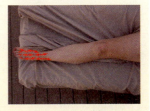

FIGURE 5.68

The Lengthwise Strokes Used in the Separation Phase for the Foot. Arrows Indicate Direction of Stroke and Colors Correspond to the Steps of Treatment.

SEPARATION PHASE (CROSS-FIBER) FIGURE 5.69 ■

☑ Choose techniques and contact points suitable to the area being worked and the depth of treatment you want to achieve (Table 5.2).

Step 1: (red)   Use deep, short, cross-fiber strokes to work the anterior foot between the lateral and medial edges. Make sure to work the whole foot between the ankle and the toes.

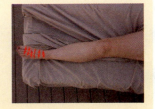

FIGURE 5.69

The Cross-Fiber Strokes Used in the Separation Phase for the Foot. Arrows Indicate Direction of Stroke and Colors Correspond to the Steps of Treatment.

REALIGNMENT PHASE FIGURE 5.70 ■

☑ Choose techniques and contact points suitable to the area being worked and the depth of treatment you want to achieve (Table 5.2).

Step 1: (red)   Use long, continuous, lengthwise strokes to work the anterior foot between the ankle and the toes.

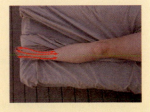

FIGURE 5.70

The Lengthwise Strokes to Be Applied to the Foot in the Realignment Phase. Arrows Indicate Direction of Stroke and Colors Correspond to the Steps of Treatment.

INTEGRATION AND CLOSING PHASE

Use a selection of appropriate closing techniques to encourage circulation to the anterior foot (Table 5.1). During this phase, it is important to include some long strokes to integrate the foot with the lower leg. Use effleurage strokes towards the core to encourage movement of blood and lymph through the area. Finish by applying range of motion movements or passive stretches to help re-educate the muscles being treated.

HOLISTIC CONNECTION

When applying firm pressure during massage, it is very common for the client to experience adjustment in their joints, especially in the vertebral column. This is very likely a good sign that the tissues are relaxing and the therapy is effective.

Many people experience excellent results from receiving regular chiropractic adjustments. Studies indicate that chiropractic therapy may be particularly effective for tennis elbow as well as chronic low back and cervical pain (Aetna InteliHealth Inc., 1996–2010). Form relationships with chiropractors so you can refer your clients for additional therapy if it is indicated. Professional relationships are also an excellent way to develop your knowledge and build your business.

TABLE 5.15	Direction of Fibers in the Muscles of the Anterior Lower Leg and Foot	
Muscle Group (from superficial to deep)	Name of Muscle	Direction of Fibers (from origin to insertion)
Lower leg	*Tibialis anterior*	proximal to distal
Lateral lower leg and foot	*Peroneus longus* *Peroneus brevis* *Peroneus tertius*	proximal to distal
Dorsal foot	*Extensor digitorum brevis*	proximal to distal
Lower leg and foot	*Extensor hallicus longus* *Extensor digitorum longus*	proximal to distal

QUICK QUIZ #10

1. Which of the following techniques are best suited for the separation phase on the muscles of the anterior neck? (Circle all that apply)
   a. Fingers technique
   b. Muscle rolling technique
   c. Straight-line flat-fist technique
   d. Palm press technique
   e. All of the above
   f. None of the above

2. Which is the correct direction for applying strokes to the Tibialis anterior during the realignment phase? (Circle all that apply)
   a. From proximal to distal
   b. From distal to proximal

   c. From medial to lateral
   d. From lateral to medial

3. It is best to use deep, short, cross-fiber strokes during the integration and closing phase for the upper arm.
   a. True
   b. False

4. Cross-fiber strokes applied to the diaphragm will run from lateral to medial.
   a. True
   b. False

SUMMARY

When applying your deep tissue massage protocol, remember the basic principles of this approach. Move slowly into the tissues following the four phases. Each phase uses a set of techniques designed to build upon the effects of the previous phase. Be aware of your body mechanics at all times to provide the best massage and to maintain your energy and posture as well. Before starting your protocol, determine if you will need any additional tools or supplies such as an extra blanket, bolsters, a heat source, etc. Pay attention to subtle cues and changes in the tissues you are treating. Remember to focus on the client and communicate throughout the protocol.

When developing your own routines, remember to be flexible and creative. The DTM protocols for any body part or set of body parts can be combined with other methods such as neuromuscular therapy, myofascial therapy, acupressure, and more.

DISCUSSION QUESTIONS

1. Why is it important to know the origin, action, and insertion of muscles you will be treating with DTM?
2. Why is it important to know the primary direction of fibers in muscles you will be treating with DTM?
3. What factors should you consider when selecting the appropriate techniques and contact points for use on the upper back, posterior shoulder, and upper arm during the Separation phase?

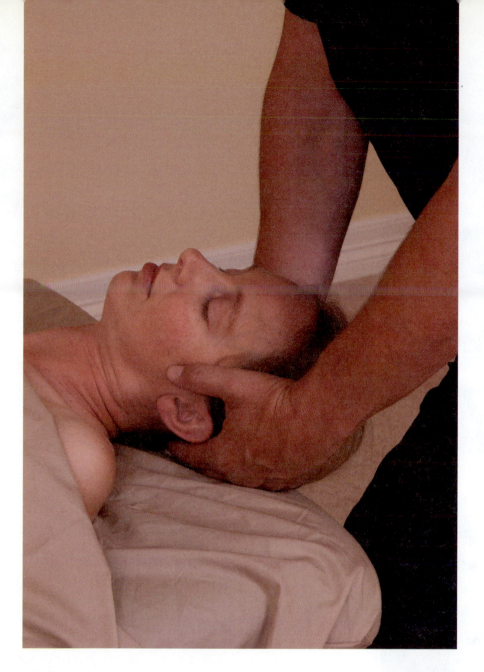

PART

3

The Neuromuscular Approach

6 A Study of Neurology

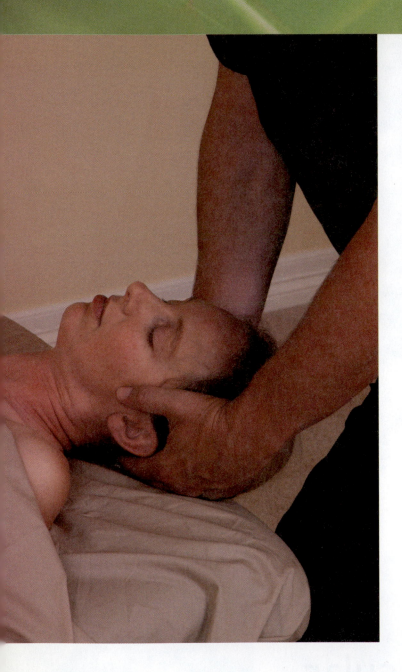

 CHAPTER HIGHLIGHTS

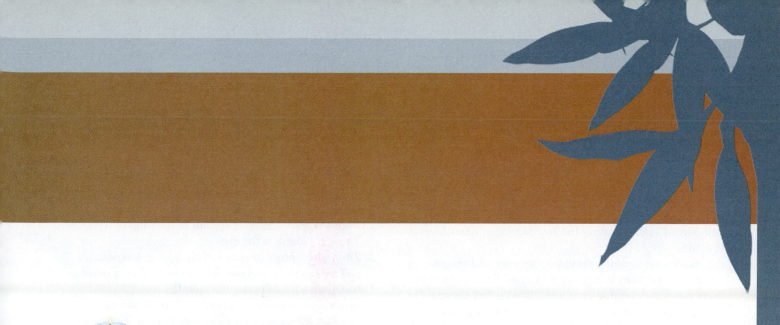

 ## CHAPTER OBJECTIVES

- Understand the classification of sensory receptors
- Examine the connections between neurology and pain
- Investigate reflexes and the law of facilitation
- Explore the formation of tonus and hypertonus

 ## KEY TERMS

SENSORY RECEPTORS

Neurology is the study of the nervous system. This includes the brain, spinal cord, and all the nerves of the body. Essential to the function of the nervous system are the sensory nerve endings, called sensory receptors, which initiate signals to the spinal cord and brain to be analyzed. An exploration of these sensory nerve endings, how they function, and how the body and mind responds to them is an important part of understanding the full picture of neurological function.

Basically, **sensory receptors** receive and respond to stimuli. A **stimulus** is any event or condition to which the body has a measurable response. Stimuli can come from changes in the environment *outside* the body, such as temperature, daylight, etc. Stimuli may also come from changes *inside* the body and can be as varied as pain, pressure, and chemical changes.

After receiving a stimulus, sensory receptors respond by sending information via signals to the spinal cord and eventually, to the brain for analysis.

DID YOU KNOW

Overstimulation of any receptor will result in the sensation of pain. Therefore, all receptors can potentially function as nociceptors. Excessive cold, heat, or pressure can be perceived as painful (Marieb, 2004).

If you have ever gotten your hands too cold on a wintry night, you may have experienced this phenomenon.

There are several types of sensory receptors in the body. In general, each sensory receptor is a specific type of nerve ending that is designed to receive a certain type of stimulus. Sensory receptors are often classified by type. There are five primary types of sensors (see Table 6.1 ■):

1. *Chemoreceptors* receive stimuli from chemicals. These are found in the nose and mouth for smelling and tasting.
2. *Photoreceptors* receive stimuli in the form of light. These are found in the eye.
3. *Thermoreceptors* respond to changes in temperature and are found throughout the skin as well as at other locations, such as inside the mouth.
4. *Mechanoreceptors* receive a variety of stimuli such as touch, pressure, vibration, and stretch. These receptors are distributed all over the body. Each type is concentrated where it is needed the most. The fingers, for example, have many receptors for touch because of the need for the hands to be especially sensitive.
5. *Nociceptors* respond to all stimuli that are either damaging, or potentially damaging, to the tissues and structures of the body. Thus, these receptors are responsible for the sensation of pain (Marieb, 2004).

Sensory receptors are found all over the body, but are concentrated where their specific type of analysis is needed most. For example, **proprioceptors** are a specialized type of mechanoreceptor that gives information about the position of the body's limbs and the body's position in space. Therefore, they are primarily located in muscles and joints. As the muscles and joints stretch and move, they stimulate the proprioceptors, giving them information about the position of the limb. (See Chapter 3 for more information on muscle spindles and Golgi tendon organs, proprioceptors that are very significant in massage therapy.)

TABLE 6.1	Five Primary Sensory Receptors	
Type of Sensory Receptor	Type of Stimuli Received	Location in Body
Chemoreceptor	• Receives stimuli from chemicals for smelling and tasting	• Nose and mouth
Photoreceptor	• Receives stimuli in the form of light	• Eyes
Thermoreceptor	• Responds to changes in temperature	• Throughout the skin as well as other locations, such as inside the mouth
Mechanoreceptor	• Receives a variety of stimuli such as touch, pressure, vibration, and stretch	• Distributed all over the body; concentrated where needed most
Nociceptor	• Responds to all stimuli that are either damaging, or potentially damaging, responsible for the sensation of pain	• Distributed all over the body

HOLISTIC CONNECTION

The use of essential oils during massage therapy is a very popular and long-standing practice. Scientific and anecdotal evidence suggests that the use of essential oils can have positive effects on our sense of well-being. A growing body of research supports the idea that the sense of smell and the application of essential oils can affect the pain response (Goubet et al., 2003; Sayyah et al., 2003). Engage the senses of your clients and explore the use of aromatherapy during massage.

DID YOU KNOW

Pacinian corpuscles also sense vibration and adapt readily to it. Think about the vibration you feel while riding in a car. As you ride you become less aware of the casual vibration of the car, even though it is still present.

Photoreceptors, are found only in the eye, as this is the only organ that is designed to take in light as information (Marieb, 2004).

Some receptors are more widely distributed. Whereas photoreceptors are only needed in the eye, other receptors, such as the pain sensing nociceptors are needed almost everywhere. Injury or pathology can occur anywhere in the body. It is important that the body is able to perceive pain everywhere because pain indicates injury or illness. The ability to locate the source of pain allows an individual to recognize and manage injury. This could even mean life or death to the individual.

Sensory Adaptation

Most sensory receptors have the ability to modify their response to a stimulus. This is called **sensory adaptation.** It is important that receptors adapt so the body can quickly and more easily adjust to common changes in the environment. Pacinian corpuscles are a common type of mechanoreceptor that adapt by becoming less sensitive when stimulated over a length of time. This receptor is responsible for sensing pressure and can be found throughout the skin, *subcutaneous* tissues, and muscles. When a person first sits down, the pacinian corpuscles, located in the buttocks and back of the legs, send signals to the brain as to the presence of the chair. However, after a few seconds the brain becomes less aware that the chair is present because the pacinian corpuscles have adapted and are no longer sending information. A continuous stimulus such as pressure from the seat of a chair does not need to be constantly sent to the brain for analysis. When the person shifts in their seat, they will become "reaware" of the chair. The shift causes a change in the pressure, and the change causes the corpuscles to adapt to the new environment.

Receptors of different types adapt at different rates. The varying rate of adaptation depends on the function of the receptor. Sensors for vibration and temperature adapt at a relatively fast rate. Nociceptors, on the other hand, do not adapt because they are the sensors for pain (Marieb, 2004). It is not beneficial for the body to adapt to a painful stimulus, as pain is an indication that damage is occurring to the tissues. Pain sends the message, "stop what you are doing and pay attention to me!" If nerves were to adapt and stop sending pain signals, then a person would likely further injure the area because they would not feel that the area is damaged.

Sensory Receptors and Pain

Interestingly, the deep receptors for pain are often found to *increase* their pain signals over time rather than adapt to pain (Cohen, 2005). This means that an old chronic injury may actually hurt worse than a fresh injury. It makes sense that the body may want to ramp up the pain signals if the area is not fully healed. It is as if the injured area is trying to shout louder to be heard. When investigating pain during massage, it is important to remember that sharp or intense pain is not necessarily caused by an acute injury. It could be an old injury that has just ramped up its signal.

Continuous pain stimulates structures called *NMDA receptors* in the spinal cord. These receptors sensitize the spinal cord to future pain impulses. Once the spinal cord is sensitized, the person becomes overly sensitive to the pain.

DID YOU KNOW

NMDA receptors also have the ability to assist nerves during the process of learning a new task. They do this by strengthening neural connections (Marieb, 2004). This is a process called facilitation. (See the discussion of facilitation later in this chapter.)

This state is called *hyperalgesia*. It is as if the brain and spinal cord have had enough, and now even a mild sensation of pain is perceived as "too much." Therapists must take into account the possibility of hyperalgesia when treating clients. What may seem like a mild injury may be much more painful to the client if it is present long enough to cause hyperalgesia. When the client is in this state, it is important to work gently and slowly. This allows the hypersensitive nerves to accept the new sensations of therapy at a pace they can tolerate.

PAIN AND NEUROMUSCULAR THERAPY

As mentioned, nociceptors are responsible for sensing pain all over the body. Pain may be classified as somatic or visceral depending upon its source. **Somatic pain** refers to pain felt in the skin and myoskeletal system (e.g., muscles, bones, and joints). *Visceral pain* arises from the organs and deep internal tissues. NMT is primarily concerned with somatic pain. It is important to note that sometimes visceral pain masquerades as somatic pain. When the kidneys are infected, for example, they can cause deep lower back pain and stiffness. Information about internal organ disease should be obtained during the health survey portion of client assessment.

Somatic pain can be further divided into superficial somatic pain and deep somatic pain. Superficial pain arises from the skin and subcutaneous tissues. Deep pain comes from the muscles, joints, and bones. According to Marieb (2004), "Deep somatic pain is more diffuse than superficial somatic pain, lasts longer and always indicates tissue destruction" (p. 494). It is important for body workers to note the depth of the pain as it can indicate which tissues are affected and which therapy will be useful for treatment.

Whether confronting superficial somatic pain or deep somatic pain, threshold and tolerance are important concepts that affect a person's experience of pain.

Pain threshold is the minimum level at which most people will become aware of a painful stimulus. This is often correlated to the level at which the tissue becomes damaged. For example, when pressure or heat is applied, most people will begin to sense the stimulus as painful at about the same level (i.e., when the tissue is being adversely affected). Pain threshold is established by averaging the experience of pain among many individuals (Marieb, 2004).

Pain tolerance is a person's subjective experience of pain. Each person has a very different interpretation of the pain they experience. This is based on their individual characteristics (Marieb, 2004). Pain tolerance is colored by the individual's gender, culture, past experiences with pain, and general attitudes toward pain. This suggests that pain can be intensified and/or lessened by the influence of the brain. Take, for example, two people from different lifestyles; one lives in a harsh environment where hard work and bodily injury are a daily norm. The other lives in an environment with very little physical stress or bodily harm. Each then stumbles while walking, causing a sprain to the lateral ankle. This is a painful situation where swelling and bruising are common. Based on the background of these individuals, it is likely they will

DID YOU KNOW

Many athletes do not experience pain during the intense activity of the game. After the game, when they turn their attention to their injuries, the pain suddenly seems to come from nowhere.

have a very different response to the pain they are experiencing. The individual with the daily exposure to harsh living will more likely have a lesser interpretation of the pain (a higher *tolerance*) even though both are experiencing the same *threshold*.

It is important to note that a person's experience of pain varies by the moment as well. An individual may sustain an injury and they will "feel" the pain differently based on the immediate circumstances. If they are injured, for example, yet they are at their favorite sporting event, the injury may "hurt less" than if they were at work. The excitement and desire to be at the sporting event "blocks" the pain to a degree. On the other hand, being at work may offer less distraction from the pain and therefore the injury "hurts more" –especially if it means going home early that day!

Based on this idea, Ronald Melzack and Patrick Wall, in 1965, developed a theory called the *gate control theory of pain*. This theory attempted to account for the mental and emotional involvement in pain perception.

According to Melzack and Wall, sensory signals travel from stimulated nerves to the spinal cord. There, they encounter a kind of "nerve gate" that can be opened or closed depending on a number of neural and chemical factors, including signals from the brain. Certain physical and emotional conditions may "open the gate" and allow the sensory signal through to the brain. On the other hand, alternate conditions may cause the gate to be closed. In this case the pain signals will not be transmitted to the brain for further action (Marieb, 2004).

DID YOU KNOW

In a study inspired by the gate control theory, an important discovery about the application of massage was made. When massage pressure was deep enough to overload the large tactile nerve fibers, they caused a reaction in the cells of the spinal cord that inhibited the transmission of pain signals. Exactly how this occurs is not clearly understood (Marieb, 2004).

QUICK QUIZ #11

1. Proprioceptors are specialized thermoreceptors that give information about limb positioning and the body's position in space.
   a. True
   b. False

2. _____ is the phenomenon that occurs as receptors become less sensitive when exposed to a continuous stimulus over a length of time.
   a. Hyperalgesia
   b. Hypertonicity
   c. Sensory adaptation
   d. Pain threshold
   e. Pain tolerance

3. Nociceptors are responsible for sensing pain all over the body.
   a. True
   b. False

4. _____ is a person's subjective experience of pain.
   a. Hyperalgesia
   b. Hypertonicity
   c. Sensory adaptation
   d. Pain threshold
   e. Pain tolerance

Sensory information is processed in the context of the individual's current mood, state of attention, state of activity, and prior experience. The integration of all this information influences whether the pain gates are opened or closed in a particular situation. Gate control theory proposes that a person's perception and experience of pain depends upon whether these gates are open or closed.

The details of the mechanisms of pain tolerance are not fully understood and gate control theory is a debated subject. However, even as a simple analogy it does provide a fairly simple sketch for understanding that mental as well as physical factors guide the brain's interpretation of painful sensations and the body's response to it. The idea that our thoughts, beliefs, and emotions affect how much pain we feel is generally an accepted concept by most researchers in this field today.

As a body worker you must be aware of these psychological controls over pain in order to better understand each client's response to their own pain. Understanding the client's tolerance helps direct the therapy towards the most suitable modalities. When applying NMT, it is important to stay within the client's pain tolerance regardless of how low the tolerance may be. If the therapy is pushed past the tolerance level, the client ends up tensing and fighting the therapy. It is important to also note that there are clients with a high tolerance for pain as well. In this case, take care to not push the tissues too far just because the client "feels no pain."

PAIN AND REFLEXES

Pain almost always triggers some sort of reflex in the body. Anybody who has ever touched a sharp object has felt how pain stimulates the reflex of pulling away. Reflexes are not limited to protecting the body from sharp objects. They actually regulate many functions in the body. Reflexes moderate activities such as blinking and swallowing, in addition to being a crucial component of myoskeletal functioning. Although reflexes of many types control numerous body systems, they all occur over a single set of neural components collectively called a **reflex arc.** A reflex arc is made of five distinct parts: receptor, sensory *neuron*, spinal cord, motor neuron, and effector (see Figure 6.1 ■).

1. The *receptor* is a nerve ending such as a nociceptor.
2. The *sensory neuron* carries the impulse to the spinal cord.
3. The *spinal cord* sends signals to the brain for further analysis and/or sends a reaction signal back to the motor neuron.
4. The *motor neuron* carries the reaction signal from the spinal cord to the effector.
5. The *effector* is the structure or tissue that will react to the stimulus. Muscles are effectors and are frequently stimulated by the reflex arc.

The simple arrangement of the reflex arc allows the body to respond quickly to the environment.

DID YOU KNOW

Although it works primarily at a subconscious level, the cerebellum plays an important role in the precise timing and coordination of muscles. The cerebellum is integral to the learning process of "muscle memory" (Marieb, 2004).

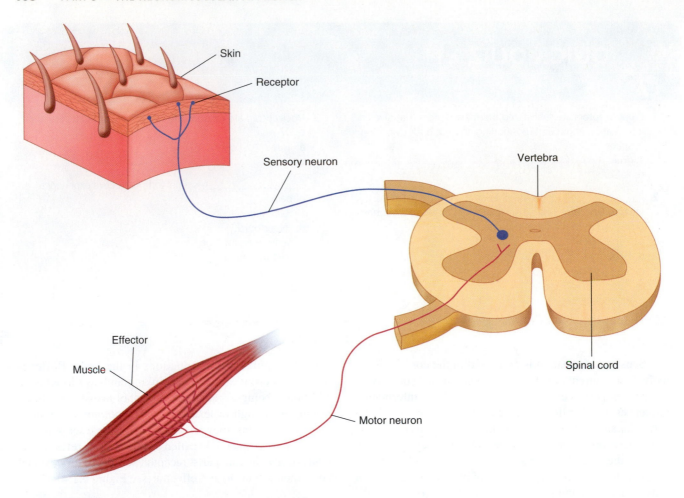

FIGURE 6.1

The Components of a Reflex Arc. The Receptor in the Skin Receives the Stimulus and Sends a Signal Along the Sensory Neuron to the Spinal Cord. The Spinal Cord Responds by Immediately Sending a Motor Signal Out Along the Motor Neuron, to the Effector (Muscle) Causing a Muscle Contraction.

Somatic Reflexes

The reflexes associated with the myoskeletal system are called **somatic reflexes.** Marieb (2004) presents two types of somatic reflexes, learned and intrinsic.

Learned reflexes are based on the experiences of the person and are not a built-in response. This type of reflex is developed when we repeat a movement over and over. It is also the process by which one learns a physical task, such as how to throw a baseball. Laymen often call learned reflexes "muscle memory" or "body memory." This is because after practicing a particular movement enough it's as if the body can perform the movement without the brain being involved. While "muscle memory" is a good analogy, it is not quite accurate to say that memory is stored directly in the muscles. However, there is a so-called learning process going on with the nerves of the muscles. The nerves learn through the process of facilitation.

Facilitation

The law of **facilitation** states that when an impulse has passed once through a certain set of neurons, it will tend to take the same course on a future occasion to the exclusion of

others. Each time it travels this path the electrical resistance will be smaller (Fritz, 2000). This means that each time a neural signal is sent to or from a particular set of muscles, the signal travels faster and more easily. It also means that over time, a less intense signal from the brain will produce the same movement (Chaitow, 2000). This is what allows us to become more and more proficient at a particular physical

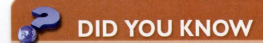

DID YOU KNOW

Facilitation of nerve pathways is like making a shortcut through a field on the way to school. The first few times you cut through, the path is full of brush, stones, etc. It is more difficult to cross. However, by walking over the same path each day, it becomes worn and easier to pass. Travel along that path is "facilitated"—or made easier—the more it is used.

task, such as throwing a baseball. The first time a person attempts to throw, they may have trouble coordinating the movements well enough to throw on target or with any speed. But each time they practice, the neural signals from the brain move faster and more efficiently, which in turn makes the muscle coordination faster and more efficient. As this happens over and over, they become proficient at throwing and it is sort of second nature to them. This is because the pathway that the impulses must travel along the nerves has been "facilitated" due to repeated stimulation. It's as though the body has cut a path along those neurons, so the signal moves very quickly and easily. This allows the muscles to move with such efficiency that it doesn't require much thought.

DID YOU KNOW

I've even seen facilitated movement patterns that linger after successful treatment in horses. The horse may present with a limp. During treatment, it is clear that there is a painful pathology so that the horse will not tolerate a complete range of motion test. After the pathology is treated, it is clear that the joint is no longer painful because the animal will tolerate complete range of motion. However, the horse may still limp. The muscles and joints are okay, but facilitation has locked the limp into the horse's way of moving. It takes further therapy and good training to replace the facilitated pattern with a healthy one.

Facilitation is good when we are properly learning new physical activities, but it can also contribute to the formation of pathological movement patterns. Injuries often cause a person to limit the movement of a limb in a certain way because it is painful otherwise. They may even have to restrict movement completely to protect the injury. Chronic restriction causes the limited movement pattern to be practiced over and over. Through repetition the nerve pathways for that pattern will be facilitated until those movements become habit. Even when the injury is healed, the body stays fixed in the old, pathological movement pattern because it has been facilitated. This reminds us that pathological movement patterns may be the result of patterns facilitated by old injuries rather than of a new or acute painful condition.

Facilitation is one of the main neurological processes behind the holding patterns and postural dysfunctions described in Chapter 2. Neuromuscular therapy uses facilitation to its advantage. It seeks to reverse the pathological pattern by re-educating the muscles to facilitate healthy positions and movement patterns.

Intrinsic reflexes (spinal reflexes) are built into our "internal wiring." They control movement and act as a protective response. Learned reflexes can be thought of as a fast connection between the *brain* and muscles. Intrinsic reflexes, on the other hand, are mainly controlled by the *spinal cord*. The brain has very little involvement aside from receiving the information that the reflex has just happened. As a result, these reflexes are also called **spinal reflexes.**

One type of spinal reflex is the withdrawal reflex or flexor reflex (see Figure 6.2 ■). It is the type of reflex that occurs when you touch a hot stove. Your body immediately

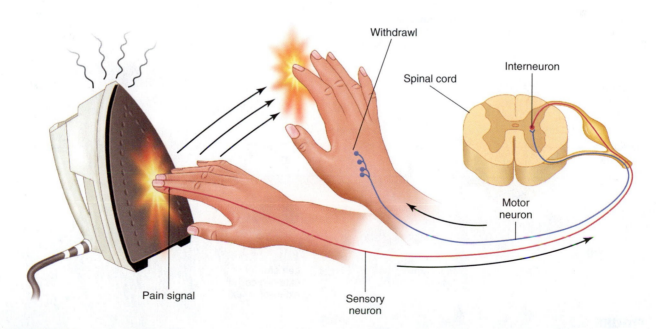

FIGURE 6.2

The Withdrawal Reflex. The Pain Signal Travels Along the Sensory Nerve to the Spinal Cord, Activating a Signal Along the Motor Nerve to Cause Withdrawal from the Stimulus.

pulls your hand away from the heated burner to protect it from getting further burned. All of this happens before you are even aware of it. The body doesn't have time to wait for the signal to reach the brain for processing. It must act immediately to protect the hand. It is much more efficient to moderate the signal at the level of the spinal cord so the reaction response can get to the muscles faster, preventing further injury.

In order for the body to send a sufficient response to withdraw, the spinal cord sends out a reaction signal that is two times the strength of the sensory signal it received (Marieb, 2004). The result is that a minor burn may cause just as vigorous a reaction as a major one. The body doesn't care if the burn is small or large; it just wants to get the hand away fast. Therefore, the spine sends out a strong motor signal that is, in a sense, an overreaction. This ensures that enough muscles are recruited to pull the entire hand and arm clear, not just the one finger that may have originally been burned.

This works very well when it is necessary to pull a body part away from something harmful such as a hot stove. However, when the pain is coming from a muscular pathology,

the body contracts all the associated muscles around the condition. This overreaction causes even more tension in the affected muscles and always complicates the original pathology. This process will be discussed in more detail later in this chapter.

Another type of spinal reflex is the crossed extensor reflex (see Figure 6.3 ■). This is a continuation of the flexor reflex. When a painful stimulus initiates the flexor reflex to withdraw a body part, the signal may cross the spinal cord and stimulate the extensors in the body part on the opposite side of the body. If, for example, you step on a sharp stone with your right foot, the flexor reflex in your right leg will pull your foot up and off the stone. Immediately, the extensors of your left leg contract to balance your body weight that has just been shifted over to it. This is a very useful protective reflex, in this case, preventing you from losing balance and falling.

Knowledge of these two reflexes helps to understand the nature of the neural response to pain and how that impacts the muscle system. No matter where the source of the pain is, it will activate the body's reflexes. Over time the pain can cause pathological tension in the muscles stimulated through the reflexes.

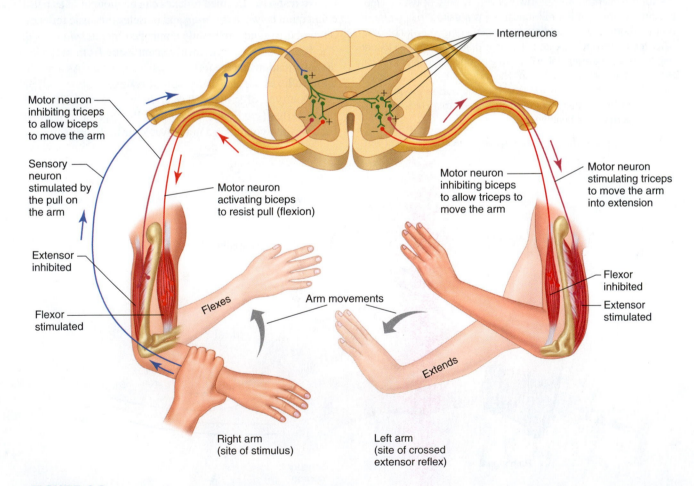

FIGURE 6.3

The Crossed Extensor Reflex in the Arms. When the Right Flexor Is Stimulated, the Right Extensor Is Inhibited. On the Opposite Side of the Body, the Left Extensor Is Stimulated While the Left Flexor Is Inhibited.

HOLISTIC CONNECTION

Moshe Feldenkrais developed the Feldenkrais method (a series of lessons in "Awareness Through Movement" and "Functional Integration"), which encourages students to discover and understand their own personal neuromuscular patterns. Students are guided verbally or with a gentle tactile cues to explore new ways of moving. Learn more about the Feldenkrais method to enhance your own well-being and to share your whole-body insights with your clients.

SPINAL REFLEXES AND TONUS

Spinal reflexes have functions other than protecting the body from getting burned by a hot stove. They are responsible for maintaining a general state of muscular contraction called **tonus.** Tonus is a sort of natural tension, which all muscles maintain at some level, at all times. It is what holds our organs, bones, and body parts in place. The level of tonus maintained by each muscle depends upon a variety of circumstances. The degree of rest, exertion, and fatigue of the muscle has an impact on the level of tonus. Tonus is regulated by proprioceptors located in the muscle.

Muscle spindles and Golgi tendon organs are the proprioceptors primarily responsible for maintenance of muscle tone as well as the smooth flow of muscle movements. When a muscle is stretched, the muscle spindles are stimulated and react by initiating a spinal reflex called the *stretch reflex* (see Figure 6.4 ■). The stretch reflex causes contraction in the agonist muscle and also causes the antagonist muscle to relax by stimulating its Golgi tendon organ. This is a process called *reciprocal inhibition* (see Figure 6.5 ■).

The Golgi tendon organ stimulates the local muscle to relax and in turn sends out a signal to the agonist muscle, causing it to contract. This is called *reciprocal activation* (see Figure 6.6 ■).

The two processes, reciprocal inhibition and reciprocal activation, are integral to the smooth flow of joint movement. As one muscle contracts it signals the opposite muscle to relax. As that muscle relaxes, it signals the other to contract. In the case of walking or running, this process allows for the

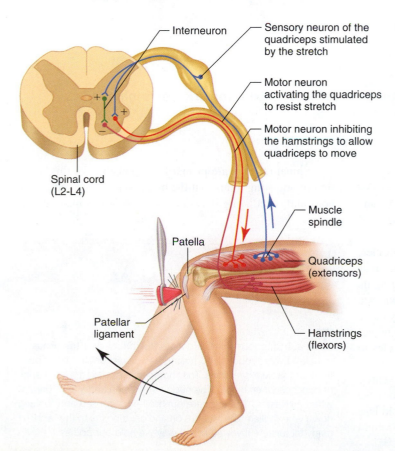

Interneuron

Sensory neuron of the quadriceps stimulated by the stretch

Motor neuron activating the quadriceps to resist stretch

Motor neuron inhibiting the hamstrings to allow quadriceps to move

Spinal cord (L2–L4)

Patella

Muscle spindle

Quadriceps (extensors)

Patellar ligament

Hamstrings (flexors)

FIGURE 6.4

The Stretch Reflex as It Occurs in the Knee and Thigh. When the Patellar Ligament Is Suddenly Stimulated, the Muscle Spindle of the Quadriceps Sends a Signal to the Spinal Cord. In Response, the Quadriceps Contract While the Hamstrings Relax, Causing the Foot to Kick Forward.

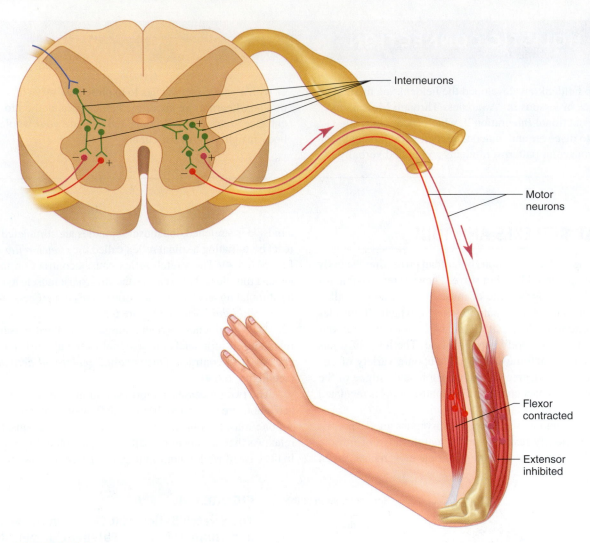

FIGURE 6.5

The Process of Reciprocal Inhibition in the Upper Arm. The Extensor (Triceps) Is Inhibited by the Contraction of the Flexor (Biceps).

rapid switching of muscle contractions from one side of the knee joint to the other. Remarkably, this process happens so fast that the muscles move smoothly and with amazing coordination. Tight muscles interrupt these two processes and may lead to distortions in movement and posture.

Tonus is maintained not only within individual muscles, but also within muscle groups. In fact, the whole muscular system is constantly maintaining, shifting, and adjusting its level of tonus. Just watch someone talking and you will see a constant adjusting and readjusting of muscles as they move their head and hands about. Every gesture or slight movement affects the rest of the body causing other muscles to adjust their level of tonus.

Even slightly tilting the head forward causes the entire length of the spinal muscles to increase their tonus to make up for the shift in weight of the head. The gluteals and legs will also have to adjust to make up for the shift in the weight of the torso.

Spinal reflexes are primarily responsible for this function of adjusting tonus, but the brain is also involved and is constantly mediating it. As the spinal reflex is maintaining

DID YOU KNOW

The subconscious mind is constantly influencing the tonus of muscles. Every thought and feeling has corresponding body positions and facial expressions. The shoulders are relaxed when happy or hunched when in fear. The neck is stiff when angry and forward when interested. The eyes are open when surprised and looking down when sullen. The list goes on and on. It points to the fact that many factors are involved in the way we hold our bodies.

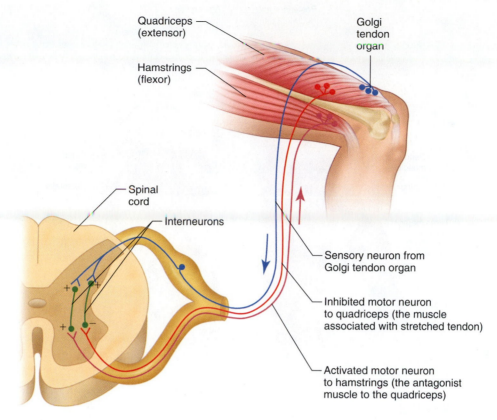

FIGURE 6.6

The Process of Reciprocal Activation in the Thigh. When the Golgi Tendon Receptor Is Stimulated, the Extensor (Quadriceps) Is Inhibited and the Flexor (Hamstrings) Is Stimulated to Contract.

normal and/or abnormal tonus, the brain monitors it and adds its own input. Therefore, tonus tends to fluctuate with emotion and thought as well. A classic example of the mind's influence on the level of muscle tone is when an individual is anxious or stressed. Often, they will unconsciously hold their shoulders high and close to their ears as they worry. Holding the shoulders high as if to protect the neck is a common posture of fear.

All of the body's muscles are in a constant flux between relaxation and contraction. It is a complex process to sit, lie down, and move through space. In fact, it requires an amazing symphony of coordination just to move the arm above the head. This action alone involves muscles from the arm, back, neck and chest. Not to mention the many muscles involved in stabilizing the rest of the torso (see Figure 6.7 ■).

SPINAL REFLEXES AND HYPERTONUS

Spinal reflexes have the ability to respond quickly and fluidly to the body's movements by adjusting tonus. However,

when subject to pathological conditions the reflex can become a problem. As described earlier, a spinal reflex is a reflex arc that runs through a set of neurons to the spinal cord, and back to the muscles. If this same set is continuously stimulated, the pathway can become facilitated and fixed. This is called the **pain reflex cycle** or the **pathophysiological reflex arc** (Fritz, 2000). Figure 6.8 ■ shows a diagram of the pain reflex cycle.

This process involves the same type of neural facilitation that occurs when learning a task. Only in this case, the nerves are "learning" to maintain a pathological level of tonus. In muscles, the pain reflex cycle leads to the chronic condition called **hypertonus**. Hypertonus is chronic, pathological tension in the muscle often caused by pain. The pain may come from an injury or inflammation. Muscles irritated due to stress or injury constantly send pain signals to the spinal cord. The cord responds by sending twice the motor output back to the muscle. This contracts the muscle further, which increases the level of irritation and thus causes even more pain signals to be sent to the spinal cord. The spinal cord reacts by again sending signals for more contraction, creating a vicious cycle.

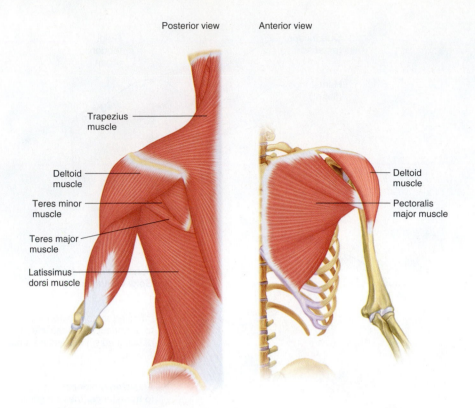

FIGURE 6.7

The Muscles Involved in the Lifting of the Arm Above the Head

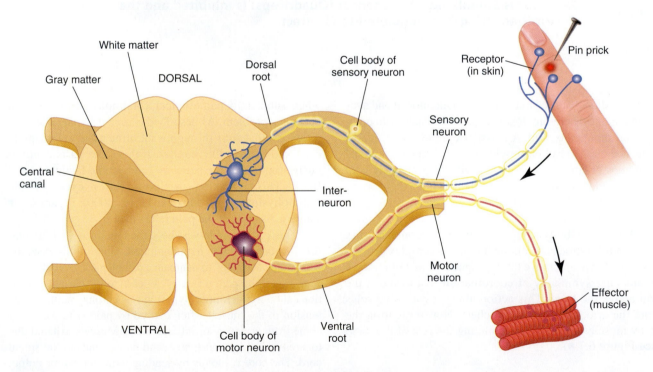

The pathway for the pain reflex arc

FIGURE 6.8

The Pain Reflex Cycle. The Pain Signal Travels Along the Sensory Nerve to the Spinal Cord, Activating a Signal Along the Motor Nerve to the Effector.

Case Study

Logan, a high school baseball pitcher, came into a clinic with a second-degree strain in the supraspinatus muscle of the rotator cuff (see Figure 6.9 ■). This is a common injury for a pitcher because each time the ball is thrown it puts strain on the rotator cuff. Logan complains of pain each time he reaches out or tries to cock his arm back to throw. This is because the supraspinatus supports the shoulder while reaching out and also will be stretched slightly when the arm is cocked back. Although the original injury was located in one muscle, by the time Logan came into clinic the muscles in his entire shoulder were tense and full of knots. The injury had spread to the surrounding muscles. In this case, the pain from the tear was continuously sent to the spinal cord. Through the reflex arc, the spinal cord signaled all of the muscles of the upper shoulder (i.e., the trapezius, levator scapula, and rhomboids) to repeatedly contract and draw back due to the pain (see Figure 6.10 ■).

This process continued over and over, increasing the tonus in the muscles of the upper shoulder. As those muscles became hypertonic, they shortened and began to pull on the injured site, causing even more pain.

The process of facilitation caused the movement pattern to be locked in to the point where it persisted past the existence of the original injury. In this case, the tear in the supraspinatus may have healed, but Logan is still suffering from the restricted pattern. This left over restricted pattern causes the pain reflex cycle to continue on.

VASOCONSTRICTION AND ISCHEMIA

The complications of hypertonicity do not end here. The condition can lead to other pathologies, such as compensation and postural dysfunction, as detailed in Chapter 2. If the muscle is hypertonic long enough, it will result in **vasoconstriction.** Vasoconstriction is the narrowing of blood vessels. This is often caused by the compression of muscles and other tissues against them. When a hypertonic muscle tightens around blood and lymph vessels, it begins to limit the flow of nutrients into the muscle, and the flow of metabolic waste out of the muscle. Metabolic wastes accumulate in the muscle and further irritate nerve endings. This causes the nerves to send more pain signals, which creates more contraction in the muscle. As this transaction between the muscle and spinal cord gains strength, a state of harmful **ischemia** is reached.

Muscles of the back

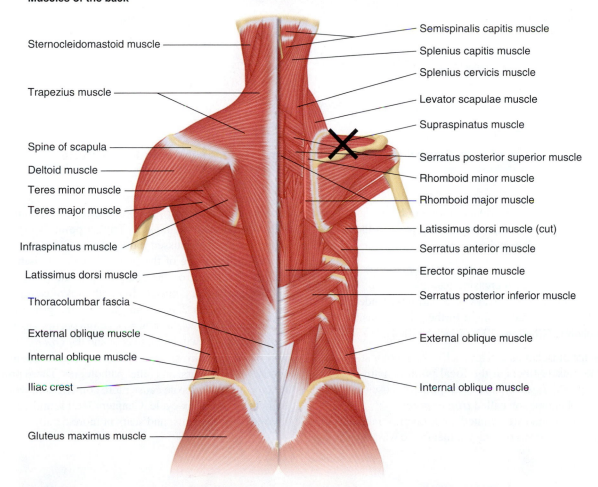

Sternocleidomastoid muscle

Trapezius muscle

Spine of scapula

Deltoid muscle

Teres minor muscle

Teres major muscle

Infraspinatus muscle

Latissimus dorsi muscle

Thoracolumbar fascia

External oblique muscle

Internal oblique muscle

Iliac crest

Gluteus maximus muscle

Semispinalis capitis muscle

Splenius capitis muscle

Splenius cervicis muscle

Levator scapulae muscle

Supraspinatus muscle

Serratus posterior superior muscle

Rhomboid minor muscle

Rhomboid major muscle

Latissimus dorsi muscle (cut)

Serratus anterior muscle

Erector spinae muscle

Serratus posterior inferior muscle

External oblique muscle

Internal oblique muscle

FIGURE 6.9

The Site of the Original Injury in Logan's Shoulder

Muscles of the back

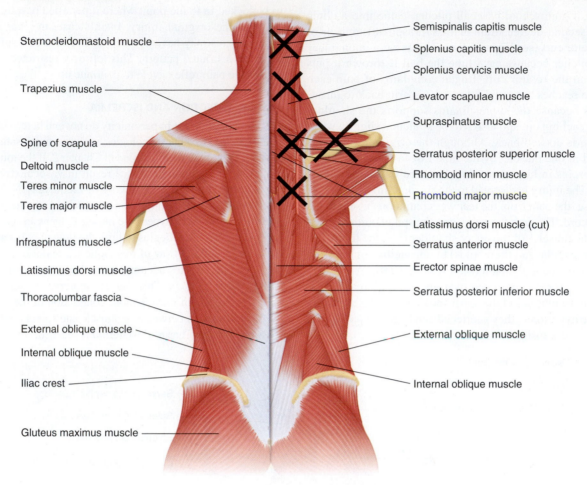

Sternocleidomastoid muscle

Trapezius muscle

Spine of scapula

Deltoid muscle

Teres minor muscle

Teres major muscle

Infraspinatus muscle

Latissimus dorsi muscle

Thoracolumbar fascia

External oblique muscle

Internal oblique muscle

Iliac crest

Gluteus maximus muscle

Semispinalis capitis muscle

Splenius capitis muscle

Splenius cervicis muscle

Levator scapulae muscle

Supraspinatus muscle

Serratus posterior superior muscle

Rhomboid minor muscle

Rhomboid major muscle

Latissimus dorsi muscle (cut)

Serratus anterior muscle

Erector spinae muscle

Serratus posterior inferior muscle

External oblique muscle

Internal oblique muscle

FIGURE 6.10

New Areas of Pain Caused by the Repeated Occurrence of the Pain Reflex Cycle

Ischemia is a focused lack of blood due to obstruction of circulation. Ischemia promotes the release of the noxious chemicals *bradykinin* and *serotonin*.

1. Bradykinin sensitizes nerve receptors to metabolic irritants, thereby increasing pain.
2. Serotonin is a powerful vasoconstrictor. Under the influence of bradykinin, it further propagates the ischemia (Chaitow, 2000; Marieb, 2004).

This stage of ischemia creates such strong motor stimulation that the muscle fibers at the focal point of pain are often drawn into *fixed spasm*. This fixed spasm of muscle fibers can lead to a phenomenon called *trigger points*.

Trigger points are irritated, taut, myofascial bands that contain excess levels of retained metabolic wastes and other noxious substances. Trigger points often manifest as tender knots or lumps in the muscle. Trigger point theory is quite complex and is discussed more fully in Chapter 7.

One final piece of the pain reflex puzzle is the effect that this cycle has on the connective tissue that surrounds and supports every muscle fiber (the myofascia). As discussed in Chapter 2, each muscle fiber and group of fibers is surrounded by fascia. When ischemia occurs, the fascia in the affected area will begin to cool and the *ground substance* will become sticky and rigid. Over time, the tissue develops *adhesions*, scars, and other pathologies. These problems in the connective tissue cause more constriction, which furthers the pain reflex cycle. Chapters 10, 11, and 12 explore myofascia, adhesions, and scars in more detail.

QUICK QUIZ #12

1. In the reflex arc, the _____ is the tissue or structure that will respond to a signal sent by a motor neuron.
   a. receptor
   b. spinal cord
   c. sensory neuron
   d. brain
   e. nociceptor
   f. effector

2. Which of the following statements are correct? Spinal reflexes: (Circle all that apply)
   a. are also called learned reflexes.
   b. often have a protective function.
   c. are responsible for the general state of tonus in the muscles.

   d. play an important part in the pain reflex cycle.
   e. All of the above
   f. None of the above

3. Hypertonicity can cause: (Circle all that apply)
   a. vasoconstriction.
   b. ischemia.
   c. trigger points.
   d. All of the above
   e. None of the above

4. Hypertonic muscles can cause vasoconstriction and ischemia, which contribute to the pain reflex cycle.
   a. True
   b. False

SUMMARY

Sensory receptors receive and respond to stimuli inside and outside of the body. There are several different types of receptors, and they are found all over the body. Sensory receptors are very important in neuromuscular therapy, especially nociceptors, which are primarily responsible for the sensation of pain.

Pain threshold and pain tolerance are important factors in a person's experience of pain. Pain tolerance indicates that the experience of pain is influenced by factors other than the presence of a pain stimulus. The gate control theory of pain attempts to explain how it is that thoughts, emotions, and past experience influence an individual's experience of pain.

Reflexes are a critical component in proper myoskeletal functioning. A reflex arc has five components: receptor, sensory neuron, spinal cord, motor neuron, and effector.

Somatic reflexes are those reflexes associated with the myoskeletal system. Learned reflexes develop when we repeat motions over and over. The law of facilitation explains the process that allows an electrical signal to travel along a neuron more quickly and easily through repetition.

Intrinsic or spinal reflexes often have a protective function and are also responsible for maintaining the overall level of tonus of the muscles. In the case of persistent pain or chronic hypertonus, these reflexes are involved in the pain reflex cycle. Vasoconstriction and ischemia also play an important role in the pain reflex cycle.

Understanding facilitation and being aware of how the body receives and responds to pain (through the pain reflex cycle) allows the practitioner to analyze and treat dysfunction and postural distortions more efficiently using the NMT approach.

DISCUSSION QUESTIONS

1. Explain the difference between pain tolerance and pain threshold.
2. What are learned reflexes? How are they learned?
3. How does ischemia cause pathology in the body?
4. How is facilitation involved in pathology?
5. Explain the role of the brain in the maintenance of muscle tone.

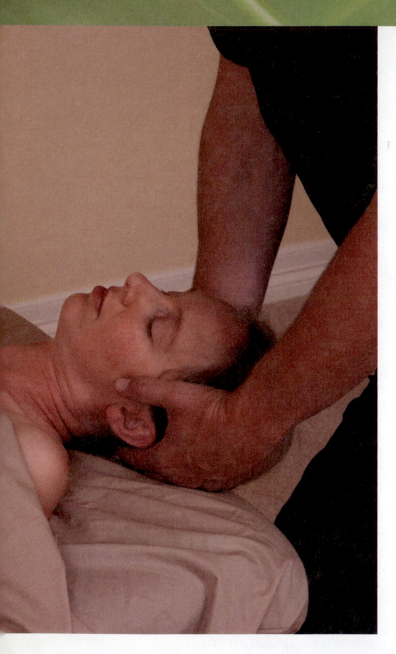

 CHAPTER HIGHLIGHTS

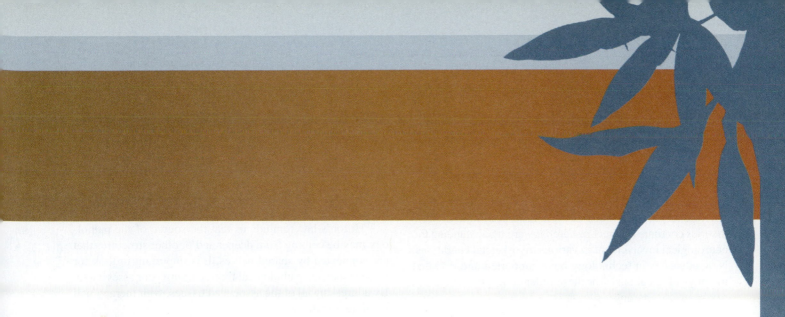

CHAPTER OBJECTIVES

- Survey the history and development of neuromuscular theory
- Consider pathology from the neuromuscular perspective
- Understand the physiology of trigger points

- Explore the phenomenon of referred pain
- Investigate the ideas behind facilitated stretching

KEY TERMS

THE FOUNDATIONS OF NEUROMUSCULAR THEORY

Neuromuscular therapy has its roots in research conducted around the turn of the century. It was during this time that physicians began studying the nerves, their distribution, and how they influence pathology. While some of these theories were established long ago, they still give insights to modern practitioners to help understand the process of injury. These theories continue to direct research toward understanding the neurological involvement in various myoskeletal conditions. New advances in technology have supported and revealed the physiological basis for these older concepts.

Hilton's Law

One of the first researchers during these early times was John Hilton (1804–1878). In 1862 Hilton wrote the classic medical text, *Rest and Pain*, still considered by some to be essential reading. He became president of the Royal College of Surgeons and is credited with a number of anatomical discoveries.

Hilton's research uncovered one of the most basic structural components of neurology. Commonly known as Hilton's law, it states: The nerve trunk that supplies a specific joint also supplies the muscles of the joint, as well as the skin over their insertions (Fritz, 2000). (See Figure 7.1 ■.) This means that, since the tissues share the same nerves, pathology in a joint can be reflected in the muscles and other superficial tissues that surround it.

For example, inflammation in a joint (such as arthritis) affects the nerves that supply it. Over time, the nerves supplying the arthritic joint will have difficulty supplying proper impulses to the skin and muscles that share it. This disrupts the function of the skin and muscles, causing new pain and pathology there. A client may seek treatment for muscle pain in the area, but in this case, the arthritis is the original cause of the pathology. The arthritis will need to be addressed to support any progress achieved through body-work. Sometimes this may require a referral to a physician for accompanying treatment.

Hilton's law reminds us that the source of the pathology may be coming from deeper and/or other structures that are connected by shared nerves. It is important to look for these associated pathological tissues during your assessment. By addressing all of the associated tissues, your therapy will be more effective.

Pfluger's Laws

Another important researcher during this time was Edward Friedrich Wilhelm Pfluger (1829–1910). He was a German physiologist and a professor at the University of Bonn. He made important contributions to the fields of embryology, physiology, electrophysiology, and muscular contraction. Through careful observation, analysis, and specific tests, Pfluger discovered a series of rules or "laws" that describe some of the body's neurological responses to pain (Fritz, 2000). These laws also describe the general progression through which pain is transmitted to the rest of the body.

- *Pfluger's Law of Unilaterality*—If a mild irritation is applied to sensory nerves, the spinal reflex (i.e., the muscle contraction) occurs typically only on the side of the spinal cord that is irritated.

Cross section of elbow joint

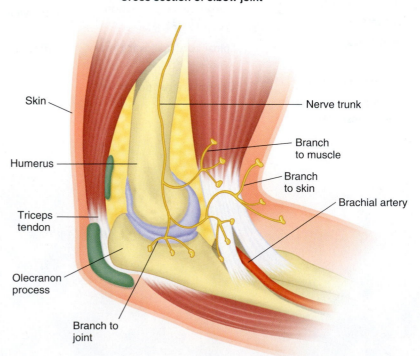

Skin

Humerus

Triceps tendon

Olecranon process

Branch to joint

Nerve trunk

Branch to muscle

Branch to skin

Brachial artery

FIGURE 7.1

The Nerve Trunk That Supports the Elbow Joint Also Supports the Muscles of the Elbow and the Skin Over the Insertions of Those Muscles.

For example, if the right shoulder has a mild irritation, only the muscles on the right side will show signs of increased tension. This is important when assessing pathology. If excessive tension is only located on one side, then we can assume the injury is relatively mild and is mainly in the local area of tension. In essence, a minor pathology will cause a limited response in the local area of the pathology.

- *Pfluger's Law of Symmetry*—If the irritation is sufficiently increased, the spinal reflex is manifested, not only on the irritated side, but also in similar muscles on the opposite side of the body.

This law describes the tendency of injuries in one limb to also manifest in the opposing limb. Using the above example, if the irritation in the right shoulder gets worse, it will cause the left shoulder to respond with tension in the same muscles. This is because nerve roots that supply each side of the body exit and enter the spinal cord between the same vertebrae.

For example, the right cervical nerve root at C5 supplies the same nerves in the right arm that the left cervical nerve root at C5 does for the left arm. (See the discussion on segment reflex massage below for clarification; see Figure 7.2 ■.) When exposed to excess pain, the NMDA receptors (described in Chapter 5) will cause the spinal cord segment to become highly sensitized. Since the nerve root for the left arm shares the same vertebral segment as the nerve root of the right arm, it makes sense that the hypersensitive cord segment may overreact and stimulate the nerves extending into both sides of the body, not just to the side of the injury.

In addition to the law of symmetry, it is also important to take into account the *crossed extensor reflex*. Through this reflex, the withdrawal from pain (i.e, contraction of the flexors) in one limb also causes the extensors of the opposite limb to contract simultaneously. For example, if you step on a sharp object with your left foot, the flexor muscles of the left leg will contract to pull away from the object. At the same time, the extensor muscles of the right leg will contract, extending the right leg to catch the weight shifted from the left. The crossed extensor reflex helps to maintain balance in this situation.

In the case of chronic pain, the law of symmetry explains that pain in the flexors of one leg can cause tension in the flexors of the opposite leg. Due to the crossed extensor reflex, pain in one leg may also cause tension in the extensors of the opposite leg. When doing assessments make sure to look for this type of associated tension in the flexors, as well as the extensors of the opposite limb.

This effect can be used to a therapist's advantage in certain situations. Stimulation, in the form of massage and rehabilitation to the *unaffected* limb, will actually increase healing in the affected limb through neural transmission across the vertebral segment. Often when a limb is immobilized (e.g., in a cast) or is too painful to treat, therapy may be applied to the unaffected side to promote healing to the painful or immobilized side (Fritz, 2000).

- *Pfluger's Law of Intensity*—The spinal reflex is usually more intense on the side of irritation. The spinal reflex on the opposite side will be generally less pronounced.

This rule compliments the law of symmetry. It simply explains that the response on the side opposite the injury will be less intense than the response on the side experiencing the source of the pain. It makes sense that you will tense up more on the injured side than on the noninjured side. During assessment this rule reminds us that the side with greater tension is probably the injured side and will require more focused treatment than the less tense, noninjured side.

- *Pfluger's Law of Radiation*—If the irritation continues to increase, it is propagated upward along the spinal cord, eventually irritating the nerves coming from the segments of the spinal cord above the level of injury.

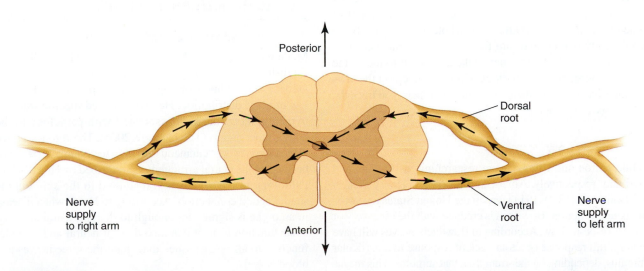

FIGURE 7.2

The Spinal Cord Segment at C5 Containing the Nerve Roots for Each Arm. This Segment Supports the Nerves Supplying the Right Arm, and Also Supports the Nerves of the Left Arm.

As discussed in Chapter 5, a chronic irritation or painful stimulus can sensitize the spinal cord to a state of *hyperalgesia*, a supersensitive condition. Over time, the irritation begins to progress upward, incrementally affecting the next highest spinal segment.

For example, a chronic hip injury will irritate the nerve roots at the low back. As the irritation progresses, the sensitization will begin to affect the segment above. In this case, the nerves of the middle back will be the next affected. Over time, this process can continue affecting each segment until the nerves of the upper back are involved. This process may even progress to the neck and eventually to the brain. The key concept here is that the progression of the neural sensitization tends to travel in an upward fashion along the vertebral column.

One reason for this is because of the structure and movement patterns of the torso. The pelvis is a relatively stable and fixed structure while the spinal cord is very flexible. The pelvis remains largely stationary as the spinal cord bends and twists, adjusting to the movements of the limbs and back muscles. As the upper torso moves, the lower torso and pelvis stabilize and support the movement. If the lower sections become painful, the body compensates by tensing the muscles of those sections as well as the next section above. The next higher section is tensed to help stabilize the painful lower section. The new section becomes affected because it is doing its own job as well as compensating for the sections below. This rule reminds us to assess as well as treat the entire vertebral column to address all radiation patterns.

- *Pfluger's Law of Generalization*—When the irritation is sufficient enough to reach the brain, the *medulla oblongata* stimulates the entire spinal cord, causing a general contraction of all muscles in the body.

This law is the culmination of the law of radiation. Once the process of radiation upward along the spinal cord progresses to the lower brain centers, they react by sending a sort of general spinal reflex that affects the whole body. Basically the whole body is recruited into the state of hyperalgesia stiffness. This overall tension may make it difficult to locate the original source of the pathology. However, keeping the laws of radiation and generalization in mind will help you trace the pathology to its source.

Bowditch's Law

While Hilton and Pfluger were researching in England and Germany respectively, American physiologist Henry Pickering Bowditch (1840–1911) was in the United States researching neural function. Bowditch is credited with the discovery of the All-or-None Law. According to Bowditch, nerves will have either a full response or a total lack of response to a particular stimulus, depending on the strength of that stimulus. This means that a nerve impulse initiated by a weak stimulus will be as strong as one initiated by a strong stimulus as long as the stimulus is above threshold. The response is all or none because neurons cannot be partially stimulated. Furthermore, if the stimulus is not strong enough, no impulse will be generated (Fritz, 2000).

This law has a couple of important implications for bodywork. First, pain from an injury or pathology will generate nerve impulses as long as the pain is above the threshold level. The severity of the pain source is not the only determinant of the level of pain felt. All that matters is that the stimulus is strong enough to cause a nerve impulse to be sent to the brain. In the brain, the stimulus will be interpreted based on the client's unique psychological and physiological makeup. For the therapist this means that whether the pathology is severe or mild is not the only basis for assessing the level of pain the client is feeling. Even small levels of pain can be "felt" by some clients as more severe than what other clients with the same level of injury may feel.

The other relevant aspect of the all-or-none principle involves the stimulation of muscle and nerve fibers by massage therapy. This law helps to explain negative responses such as guarding. If the treatment (even if it is intended to be gentle) is strong enough to cause contraction (over the threshold) in the muscle fibers, the muscle will contract or guard even if the client is trying not to. In this case the muscles are stimulated by massage into increased tension. NMT practitioners work just under this threshold or use therapies such as facilitated stretching to temper or even suppress this threshold.

This law reminds us that therapy doesn't need to be aggressive to produce a strong effect. The use of very gentle and subtle techniques to influence nerve and muscle tissue is also effective. The therapy doesn't have to be intense to have an effect. It just has to be strong enough to generate a response in the nerve or muscle fibers, and the body will respond maximally.

THE MODERN HISTORY OF NEUROMUSCULAR THERAPY

Research and Discoveries in Neurology

Modern researchers such as Sir Henry Head (1861–1940), an English scientist and physician, expanded on the work of his predecessors. While working with concepts such as Hilton's law of nerve distribution, Head discovered specific zones of hyperalgesia on the skin associated with pathology in the body's inner organs (Turchaninov, 2006). These zones, called "Head's zones" or "cutaneous zones" (see Figure 7.3 ■), exist because of the neural arrangement described by Hilton's law. Pathology in the organs is transmitted to the skin via the shared neural connection. According to Head, when disease in an organ is significant enough to disrupt neural and vascular function to it, it can also disrupt neural and vascular function to all other tissues that share the same nerves and blood vessels.

For the bodyworker the implications are simple. Sometimes pathology found in the superficial tissues such as the muscles, skin, and connective tissue has a cause that arises from the organs and not the myoskeletal system.

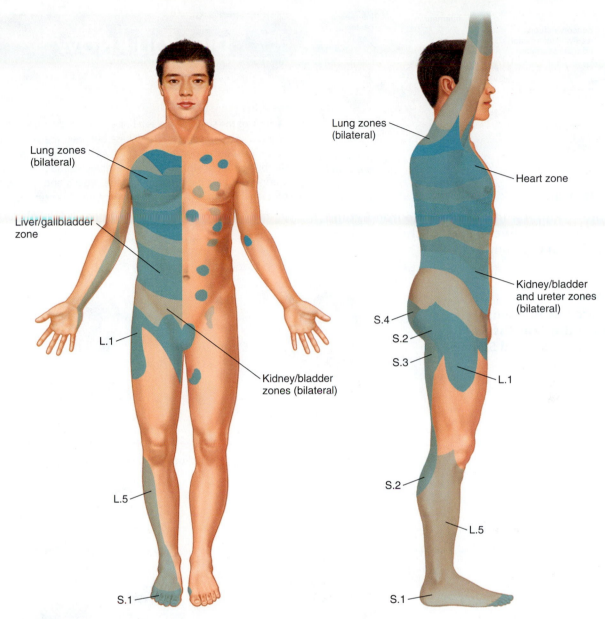

Lung zones
(bilateral)

Liver/gallbladder
zone

L.1

L.5

S.1

Lung zones
(bilateral)

Heart zone

Kidney/bladder
zones (bilateral)

Lung zones
(bilateral)

Heart zone

Kidney/bladder
and ureter zones
(bilateral)

S.4

S.2

S.3

L.1

S.2

L.5

S.1

FIGURE 7.3

Indicated by the Various Areas of Shading, Head's Zones Are Areas on the Skin Which Reflect Pathology in Associated Organs That Share the Same Nerve Root.

Head's discovery gave insight into another important structural aspect of the nervous system. That is the segmented nature of neural distribution. Professor A. Sherbak, one of the founders of Russian physiotherapy, expanded on Head's work. Sherbak developed the Russian system called *segment reflex massage* (Turchaninov, 2006).

A cornerstone of segment reflex massage is the understanding of the unique distribution of nerve pairs. Between each vertebra extends a pair of nerves—one sensory and one motor (see Figure 7.4 ■). Each pair of nerves supplies mainly the segment of the body which extends laterally from the specific vertebra. While there is some overlap in the segments, it is fair to say that all the organs, tissues, etc., that are contained in each segment are primarily supplied by the nearest

pair of nerves extending from the left and right sides of the vertebral column. The arms and legs are segmented parallel to their axis (Figure 7.4).

The segmentation of the body's nerve distribution is reflected in the **dermatomes** of the skin. Dermatomes are the sensory areas in the skin associated with individual spinal nerve pairs (see Figure 7.5 ■). They provide a superficial map of the spinal nerve segments and are used for assessment in segment reflex massage. Since the skin is the end point of the nerve branches, it will reflect the health of the nerve pair all the way to the root (the vertebral column). If there is pathology present in any organ or tissue along the path of the nerves, it can eventually show up as pathology in the skin (Turchaninov, 2006). Modern practitioners use the dermatomes of the

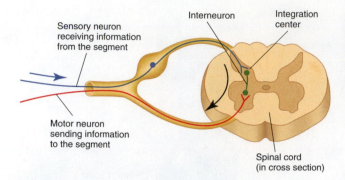

Sensory neuron receiving information from the segment

Interneuron

Integration center

Motor neuron sending information to the segment

Spinal cord (in cross section)

FIGURE 7.4

A Motor Neuron and a Sensory Neuron Extend from the Area Between Each of the Vertebrae in the Spinal Column.

DID YOU KNOW

Think of the spinal nerve as a horsetail extending from the sides of your vertebral column. At its base between the vertebrae, the nerve fibers are all bunched together. As the fibers extend out into the body, they feather out like the many strands of a horsetail. The nerve fibers pass through all the organs and tissues of the segment. The ends of each strand reach into the skin and become the skin's senses.

FIGURE 7.5

Dermatomes Are Sensory Areas in the Skin Associated with Individual Spinal Nerve Pairs.

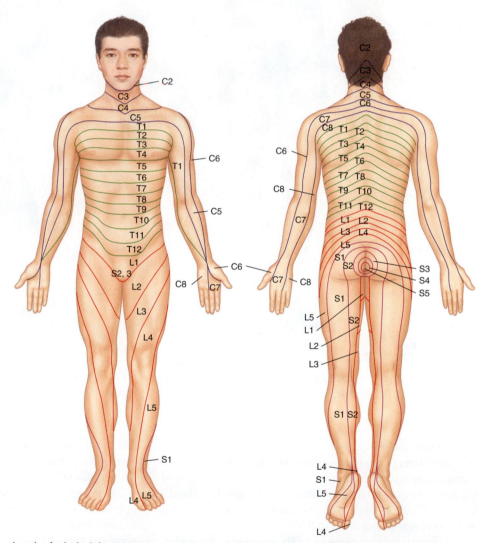

Levels of principal dermatomes			
C5	Clavicles	T10	Level of umbilicus
C5, 6, 7	Lateral parts of upper limbs	T12	Inguinal or groin regions
C8, T1	Medial sides of upper limbs	L1, 2, 3, 4	Anterior and inner surfaces of lower limbs
C6	Thumb	L4, 5, S1	Foot
C6, 7, 8	Hand	L4	Medial side of great toe
C8	Ring and little fingers	S1, 2, L5	Posterior and outer surfaces of lower limbs
T4	Level of nipples	S1	Lateral margin of foot and little toe
		S2, 3, 4	Perineum

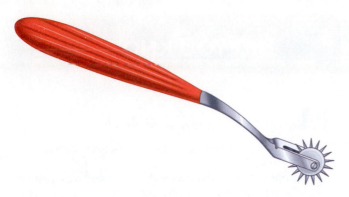

FIGURE 7.6

A Rolling Pinwheel Used to Assess the Sensitivity of the Dermatomes

skin to assess the presence of nerve compression at the root. The therapist will check for any increase or decrease in sensitivity in the skin by rolling a pinwheel of needles along the dermatomes (see Figure 7.6 ■). If any numbness or increased sensitivity is noted, the nerve that supplies that dermatome is checked for compression all the way to the root.

Another of Head's contributions to the field of neuromuscular therapy was the observation that, when a painful stimulus is applied to an area of low sensitivity that connects with an area of higher sensitivity, the pain is felt where there is higher sensitivity rather than in the area of lower sensitivity (i.e., where the stimulus was applied; Turchaninov, 2006).

This rule, called Head's law, describes a very important phenomenon in neurological function. Although the nervous system infuses all tissues of the body, it doesn't apply the same level of sensitivity to them. The sensitivity varies depending on the function of the structure. For example, the hand has about

five to ten times the nerve endings as the forearm. As a result, the hand is much more sensitive. In a sense, the brain is much more informed about the hands than the forearm.

According to this rule, a person may feel pain in the hand when the injury is actually farther up the arm. This is because the hand and arm share the same nerve roots and branches, but the hand is far more sensitive than the arm. This is significant for massage therapists as it explains that sometimes, the area where the pain is felt most by the client may not be the source of that pain.

One of the most common examples of this phenomenon is sciatic nerve compression. A client may complain of pain or "pins and needles" in the feet. However, assessment reveals little or no pathology in the feet. It is likely that the pathology is from compression of the nerve at the hips and/or low back. The feet have a higher sensitivity than the hips, so most of the sensation for the client occurs in the feet. This rule reminds us that it is important to trace the entire nerve, from root to branch, to find all of the pathology.

Research and Discoveries in Other Health Fields

Some important discoveries that influenced neurology came from other areas of research. Hugo Schulz (1853–1932) was a German pharmacologist and a professor at the University of Greifswald. He studied under Edward Friedrich Wilhelm Pfluger and also researched toxicology with Dr. Rudolf Arndt (1835–1900). Together they discovered the Arndt–Schultz Law, which states that moderate or low-level stimuli *activate* physiological processes while very strong stimuli *inhibit* them (Fritz, 2000).

Even though this phenomenon was discovered in the field of toxicology, it also applies to bodywork. Strong stimulation, along the lines of deep pressure with long duration, tends to be sedating to the nerves and muscles. Light

QUICK QUIZ #13

1. Which of the following statements are correct?
   a. Pathology affecting the nerves in a joint can be reflected in superficial tissues surrounding it.
   b. If the excessive tension is only located on the originally affected side, you can assume the injury is relatively mild and has not progressed.
   c. If a limb is too painful to treat, therapy on the unaffected side may promote healing through the crossover effect.
   d. Increasingly painful stimuli will incrementally affect the next lowest spinal segment until it reaches the pelvis.

2. The law of _____ explains that the side of the body with more tension is probably the side that has the original injury.
   a. facilitation
   b. intensity
   c. generalization
   d. radiation
   e. symmetry

3. Head's law explains that pain may be felt in the hand, even though the injury may be farther up the arm, because the hand is a more sensitive area.
   a. True
   b. False

4. Light stimulation tends to be sedating, while strong stimulation tends to encourage function.
   a. True
   b. False

stimulation, in the form of superficial strokes of a short duration, tends to invigorate the nerves and muscles and encourage function.

For example, when a muscle is in spasm, deep, slow work is more appropriate. The deep, slow pressure will relax the muscles and stretch the fibers to a better resting length. Conversely, when a muscle needs neural stimulation (in the case of weakened, overstretched muscles), lighter, shorter strokes are used to help stimulate neural function. The use of light, short strokes stimulates excitation in the nerves causing contraction of the muscle and increasing its general tonus.

THE MECHANICAL-EMOTIONAL CONNECTION

An important characteristic of the neuromuscular model is that it considers the mental-emotional as well as the mechanical contributions to dysfunction. Life can take its toll on our bodies. Not only does the body endure the impact of the physical world, but it also reflects our inner emotions, feelings, and perceptions. It is generally easy to understand the effects of physical injury. Injuries can cause pain, which causes the body to tense up. Over time, this leads to limited range of motion and a host of other postural problems. However, a person's mental state can impact the body in much the same way.

Take, for example, the case of Spencer, a "stressed out executive" sitting in a meeting where his department is reporting a poor performance for the third quarter in a row. As he listens to the anger in his boss's voice, he ducks his head and pulls his shoulders high to his ears. This is a classic protective posture that people often exhibit when they are defensive or fearful. Spencer leaves the meeting, but the emotion stays with him and so does his protective posture. After three quarters of declining profits, he has spent so much time hunched into this posture that he begins to develop a full-blown, fixed postural distortion. What was once an emotional response has now become fixed into his physical structure. According to NMT, pathology is almost always both mechanical and emotional in nature. Neuromuscular therapists consider the origins of a

DID YOU KNOW

Mechanical stress can come in the form of:

Trauma—such as bruises, contusions, fractures, sprains and strains.
Improper body mechanics—including chronic poor posture and bad *ergonomics* at work, sports, etc.
Chronic overuse—during work, sports, and hobbies, especially if the activity is one-sided (such as tennis).

Psychological stress can come from a huge variety of sources. Some of the most common sources are from:

1. the work place
2. relationships
3. elder/child care
4. money problems

client's pathology, as it may give clues about the type of compensation that is occurring.

THE FIVE CATEGORIES OF PATHOLOGY

Although there are as many manifestations of myoskeletal pathology as there are people experiencing it, neuromuscular theory has narrowed the possible expressions to five common conditions or complications.

1. *Nerve compression or entrapment*—Pressure on nerves can be caused by soft tissues (e.g., muscles, tendons, ligaments, fascia, etc.) and hard tissues (e.g., bone or cartilage). Nerves run over, under, and through every tissue, structure, and muscle. If there is muscular tension present for any reason, it is common for the nerve to be caught and/or compressed between the tense structures. When a nerve becomes compressed,

HOLISTIC CONNECTION

The "mind-body connection" refers to the fact that our bodies respond to what we are thinking as well as how we are feeling and acting. The muscle tension you are treating is very likely connected to emotional tension the client has experienced. Be aware of the mind-body connection and realize that your therapy will make a difference in your client's emotional well-being.

Encourage your clients to reduce emotional stress with relaxation techniques on their own. Clients may express interest in exploring the emotions underlying their tension. By being ready to recommend counselors, psychologists, or support groups if asked, you will help your clients to achieve overall well-being.

it cannot transmit signals to the spinal cord effectively. This can lead to a sensation called **paraesthesia.**

Paraesthesia is often described as "pins and needles" but can be defined as any abnormal nerve sensation such as tingling and burning (Werner, 2005). Paraesthesia will be present in moderate to severe nerve compression. If the compression is severe or is present long enough to cause degenerative changes to the nerve, then numbness will result. Generally, paraesthesia will be the first chronic symptom and then numbness follows (Turchaninov, 2006). This is important because it suggests that when numbness occurs, the pathology is worse or has been present for a long time. In either case, both sensations activate the pain reflex cycle and contribute to the *pathophysiological* response.

2. *Postural distortion*—When the bones are in proper alignment, the spine and the hips are centered so the body's weight is balanced between both legs. When properly aligned, the body has to use very little effort to maintain the proper level of tonus required to hold the body in correct posture. When the body's alignment deviates from the correct position towards the front, side, or back, the posture is categorized as distorted. Injury, compensation, and systemic postural distortions (as described in Chapter 2) cause changes in shape, structure, and movement patterns. As the body tilts, bends, and curves around injury, it forces the muscles to do more of the work instead of using the bones for support. This causes the muscles to be overworked and can cause damage.

3. *Nutritional deficiencies*—Muscles in spasm constrict the blood supply, effectively cutting off the supply of nutrients to the tissues. Without the nutritional building blocks for repair, the process of healing is slowed. Well-nourished, well-hydrated, healthy tissues resist dysfunction.

Sometimes, a lack of certain nutrients can be the cause of spasm or dysfunction in the first place. Take calcium deficiency, for example. Calcium is a critical component in the biochemical reaction that causes muscle contraction. A lack of calcium can cause an interruption in this process, leading to problems such as malfunction and spasm. Relief for this deficiency is often as simple as including more calcium in the diet.

DID YOU KNOW

Due to the important connection between various nutrients and muscle contraction, it is often recommended that individuals take supplements such as calcium, magnesium, and potassium before bed to help prevent nighttime leg and foot cramps.

Two other common nutrients involved in spasm are potassium and magnesium. A deficiency of either of these nutrients has the potential to shut down the normal function of muscle contraction and relaxation. Other nutritional deficiencies may be more complicated, but are always important to consider. If nutritional deficiency is suspected, a referral to a doctor or nutritionist may be recommended.

4. *Biomechanical dysfunction*—This is a catchall term for all pathologies of the myoskeletal system. Everything, from the body's response to stress to work habits, sports, and injuries, can cause biomechanical dysfunction. All of life's activities place demands on the body. When those demands become overwhelming, dysfunction and pathology may develop. For example, pathology may arise from standing for long periods, and even the way we sleep can have adverse effects.

5. *Trigger points*—**Trigger points** are perhaps one of the most important pathologies that NMT addresses.

THE DISCOVERY OF TRIGGER POINTS

The underpinnings of trigger point theory began in the work of Dr. Stanley Leif and Boris Chaitow. Dr. Leif was a trained naturopath and chiropractor who, in 1925, established his own healing center in Hertfordshire, England. His center focused on a holistic health approach including diet, exercise, stretching, massage, and bone manipulation. Boris Chaitow, a cousin of Dr. Leif's, was a trained chiropractor and worked as Dr. Leif's assistant. Together they discovered certain pathologies in the muscle, which they termed "lesions."

HOLISTIC CONNECTION

Nutrition is extremely important to every aspect of health, including the myoskeletal system. Maintaining a wholesome fresh-food diet will keep you healthy. It will also help your clients to overcome injuries. Recommending a nutritionist for your clients will help build your professional relationships and will enhance the effects of your therapy.

A "lesion" was considered to be any irregularity or inconsistency in the muscle and its associated tissues that gives rise to pain. Leif and Chaitow discussed four conditions commonly associated with the presence of these lesions:

1. *Congestion of the local connective tissues*—The congestion is caused by the lack of circulation of blood and lymph through the area. It allows the ground substance of the connective tissue to cool, thicken, and form *adhesions*. (See Chapter 8 for more about adhesions.)
2. *Disturbance of the acid/base (pH) balance of the connective tissues*—The lack of circulation causes a build up of metabolic waste in the tissues. One such waste product is carbon dioxide, which is acidic.
3. *Fibrous infiltrations*—If the muscle is sufficiently damaged or irritated, the connective tissue will begin to grow fibrous connections (essentially scars) in the tissue. This is an effort to hold the area still to prevent more damage. Fibrous connections have a ropelike feel in the muscle.
4. *Chronic muscular contractions*—This condition may be the cause and/or the result of lesions. Chronic muscular contractions can initiate the formation of lesions by slowly breaking down and pulling the tissues apart. Or, as a lesion forms, it may be compounded by the constant pulling of a chronically contracted muscle. This may cause the surrounding muscles to then chronically contract in an effort to compensate for the injury (Chaitow, 2000).

These four conditions have become the foundation for trigger point theory, which is one of the hallmarks of neuromuscular therapy.

Trigger Point Theory

In the late 1940s and early 1950s Dr. Janet Travell began to study the relationship between pain and chronic conditions of the muscle and related tissues. Dr. Travell was very well known and respected; in fact, she was John F. Kennedy's physician during his presidency. She coined the term "trigger points" ("TrPs") and studied their connection to myofascial pain syndromes.

In the 1980s and 1990s, Dr. Travell wrote the classics, *Travell & Simons' Myofascial Pain and Dysfunction: The Trigger Point Manual, Volumes 1 & 2* with her colleagues David Simons and Lois Simons. These two books are still used by body workers all over the world as basic texts for understanding and treating this unique pathology.

Dr. Travell describes a myofascial trigger point:

A hyperirritable spot in skeletal muscle that is associated with a hypersensitive palpable nodule in a taut band. The spot is painful on compression and can give rise to characteristic referred pain, referred tenderness, motor dysfunction, and autonomic phenomena. (Simons, Travell, and Simons, 1999, page 5)

In more simple terms, trigger points are knots in the muscle. When pressed, they are tender or cause tenderness in another muscle group. Trigger points also affect the neurology of the muscle, causing distortions in the proprioceptors that leads to problems in the muscle's ability to relax and contract.

THE FORMATION OF TRIGGER POINTS

According to Dr. Travell (Simons, Travell, and Simons, 1999), there are roughly six factors that contribute to the formation and perpetuation of trigger points.

- *Mechanical stresses*—Physical asymmetry, muscular stress, poor ergonomics, poor posture, and prolonged immobility can all contribute to overtaxed and/or depleted muscles.
- *Nutritional*—Common examples include low levels of vitamins B1, B6, B12, vitamin C, magnesium, calcium, potassium, iron, and some trace minerals. All tissues, including the myofascial structures, need these nutrients to function properly.
- *Metabolic and endocrine (hormone and glandular) deficiencies*—If the metabolism and/or hormonal profile becomes imbalanced, the body's ability to heal and cope with injury is compromised.
- *Psychological factors*—Depression, tension, and anxiety all effect the subconscious physical expression. These mental conditions tax the system and slow healing.
- *Chronic illness*—This may include viral or bacterial infection, unhealed wounds, parasitic infestations, and other chronic diseases. When the body is fighting a chronic bronchitis, for example, it has fewer resources for healing other injuries.
- *Other factors*—Many conditions, from allergies to impaired sleep, contribute to the formation of TrPs.

Modern Research and the Energy Crisis

Modern research has developed the **energy crisis hypothesis** to describe the process of trigger point formation. In order to understand this hypothesis, it is important to review basic muscle structure and discuss how a muscle contracts.

A muscle is made up of bundles of thousands of muscle fibers called fascicles. Muscle fibers are long cylindrical cells that run the length of the muscle. Each muscle fiber is made up of bundles of myofibrils. When viewed from the ends, the bundled myofibrils of the muscle fiber resemble the bundled fibers of a rope (see Figure 7.7 ■).

Each myofibril is made up of small sections called **sarcomeres.** Sarcomeres are short segments which lie end to end to make up the length of the myofibril (see Figure 7.8 ■).

Each sarcomere is made up of groups of two types of myofilaments made of the proteins **myosin** and **actin.** Myosin filaments are thicker and are located between two thinner actin filaments. These filaments are the contractile structures of the muscle.

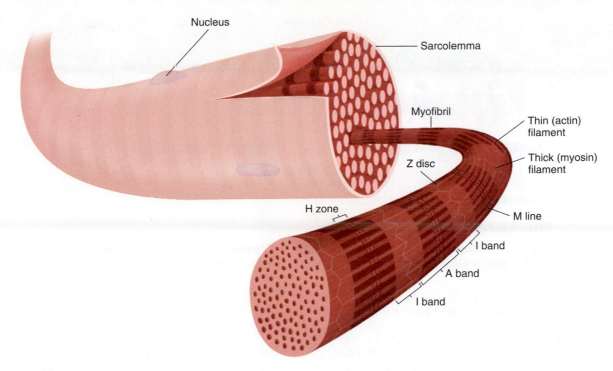

FIGURE 7.7

A Cross-Section View Shows the Bundle of Myofibrils Which Make Up a Muscle Fiber.

When a muscle receives a neural impulse to contract, it stimulates the release of calcium. This causes the myosin filament to attach to the actin filament via cross-bridges located on the myosin filament. The cross-bridge is a chemical binding site that acts like a kind of arm that reaches out to pull the actin filament along the myosin (see Figure 7.9 ■). As the myosin cross-bridges pull the actin filaments along, the two ends of the sarcomere are drawn closer to each other (see Figure 7.10 ■).

The net result of all the sarcomeres contracting in the fibers is the contraction of the entire muscle. In order to release the contraction, the body uses energy derived from *ATP* (an energy storage molecule) in the muscle. Energy from ATP is needed to reabsorb the calcium used to initiate the cross-bridge for contraction. When the calcium is

absorbed, the cross-bridge is released and separates the myosin and actin filaments. This releases the contraction in the sarcomere and relaxes the muscle. As long as calcium is present, the filaments will continue to make cross-bridges and contract the sarcomere. When a biomechanical dysfunction causes ATP (stored energy) to be depleted, an "energy crisis" exists. If there is not enough ATP available, the muscle cannot reabsorb the calcium and cannot release its contraction. This becomes a chronic contraction at that site and develops into a trigger point.

TRIGGER POINT ONSET

Depending on the cause, trigger points may develop in two ways. They may have a sudden onset where they form

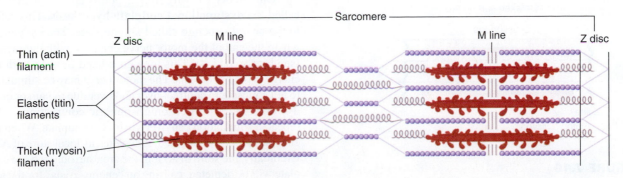

FIGURE 7.8

Each Myofibril Is Made of a Series of Sarcomeres Lying End to End.

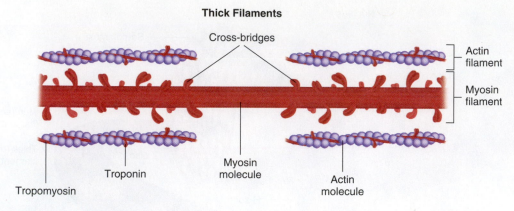

Thick Filaments

Cross-bridges

Actin filament

Myosin filament

Troponin

Myosin molecule

Actin molecule

Tropomyosin

FIGURE 7.9

Myosin Filaments Have Projections Called *Cross-Bridges* Which Attach to the Actin Filaments During a Muscle Contraction.

quickly. They may also develop over time, having a gradual onset.

- Sudden onset usually occurs when there is an acute trauma, such as a sudden exposure to cold, localized infection, spasm, or some other acute condition that causes an overload of a myofascial structure.
- Gradual onset is usually the result of an overload of a muscle over an extended period. General stress from life (work, commuting, personal relationships, etc.), can cause focused tension in muscles. Tension may be seen anywhere, from head to toe and in the limbs, hands, and feet. It seems postural muscles, such as the erector spinae, are especially vulnerable, as these muscles are always holding high levels of tonus in the form of isometric contractions.

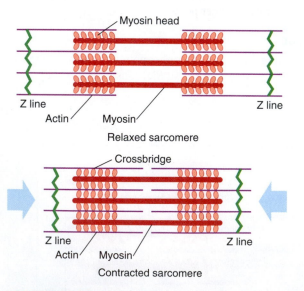

Myosin head

Z line

Actin   Myosin

Relaxed sarcomere

Crossbridge

Z line

Actin   Myosin

Contracted sarcomere

FIGURE 7.10

During a Contraction, the Two Ends of the Sarcomere Are Pulled Closer Together.

Trigger Points and Chronic Isometric Contractions

An **isometric contraction** is a type of contraction where the muscle tightens but does not move the body part to which it is attached. The body uses isometric contractions to stabilize joints and hold itself in posture. Most muscles, especially postural muscles (e.g., back muscles), are constantly holding at some level in a range of isometric contraction.

The head weighs roughly 8 to 10 pounds and sits atop the very flexible cervical vertebral column. As we move about, changes in the position of our head call for dynamic shifts in the level of isometric contraction of the neck muscles.

When the posture is healthy and balanced, the muscles can maintain these normal levels of contraction without developing trigger points or other pathology. However, when the posture is distorted, even to a small degree, some muscles are forced to increase their contractions to resist the unusual stresses placed upon them by incorrect posture. This increased level of contraction (even if it is in just a few muscles) can develop into a chronic isometric contraction as the muscles work to hold their position. With time, this overloads the muscles, causing trigger points. Trigger points tend to form in specific sections of the muscle or on specific fibers rather than encompassing the whole muscle.

One theory for why trigger points are so localized is called the **dysfunctional endplate hypothesis.** This refers to the neural structure called an **endplate.** The endplate is where the end of the motor nerve connects with the muscle (see Figure 7.11 ■). This idea goes hand in hand with the energy crisis hypothesis. The motor nerve may be stimulated to tell a muscle to contract over and over due to pain or other dysfunction such as chronic isometric contractions. This repeated stimulation can overwhelm the endplate. When the endplate becomes overused, it depletes its local store of ATP. Eventually, the store of ATP in the area surrounding the endplate will be depleted, causing an "energy crisis" for the sarcomeres closest to the endplate. These sarcomeres are the ones most likely to develop trigger points.

Neuromuscular Junction

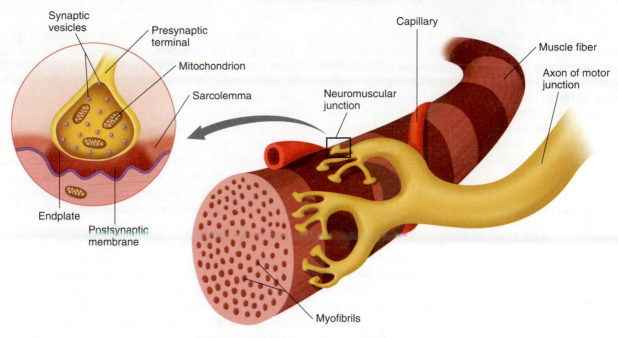

- Synaptic vesicles
- Presynaptic terminal
- Mitochondrion
- Sarcolemma
- Endplate
- Postsynaptic membrane
- Capillary
- Muscle fiber
- Axon of motor junction
- Neuromuscular junction
- Myofibrils

FIGURE 7.11

The Endplate of a Motor Nerve Is the Area Where It Connects to a Muscle.

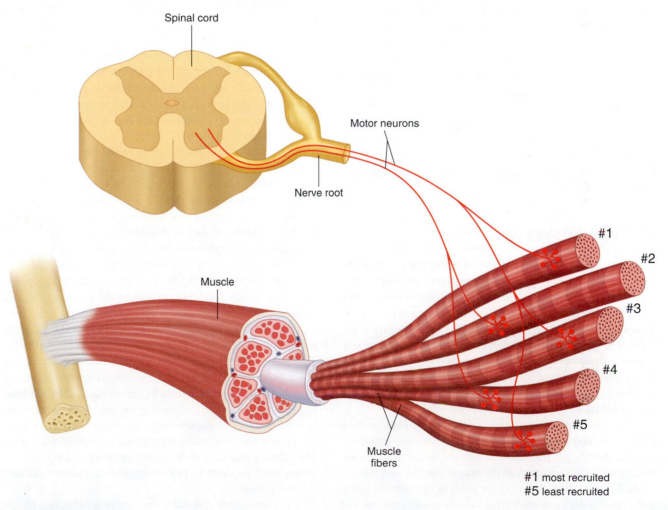

- Spinal cord
- Motor neurons
- Nerve root
- Muscle
- Muscle fibers
- #1
- #2
- #3
- #4
- #5
- #1 most recruited
- #5 least recruited

FIGURE 7.12

A Simplified Diagram of a Muscle Containing Five Muscle Fibers.

The uneven distribution of nerves on the muscle also influences the location of trigger points. Some neuromuscular junctions are more active than others due to facilitation. This allows a particular muscle to contract only the number of muscle fibers needed for a particular action. Take for example, a simplified muscle with only five fibers (see Figure 7.12 ■). When something light is picked up, only fibers 1 and 2 are recruited to lift the object. When a heavier object is picked up, fibers 1, 2, and 3 are recruited. A heavier object recruits 1, 2, and 3, as well as fiber 4. When an even heavier object is lifted, all fibers are recruited together (1, 2, 3, 4, and 5). Based on this example you see that fibers 1 and 2 are constantly being used while fibers 3, 4, 5 are only recruited when heavier lifting is needed. Even small changes in posture can have a big impact on a muscle, especially the fibers that are always recruited. Those fibers that are always recruited (fibers 1 and 2 in the example) become chronically overused and are most likely to become overloaded and form trigger points.

This helps explain why we often find trigger points in the same locations on many different clients, especially those with the same professions or hobbies. Most of us spend a great deal of our time at our jobs and doing specific hobbies. Our jobs and lives require us to hold our bodies in specific ways. Each job has demands that cause us to adjust our posture, causing new patterns of isometric contractions. These new patterns can overload specific parts of our muscles. Those overloads consistently show up as trigger points in the same locations. Experienced body workers can often tell a lot about a client's profession or hobbies based on the posture and specific trigger point patterns they present. A cab driver presents very different patterns than a food server. Each job places different demands on our bodies, so our bodies react to those demands by developing pathology such as trigger points.

TRIGGER POINTS AND PAIN

One of the most interesting features of trigger points is the type of pain they can cause. Trigger points are responsible for local pain, that is, pain surrounding the trigger point. Often the client describes this as a dull and/or aching type of pain. If words like throbbing, shooting, tingling, or electrical are used, it is likely that some other underlying vascular, neural, and/or inflammatory condition exists and should be investigated. The intensity of local pain varies from mildly uncomfortable to incapacitating, depending on the level of pathology and its location.

Trigger points also activate a very unique phenomenon called **referred pain.** This is a pattern of pain that manifests around the trigger point and in remote areas that are not mechanically associated with the muscles containing the TrP itself. That is to say that a trigger point in one muscle group can create pain in an entirely different muscle group. For example, a trigger point in the sternocleidomastoid (one of the neck muscles) can give rise to pain on the top of the head.

Therapists have been able to correlate the most common trigger point locations with the areas where referred pain is most likely to occur (**referral zones;** see Appendix 2). There is almost always a referred pain pattern found in the local muscles surrounding the one containing a trigger point. This pattern is called the primary referral zone. Then there are referral patterns in remote muscle groups called the secondary referral zones. The patterns of referred pain are remarkably predictable. This predictable referral pattern can be used to assist in locating trigger points. After investigating the primary referral zone for trigger points, you should then look to the common secondary referral zones for additional TrPs.

Referred pain can occur outside of these common patterns, so it is important to be flexible in your assessment. If you press a trigger point, the client may feel pain arise in an area that is not a commonly associated referral zone for that muscle. It is still safe to assume that this is referred pain associated with the trigger point and should not be dismissed. This information is valuable and should be used in assessment and treatment.

The Mechanism of Referred Pain

Janet Travell (Simons, Travell, and Simons, 1999) discusses the importance of referred pain throughout her writings. In fact, according to Dr. Travell, the presence of referred pain is one of the determining factors for the positive diagnosis of trigger points. However, the mechanism behind referred pain is somewhat of a mystery. Just how an active trigger point in one muscle group causes generalized pain in distant areas has been the subject of much study. Researchers have created many theories to explain the process.

One plausible explanation is called the **convergence-projection theory** (see Figure 7.13 ■). A nerve root extending from a segment of the vertebral column receives information from many different muscles. This is because many peripheral nerves converge on that same nerve root. Under normal conditions the nerve root is able to handle all of the sensory input passing through it and the brain is able to correctly interpret from which muscles the information is coming.

However, when a muscle contains a painful trigger point, it will repeatedly send pain signals to the shared nerve root causing a sort of traffic jam at the root. When the brain tries to interpret the signals, it may become confused by all of the sensory information coming into the common pathway. This may cause the brain to assign pain to other muscles that share the same root as the muscle containing the offending trigger point. In other words the brain has a difficult time telling which muscles are causing the pain so it guesses and gets some right and some wrong. The brain in effect projects the pain from one muscle onto another (Muscolino, 2009). This theory explains most of the primary (local) referral zones but falls short in explaining the secondary (distant) referral zones.

The secondary referral zones are best explained by the theory called the **spinal cord spillover theory** (see Figure 7.14 ■). This theory proposes that interneurons may

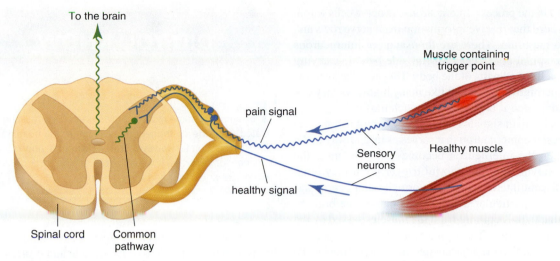

FIGURE 7.13

A Diagram Showing the Sensory Nerves from Two Muscles Converging on the Same Nerve Root. Both Muscles Share the Same Connection to the Spinal Cord. According to the Convergence-Projection Theory, Pain from a Trigger Point in One Muscle Can Be Interpreted by the Brain as Pain Coming from Another. This Is Because the Signals Intermingle at the Nerve Root.

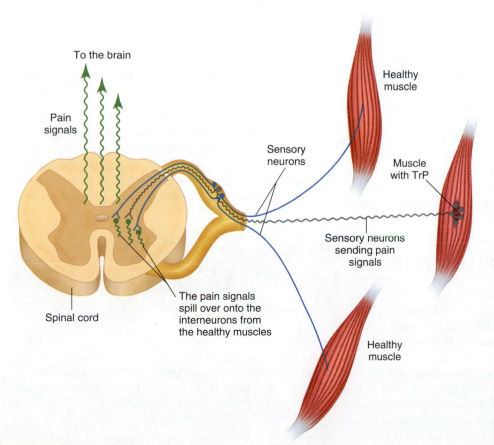

FIGURE 7.14

This Diagram Shows a Very Strong Pain Signal Sent from a Trigger Point in a Muscle. According to the Spillover Theory, the Strong Signal May Overwhelm the Interneuron in the Spinal Cord. The excessive Pain Signal "Spills Over" to Adjacent Interneurons That Carry Information from Other Parts of the Body. The Brain Registers Pain Signals Coming from Both Sets of Interneurons and Interprets That There Is Pain in Both Parts of the Body.

be involved in the process. Interneurons are nerve cells within the spinal cord that receive information from nerve roots and carry it to the brain. There are thousands of interneurons within the spinal cord. They all run side by side carrying information from all parts of the body. They are like an information superhighway, and just like many highways they can become congested if they have too much traffic.

Excessive pain signals from a trigger point in a muscle may congest the interneuron that serves as its pathway to the brain. When the interneuron becomes overwhelmed, the excessive signal from the painful trigger point may jump over to adjacent interneurons that normally don't carry signals from that particular muscle. This causes the brain to interpret that pain is coming from the muscles served by the adjacent interneurons. The signal from the trigger point is said to "spill over" to the adjacent interneurons, confusing the brain in the process (Muscolino, 2009).

Perhaps some of the most well known research on referred pain comes from Irwin Korr. He conducted studies using measurements of electrical resistance in the paraspinal muscles. He discovered that spinal segments could be stimulated into a rise in neurological activity. In fact, when sufficiently overstimulated by pain signals, spinal segments can be sensitized in such a way that they will overreact by responding to any stimulation, even light stimulation, as if it were painful. Korr's experiments seem to validate these theories that pain stimulation, if sufficient, overloads the nervous system. When the system is overloaded the brain has a difficult time reading the signals, which leads to the phenomenon of referred pain.

Pfluger's laws of radiation and generalization describe the phenomenon of referred pain in another way. Through radiation and generalization, a hypersensitive spinal cord segment will become over-reactive, responding with excessive output that will recruit more spinal segments. As new spinal segments are recruited, they become potential sites for referred pain. The excessive output from the irritated spinal segment propagates to higher and higher centers in the central nervous system until the brain sends out general pain signals. The general pain signals may affect the whole body or just large, generalized areas. These large, generalized areas have come to be known as referral zones.

For a list of muscles and their common referral zones, refer to Chapter 9.

CLASSIFICATIONS OF TRIGGER POINTS

Myofascial trigger points are categorized in several different ways because there are several different important characteristics to consider when assessing this pathology.

First, trigger points may be classified depending on their location within a muscle. Trigger points can be present anywhere on the muscle and related connective tissue structures, but they most often appear in the belly of the muscle. That is because this area has the most neuromuscular junctions (endplates). Trigger points found here are called **central trigger points.** These trigger points are considered the most

DID YOU KNOW

For simplicity, some modern practitioners classify secondary, associated, and satellite trigger points all under the heading of "satellite" trigger points. However, Travell's categorization (according to a variety of locations) is valuable for keeping track of all the possible places one might find trigger points.

important to treat. This is because tension in the belly of the muscle pulls on the ends of the muscle and is often the cause of trigger points that develop there. Those trigger points found closer to the attachment sites of the muscle are called **attachment trigger points.** These trigger points may be caused by central trigger points, but they can develop on their own as well. Trigger points are also classified as being either active or latent.

1. *Active trigger points*—These are TrPs that are currently causing pain and/or dysfunction of the muscle. Whether the client is at rest or moving about, these trigger points are actively painful. All trigger points are considered active trigger points when causing pain during normal activity.
2. *Latent trigger points*—These are TrPs that are painful only when pressure is applied. A client may not even know this area is painful until it is touched.

Trigger points are categorized by their location within the muscle, by their level of activity, and lastly by their relationship to each other.

1. *Primary trigger points*—These are TrPs that are caused directly by acute or chronic overload, or injury. They are often found in the prime-mover (*agonist*) of a particular action. Sometimes these are the most painful and the largest TrPs a client will have and sometimes not. The distinguishing characteristic

DID YOU KNOW

The cold spray and stretch technique consisted of passively stretching the affected muscle while spraying it with a steady stream of Freon. The coldness of the Freon distracts the nervous system from the pain of the trigger point. This allowed Travell to stretch the muscle releasing the trigger point.

is that they are found in the muscles that are directly affected by the overload or injury. Because they are a direct result of the injury, primary trigger points are the first trigger points to show up.

2. *Secondary trigger points*—These are TrPs that are activated in *synergist* and/or *antagonist* muscles of the one containing the primary trigger point. As the restriction progresses from the primary trigger points, other associated muscles become overloaded. Let's say the biceps have become injured and have developed trigger points. The trigger points shorten the biceps and restrict their range of motion. Over time, this causes the triceps, on the opposite side of the elbow (the antagonist), to become stressed and develop secondary trigger points.

3. *Associated trigger points*—These are TrPs that are activated as a result of compensation. Once the agonist and antagonist and/or synergists are sufficiently overloaded, the surrounding structures develop trigger points. Using the example above: Once the biceps (agonist) and triceps (antagonist) become affected, their restriction will cause the shoulder to become overloaded. Supporting muscles of the shoulder, such as the trapezius, will then present with associated trigger points.

4. *Satellite trigger points*—These are TrPs that develop in the referral zone of the primary TrP. A referral zone is a distant area that presents with pain or discomfort as a result of a trigger point in a muscle in the acutely affected area.

Even though we see common patterns of trigger point development, they can develop anywhere in the body. They will show up anywhere that has slightly shifted from normal balance or anywhere there is a large amount of mechanical and postural stress. It is important to consider many factors when looking for the formation of trigger points because all aspects of our lives, jobs, emotions, lifestyles, etc., have an effect on our posture. It is important to search all the myoskeletal structures around a distortion or pathology to

DID YOU KNOW

A hallmark of the early form of PNF, developed by Voss and Knott, was rotary diagonal movement patterns of the limbs. These patterns were designed to re-educate the nervous system. They incorporated a type of movement called "cross-crawl." The technique repatterns and stimulates the right and left hemispheres of the brain by forcing both sides of the brain to work together.

The technique begins with the therapist moving one of the client's legs as well as the arm on the opposite side. Then, the movements are switched to the opposite leg and arm. Cross-crawl has been successfully used to treat infants with neuromotor damage.

note all of the possible trigger points. The role of the client's overall posture will influence the function of their neuromuscular system.

GENERAL TREATMENT OF TRIGGER POINTS

Dr. Travell primarily treated trigger points using a "cold spray and stretch" technique and/or injecting the trigger points with lidocaine. While these two treatment techniques are beyond the scope of most modern body workers, there are a host of other distraction, stretching, and manual techniques available. These and other direct methods of treating trigger points will be discussed in the next chapter.

Dr. Raymond Nimmo D.C., a contemporary of Dr. Travell's, also studied the relationships between muscle knots and pain. He independently discovered the same relationship between points of sensitivity and myoskeletal dysfunction. He called these points "noxious generative points" or "noxious pain points" (Chaitow, 2000).

Dr. Nimmo created a manual technique for treating the points instead of using injections. His technique is called the "five-second compression technique." The idea behind the method was that applying pressure on the area for five seconds would temporarily stop blood flow. When the pressure was released, it would result in an increased blood flow to the point. While the mechanism behind the technique has since been re-evaluated (Simons, Travell, & Simons, 1999), similar trigger point pressure release techniques are effective and applicable for today's body workers. Variants of the technique are commonly used today.

Regardless of which technique they used to treat trigger points, Dr. Nimmo and Dr. Travell both approached the pathology with the same goals in mind:

1. To eliminate the chemical buildup in the trigger point
2. To increase circulation to the ischemic area

DID YOU KNOW

Paul St. John is one of the most prominent therapists to focus on posture, postural evaluation, and pelvic stabilization as cornerstones of NMT theory. In the 1970s, St. John developed his unique style called the St. John method of neuromuscular therapy. He emphasizes the positions of the pelvic and shoulder girdles as the keys to balancing the body. He also calls attention to the idea that the entire body is always involved in every movement and therefore the entire body must always be considered when looking for trigger points.

By releasing the waste buildup in the tissues, the blood vessels are free to bring nutrients and hydration to the tissues. This is essential to healing the structures.

The Role of Facilitated Stretching in Neuromuscular Theory

Facilitated stretching (FS) is perhaps one of the most significant contributions to neuromuscular theory and application. Facilitated stretching includes a broad range of techniques that use specific neural reflexes to cause muscles to relax and lengthen.

Facilitated stretching has its roots in a system called proprioceptive neuromuscular facilitation (PNF). PNF originated in the field of physical therapy in the 1950s and was formalized for use in spinal cord injuries and strokes by Margaret Knott and Dorothy Voss. In 1968 they cowrote the book *Proprioceptive Neuromuscular Facilitation: Patterns and Techniques* (Knott & Voss, 1968). There are many elements to PNF. One distinguishing feature is its use of a maximum contraction of the muscle being treated, followed by a stretch of that same muscle (Turchaninov, 2006).

Borrowing from the research behind PNF, Dr. T. J. Ruddy, an osteopath, developed a technique called **resistive induction.** Resistive induction makes use of the fact that when a muscle undergoes an *isometric contraction*, it experiences a subsequent period of relaxation. This is called **postisometric relaxation (PIR).** During this period, the muscle can be stretched (Turchaninov, 2006).

Dr. Fred Mitchell, also an osteopath, with Dr. Karel Lewit built on Dr. Ruddy's work by further developing the use of postisometric relaxation in stretching. Mitchell named his system "muscle energy techniques" (METs) because they required the client to actively contract the muscle during the technique. Dr. Leon Chaitow, an osteopath and son of Boris Chaitow, seized on the ideas of Dr. Mitchell and Dr. Lewit and popularized PIR as well as a host of other techniques that use the same principles. These techniques use the body's natural responses to stretches and contractions to achieve lengthening of muscles. Dr. Chaitow released two important books, *Muscle Energy Techniques* (Chaitow, 1999) and *Modern Neuromuscular Techniques* in 1996 (Chaitow, 2000). During this time, noted sports therapist (and one of my teachers) Robert McAtee developed a book called *Facilitated Stretching* (McAtee, 1999). In this book, McAtee describes the use of PNF stretching for the modern therapist.

THE PHYSIOLOGY OF FACILITATING LENGTH

Facilitating length is often confused with stretching a muscle. While there are some similarities, for our purposes, stretching a muscle is different than lengthening a muscle. Stretching is the result of mechanical force applied to elongate the muscle and pull apart connective tissues. This is the type of stretching we are all familiar with to warm up the muscles.

The lengthening of a muscle is more of a neurological response. The muscle is relaxed by using indirect methods

QUICK QUIZ #14

1. Trigger points are knots in the muscle which: (Circle all that apply)
   a. are tender when compressed.
   b. give rise to referred pain when compressed.
   c. are formed as a response to emotional stress.
   d. are formed as a response to nutritional deficiencies.
   e. All of the above
   f. None of the above

2. The surface area over a trigger point is often warmer and darker in color than the surrounding tissue.
   a. True
   b. False

3. Referred pain: (Circle all that apply)
   a. occurs in very unpredictable patterns.
   b. is a sharp stinging pain in the local area of a trigger point.
   c. is not a clear indicator of the presence of a trigger point.
   d. was the main focus of research of Margaret Knott and Dorothy Voss.
   e. All of the above
   f. None of the above

4. Lengthening of muscles can be achieved by stimulating neurological structures using the techniques of facilitated stretching.
   a. True
   b. False

5. Nerve compression or entrapment of nerves may be caused by: (Circle all that apply)
   a. muscles.
   b. bone.
   c. cartilage.
   d. paraesthesia.
   e. All of the above
   f. None of the above

6. When a muscle undergoes an isometric contraction: (Circle all that apply)
   a. it is followed by an increase in paraesthesia.
   b. it is followed by a period of relaxation.
   c. it is followed by postisometric relaxation.
   d. it is followed by a period when the muscle is more receptive to being stretched.
   e. All of the above
   f. None of the above

which stimulate neurological structures in specific ways that cause lengthening. Many techniques manipulate the muscle spindles and Golgi tendon organs, stimulating reciprocal inhibition and reciprocal activation, which influence the length of a muscle. Other techniques influence proprioceptors and other neural structures such as the brain and spinal cord to facilitate the neurological response. While it is important to stretch and mechanically separate tissues and break down adhesions, the tension created by the neurology of the muscle should also be addressed.

SUMMARY

Researchers investigating neurology at the turn of the century laid down important principles that still guide the practice of neuromuscular therapy today. The neurological laws proposed by Hilton, Pfluger, Bowditch, Head, and Shultz provide the starting point to understanding and treating physical conditions from a neurological perspective.

Several individuals have made important contributions to modern neuromuscular theory and practice. Boris Chaitow, Stanley Leif, Janet Travell, and Leon Chaitow are a few of those who formulated theories, conducted studies, and designed the treatment modalities that influence today's NMT. Among the most salient concepts are trigger point theory and facilitated stretching (FS).

The neuromuscular model takes into account both the physical and the emotional factors that cause dysfunction in the myoskeletal system. NMT seeks to understand the origins of pathology in order to treat and heal it. Some common roots of pathology include physical injury, improper body mechanics, and emotional stress. The neuromuscular model lists nerve compression, postural distortion, nutritional deficiencies, biomechanical dysfunction, and trigger points as the main categories of neuromuscular pathology.

Trigger points are responsible for a large amount of dysfunction, so they are a primary focus of NMT. Trigger points are focused points of hyperirritability. Trigger points are activated by a number of pathological conditions, such as nutritional deficiencies and mechanical dysfunction. The energy crisis hypothesis and chronic isometric contraction are also important concepts explaining the formation of trigger points.

Trigger points are responsible for local pain and referred pain. Understanding the mechanism and patterns of referred pain is essential to assessing and locating trigger points. There are several types of trigger points that are categorized according to which tissues and structures they affect.

Facilitated stretching includes a broad range of techniques that take advantage of neurology to cause muscles to relax and lengthen. Ruddy is credited with developing a technique called *resistive induction*. Mitchell, Lewit, and Leon Chaitow further expanded this strategy as they created and popularized the methods known as *muscle energy techniques*.

DISCUSSION QUESTIONS

1. Explain how Hilton's law is important to massage therapists.
2. Using Pfluger's laws, explain how pathological muscle tension can spread through the body.
3. Describe four conditions commonly associated with the presence of trigger points (lesions).
4. How is the effect of the emotions on posture important to NMT?
5. How does nerve compression contribute to the pain reflex cycle?
6. How is referred pain important to NMT therapists?

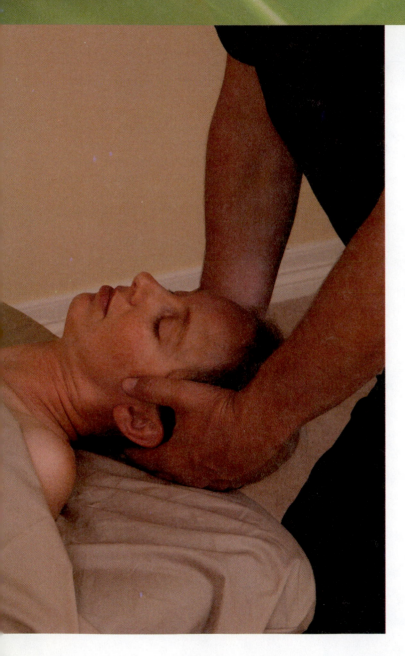

8 The Techniques of Neuromuscular Therapy

CHAPTER HIGHLIGHTS

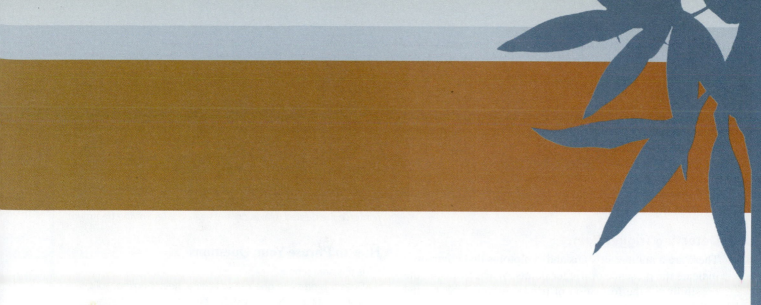

CHAPTER OBJECTIVES

- Understand the principles of neuromuscular therapy
- Learn to perform the direct neuromuscular techniques
- Discern three types of muscle contraction
- Recognize the three barriers to joint movement

- Learn to perform the indirect neuromuscular techniques
- Explore the five stages of neuromuscular treatment
- Identify the cautions and contraindications for neuro-muscular therapy

KEY TERMS

Trigger point pressure
    release *141*

Isometric contraction *145*

Isotonic contraction *145*

Range of motion
    (ROM) *145*

Anatomic barrier/absolute
    end range *145*

Physiologic barrier *146*

Pathologic barrier *146*

Comfort barrier *146*

Joint end feel *146*

TREATMENT USING NEUROMUSCULAR THERAPY

Neuromuscular therapy emphasizes the treatment of entire structures, not just locally affected areas. You should begin by identifying postural distortions that are involved in the client's pain patterns. Note all areas of compensation. Once the major structures are noted, it is important to find all of the involved trigger points.

Detecting Trigger Points

There are a number of signs and symptoms that commonly indicate the presence of trigger points. When assessing the possibility of the formation of trigger points, look for the following:

- **Restricted movement, stiffness in the muscle or joint (hypertonicity)**—This is because the trigger point holds the muscle in contraction, causing the joint to feel stiff.
- **Weakness in specific muscles**—There is a principle known as the *length tension relationship curve* that describes a muscle's tendency to weaken when in prolonged contraction (as is caused by a trigger point).
- **Passive or active stretching that causes pain**—Muscles usually hurt the most at the site of a trigger point. However, the tension caused by the trigger point can cause pain at the attachments or anywhere along the muscle when stretched.
- *Subcutaneous* **tissues feel coarse, granular, ropy, or knotty**—The skin or subcutaneous tissues will be affected from the lack of nutrient supply due to the ischemia.
- **"Jump sign"**—The client jumps when pressure or a stretch is applied. This is due to guarding from the pain. If the pathology is severe, it may cause the client to completely pull away from the pressure; often this is involuntary.
- **Deep tenderness and/or** *paraesthesia* **(i.e., numbness, pins and needles, tingling, and/or hypersensitivity)**—This results when tense muscles compress nerves.
- **Surface area is colder than surrounding tissue**—This is due to ischemia (lack of blood flow) caused by compression of tense muscles on blood vessels.

- **Changes in the color of the tissues**—Usually pale due to ischemia.
- **Changes in the thickness of muscles**—The classic feeling of trigger points is that they are like "knots," or lumps, in the muscle layers. Sometimes they even feel like stones in the muscle. This is due to the hardening of the ground substance in the muscle.
- **Taut, palpable bands in affected muscle**—Central trigger points may pull on both ends of the muscle causing the whole band to become taut.
- **Pressure**—Pressure gives rise to local pain (hyperirritability) and/or referred pain.
- **Local "twitch response"**—When snapping or rolling the fingers across the grain of the muscle with a suspected trigger point, there is a visible twitch in the muscle.

Once the trigger points are located, the targeted soft tissues will be treated to promote structural change and balance in the muscles and posture. To achieve this balance, with NMT you will use a combination of strategies which release trigger points, lengthen muscles, and re-educate the nervous system.

Some forms of bodywork (e.g., deep tissue massage) focus treatment primarily on the muscle bellies. Dr. Travell, Dr. Simons, and Dr. Turchaninov identified trigger points along the entire length of the muscle as well as its tendons and bony attachments. Therefore, the techniques of NMT were developed to treat all of these structures.

Modern therapists borrow from many systems and techniques. Those showcased here are considered by many to be the foundation of NMT therapy.

THE TECHNIQUES OF NEUROMUSCULAR THERAPY

NMT approaches the treatment of trigger points and other muscular tensions with direct methods and indirect methods. You may work directly on the site of pathology using any of three forms of **trigger point pressure release** (formerly known as *ischemic compression*) and/or by using stripping strokes. You may indirectly treat local pathology, as well as address multiple restrictions, by using forms of facilitated stretching. While the direct and indirect techniques are often used independently, they are extremely effective when combined together. Commonly, the specific trigger points are addressed first using a direct method, then the entire muscle is released to both lengthen and re-educate the muscle using a facilitated stretching technique found in the indirect method section.

The Direct Methods

TRIGGER POINT PRESSURE RELEASE (ALSO CALLED *MANUAL PRESSURE RELEASE*)

There are three slightly different variations to the basic trigger point pressure release technique. The differences are subtle but are significant and provide an opportunity to tailor your treatment to the individual client. The basic method is the same and the physiology behind the variations is the same.

- **Physiology behind the technique:** The formation of trigger points involves processes explained by the energy crisis hypothesis (described fully in Chapter 7). The *actin* and *myosin* filaments of a muscle fiber attach to one another to create a contraction. Under normal circumstances the attachment bond is broken to release the contraction. In the case of trigger point pathology, the actin and myosin filaments

are unable to release. They are effectively "stuck" together, which maintains the chronic contraction (see Figure 8.1 ■). When gentle pressure (compression) is applied directly to the area, it helps to release these stuck filaments by helping to separate the bond between them (Simons, Travell, and Simons, 1999). In addition, the slow constant pressure causes the release of endorphins and enkephalins, which are morphinelike substances that the body uses to mitigate pain and relax muscles (Chaitow, 2000).

VARIATION 1—PROGRESSIVE PRESSURE

This variation is often useful for newer therapists as it gives a measured guideline for pressure based on feedback from clients. It is also good to use this variation with clients who tend to want to participate in the therapy or for those who are less inclined to speak up on their own regarding any discomfort.

This variation is good to use on harder knots, less sensitive areas, or more robust clients.

- **Procedure (Figures 8.2 ■ to 8.5 ■):**
  1. Using the thumbs, fingers, knuckles, or elbows, press the trigger point until a slight discomfort arises in the referral zone, or in the local area. Have the client use a scale of 1–10 to describe the level of discomfort. One is little or no discomfort, and ten is too much. The pressure applied should reach a 2 or a 4, but not pass a 6 on the scale.

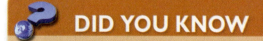

DID YOU KNOW

When working with the direct methods, it may be helpful to shorten the muscle you are treating. This helps to relax the muscle and prevents guarding, making the therapy more effective. For example, you can bend the elbow to shorten the biceps. This will make it more relaxed and more receptive to therapy.

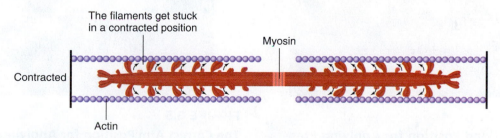

The filaments get stuck in a contracted position

Myosin

Contracted

Actin

FIGURE 8.1

When the Bond Between the Myosin and Actin Filaments Is Unable to Release, the Filaments Become "Stuck" in the State of Contraction.

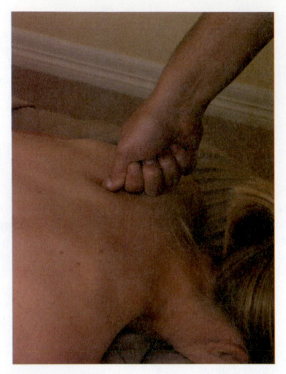

FIGURE 8.2
The Correct Hand Position for Applying Pressure with the Thumb During the Trigger Point Pressure Release Technique.

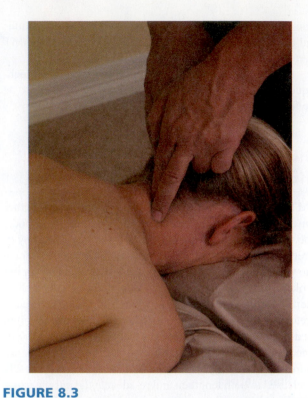

FIGURE 8.3
The Correct Hand Position for Applying Pressure with the Fingers During the Trigger Point Pressure Release Technique.

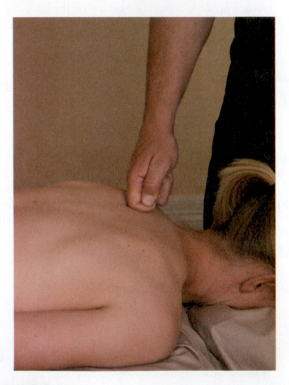

FIGURE 8.4
The Correct Hand Position for Applying Pressure with the Knuckles During the Trigger Point Pressure Release Technique.

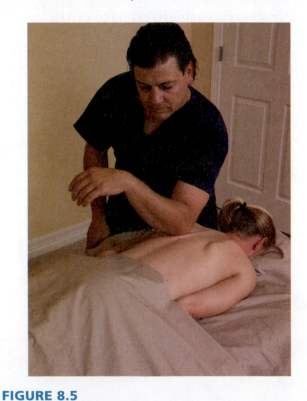

FIGURE 8.5
The Correct Arm Position for Applying Pressure with the Elbows During the Trigger Point Pressure Release Technique.

2. Hold the trigger point consistently at the level of 2 or 4 until the local or referred discomfort diminishes (i.e., less than a 2 or 4). *Note:* The discomfort should begin to diminish by a count of 12 seconds. If the discomfort does not diminish, release your pressure, and try again. This time use lighter pressure, taking the pressure to a level of 1 or 2, and hold there until it diminishes.

3. When the discomfort diminishes, press deeper into the trigger point, until the slight discomfort comes back to a level of 2 or 4 and hold again until it diminishes.

4. Repeat this process as many times as needed.

5. You can keep working deeper into the trigger point many as 4 or 5 times or as few as 1 or 2. Consider these factors as to how deep you should go and when you should stop treating the trigger point:
   a. Stop if pressing deeper would be too painful.
   b. Stop when you are unable to work deeper, such as when treating a shallow area

VARIATION 2—BARRIER RELEASE

This variation is good for therapists who have well-developed skills for palpating tissues. It works well with clients who are less interested in talking during massage. It is also good to use on harder knots, less sensitive areas, or more robust clients.

- **Procedure (Figures 8.2 to 8.5):**
  1. Using the thumbs, fingers, knuckles, or elbows, press the trigger point until you feel a "barrier," or a slight resistance in the tissues.
  2. Hold the trigger point consistently until you feel the barrier soften (i.e., the resistance diminishes). This usually occurs after a few seconds.
  3. When the barrier softens, increase the pressure into the trigger point, until another barrier is reached.
  4. Repeat this process as many times as needed until the trigger point is sufficiently diminished.
  5. You can keep working deeper into the trigger point many as 4 or 5 times or as few as 1 or 2.

VARIATION 3—INTERMITTENT PRESSURE RELEASE

This variation uses a release of pressure several times during the process. This slightly changes its effect on the nervous and vascular systems. In this case, the nervous system gets a break from the pressure. This may be desirable in situations where there is a significant amount of pain or for more sensitive clients. The intermittent release of pressure is gentler on the blood vessels, which is useful when treating sensitive areas like the neck.

- **Procedure (Figures 8.2 to 8.5):**
  1. Using the thumbs, fingers, knuckles, or elbows, press the trigger point until discomfort arises in a referral zone, or in the local area. Have the client use a scale of 1–10 to describe the level of discomfort. One is little or no discomfort, and ten is too much. The pressure applied should reach a 2 or a 4, but not pass a 6 on the scale.

  2. Hold the trigger point consistently at the level of 2 or 4 until the local or referred discomfort diminishes. *Note:* The discomfort should begin to diminish by a count of 12 seconds. If not, restart with lighter pressure (up to a 1 or 2 on the scale).

  3. When the discomfort diminishes, release the pressure but keep contact with the point for 1 to 2 seconds. Then press back into the trigger point, until the discomfort arises to a level of 2 or 4, and hold again until it diminishes. The main difference between this technique and the progressive pressure technique is that here the pressure is released for 1–2 seconds before applying further pressure. You can keep working the point many as 4 or 5 times or as few as 1 or 2. The number of repetitions depends on a few factors:
     a. Stop if pressing deeper would be too painful.
     b. Stop if you are unable to work deeper such as when treating a shallow area.

- **Special considerations for all variations of trigger point pressure release:**
  ○ Best for central trigger points.
  ○ Save your hands: Use elbows for large muscles, knuckles and thumbs for medium muscles, and fingers for small muscles.
  ○ Depending on the size of the muscle, its level of tension, and the length of time it has been present, you may or may not be able to release the trigger point in one session. Multiple sessions may be required.
  ○ Sometimes while applying pressure, the muscle and the discomfort just seem to release all at once. When this occurs, it is not necessary to continue applying pressure; just move to the next stage of treatment.
  ○ It is important to work on the lighter side of pressure because the goal is to release the tension, not to break down fibers. If the client is holding her or his breath or is resisting, you may be pressing too hard.
  ○ Even though the pressure may be light, use your body weight to lean into the technique whenever possible. Using weight instead of your muscles saves your energy and causes less wear and tear on your muscles and joints. When using your body weight, the pressure is more even and easier for the client to accept.
  ○ Have the client breathe out when applying the pressure as it helps the client to mentally focus and relax into the therapy.

STRIPPING STROKES (SOMETIMES CALLED *DEEP-STROKING MASSAGE*)

● **Physiology behind the technique:** This technique causes an increase in blood flow to the ischemic tissues around the trigger point. The increase in blood flow brings nutrients to the site, helping to resolve the energy crisis caused by the trigger point. Deep strokes along the length of the muscle help to stretch and separate the frozen myosin and actin filaments, releasing the tension in the trigger point.

● **Procedure (Figures 8.6 to 8.8):**

  1. Using the thumbs (Figure 8.6 ■), fingers, knuckles (Figure 8.7 ■), or elbows (Figure 8.8 ■), perform short, moderately deep strokes (not enough to cause guarding) right over the trigger point. Have the client use a scale of 1–10 to describe the level of discomfort. One is little or no pain, and ten is too much. The pressure applied should reach a 4 or a 6, but not pass an 8 on the scale.
  2. The strokes should be performed primarily along the direction of the muscle fibers; however, it is useful to work cross-fiber as long as you don't overstress the muscle.
  3. Apply the strokes at a moderate pace, about 1 to 2 seconds per stroke.
  4. You may apply 30 to 60 strokes per trigger point.

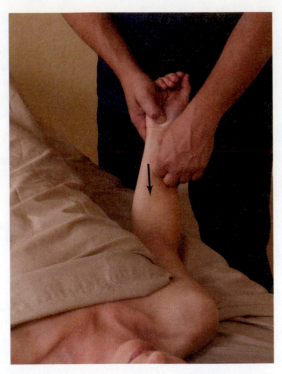

FIGURE 8.7

The Correct Position for Applying Pressure with the Knuckles During the Stripping Stroke Technique. The Arrow Shows the Direction of the Stroke.

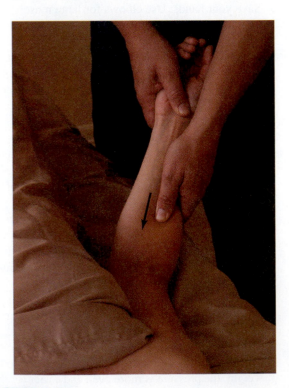

FIGURE 8.6

The Correct Position for Applying Pressure with the Thumbs During the Stripping Stroke Technique. The Arrow Shows the Direction of the Stroke.

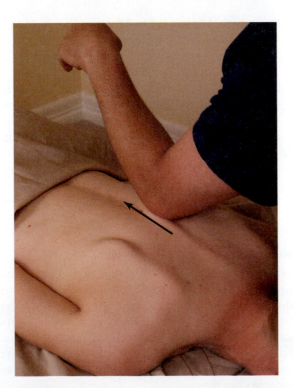

FIGURE 8.8

The Correct Position for Applying Pressure with the Elbow During the Stripping Stroke Technique. The Arrow Shows the Direction of the Stroke.

5. The number of strokes depends on a few factors:
   ○ Stop when the client no longer feels discomfort at the site.
   ○ Stop when the knot diminishes.
   ○ Stop before the muscle becomes overstressed.

- **Special considerations:**
  ○ This technique is good to use in the case of *myogelosis*, or thick hardened trigger points.
  ○ This technique works well for attachment and central trigger points.
  ○ Save your hands: Use elbows for large muscles, knuckles and thumbs for medium muscles, and fingers for small muscles.
  ○ Depending on the size of the muscle, its level of tension, and the length of time it has been present, you may or may not be able to release the trigger point in one session. Multiple sessions may be required.
  ○ Sometimes while applying the strokes, the muscle and the discomfort just seem to release all at once. When this occurs, it may not be necessary to continue applying the strokes; just move to the next stage of treatment.
  ○ It is important to work within the medium range of pressure, as the goal is to relax the muscle as well as to break down fibers. If the client is holding his or her breath or is resisting, you may be pressing too hard.
  ○ Use your body weight to lean into the technique whenever possible. Using weight instead of your muscles saves your energy and causes less wear and tear on your muscles and joints. When using your body weight, the pressure is more even and easier for the client to accept.
  ○ Have the client breathe out when first applying the strokes, as it helps the client to mentally focus and relax into the therapy.

The Indirect Methods

FACILITATED STRETCHING

Facilitated stretching includes a very versatile group of techniques that can be used in a wide range of circumstances. These techniques indirectly treat trigger points by facilitating length in the muscle and releasing tense tissues. They are also used to re-educate the muscles to a new resting length after administration of other techniques. Facilitated stretching techniques are especially effective because they manipulate the nervous system, causing the muscle to relax so that the tissues can be lengthened further. Once the muscle has been lengthened, it can "learn" a new resting length that is beyond that which can be achieved with simpler forms of stretching.

The Foundations of Facilitated Stretching   Before the actual techniques can be explained, it is essential to introduce some basic terms and concepts that are used in the discussion and application of these techniques.

MUSCULAR CONTRACTIONS

Facilitated stretching uses the different types of muscle contractions to manipulate neuromuscular processes and lengthen the muscle. There are three types of muscular contractions that are used during facilitated stretching.

1. **Isometric contraction**—The muscle contracts but produces no movement at the joint, only effort. When a person flexes a muscle and holds it (as in a "show me your muscle" pose), the contraction is isometric.
2. **Isotonic contraction**—The muscle contracts and produces movement at the joint. Isotonic contractions occur when moving a limb, such as bending or extending the arm.
   There are two types of isotonic contraction:
   a. Concentric contraction—The insertion moves closer to the origin, thereby shortening the muscle. For example, bending/flexing the elbow when lifting an object shortens the biceps.
   b. Eccentric contraction—The insertion moves away from the origin, lengthening the muscle as it is contracting. When straightening the elbow to put down an object, the biceps contracts to resist the weight, but also lengthens to allow the object to be put down.

BARRIERS TO JOINT MOVEMENT

Facilitated stretching is used to lengthen muscles. This translates to an increase in the **range of motion (ROM)** of a joint. The range of motion of a joint is the extent of its movement through flexion and extension. The ROM of a joint may be limited by several factors. It is important to understand and be able to discern these different barriers in order to properly perform facilitated stretching techniques. There are four types of barriers to joint movement:

1. **Anatomic barriers**—These are limits in the range of motion that are determined by the shape and fit of the bones at the joint. The anatomic barrier of a joint is also called the **absolute end range.** The way the proximal end of the olecranon process fits into the distal end of the humerus is an example of an anatomic

DID YOU KNOW

I often surprise my students because even while I am laying face down receiving massage, I can tell when they are using proper posture and body weight. When they use proper technique, it feels stronger, more stable, and easier to accept. When they use their muscles to apply pressure, they are shaky and apply less pressure.

barrier. The olecranon essentially locks in against the humerus, preventing any further extension of the joint (see Figure 8.9 ■).

2. **Physiologic barriers**—These are limits in the ROM that are determined by normal, protective nerve and sensory function. This barrier occurs just before the absolute end range of the joint. When a joint is reaching its end range, or when the tissues reach a full stretch, the muscles of the body will resist further movement in order to protect the joint. This barrier protects all joints.

3. **Pathologic barrier**—This is a neurological change due to pathology. This translates as stiffness, pain, or a "catch" in the joint. The natural neural functions that maintain the protective physiologic barrier may adapt in the case of injury, restriction, trigger points, etc. The joint's range of motion will be reduced to restrict movement and protect the joint. A pathologic barrier almost always limits the action at the joint of an injured limb. If this becomes chronic, the tissues themselves will become fixed in a shortened position. Pathologic barriers may be caused by arthritis or non-muscular conditions. Keep this in mind as you perform your assessment.

4. **Comfort barrier**—When moving a client's body into a passive stretch, this is the first point of resistance, just short of the perception of any discomfort. This is the barrier that is used to guide the performance of most facilitated stretching techniques. Over time, facilitated stretching techniques help to reset the pathologic barriers and bring the joint movement back to the normal physiologic barriers.

ASSESSING BARRIERS

In order to perform facilitated stretching techniques, it is important to assess the type and quality of the range-of-motion barrier. The quality of the end of the range is called **joint end feel.** When assessing joint end feel, bring the client through the passive stretch and notice how it feels when the end is reached. There are two basic types of joint end feel:

1. *Soft end feel*—This occurs when the normal physiologic barrier of the muscle is reached. It feels like the movement is restricted, but the joint still retains a little springiness to it.

2. *Hard end feel*—This occurs when the pathologic barrier is reached. Here the client is injured, and the joint

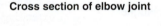

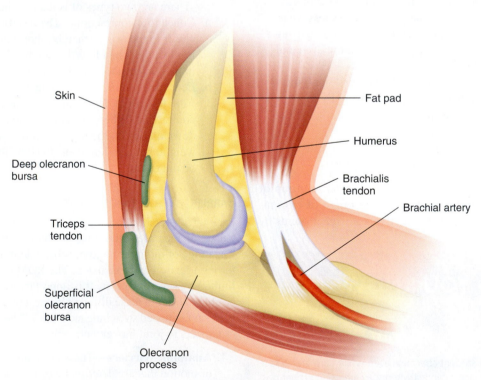

FIGURE 8.9

A Diagram of the Elbow Joint Showing How the Olecranon Process and the Humerus Fit Tightly Together to Form the Anatomic Barrier.

is restricted. Typically, when the end of the range is pathological, there is no feeling of residual springiness. There may be binding that feels like a jammed drawer.

General Principles for Performing Facilitated Stretching

Prepare the Tissues   It is very important that the area be warmed up prior to performing facilitated stretching techniques. Connective tissue is very inelastic when cold or cool. As with all stretches, FS elongates connective tissue as well as muscle tissue. Warming the area first allows the connective tissue to be more receptive to change. Light massage modalities or an application of moist heat may be used to prewarm tissues.

Establish the Correct Position for Stretching   Make sure you are positioned to allow yourself space to move the joint through its full range of motion. Take a moment to discern the best way to position the client to allow a full ROM of the area being stretched. Keep in mind that it may be necessary to have the client turn over to stretch a particular area.

Generally, it is easier to lift the limb than it is to push it toward the table. For example, to stretch the anterior chest, it is best to have the client in the prone position, with the muscles of the anterior chest in contact with the table. The arm can then be easily lifted to create the stretch (see Figure 8.10 ■). If the client were supine, the arm would have

to be pushed toward the floor and the presence of the table would interfere with the stretch (see Figure 8.11 ■).

Use Proper Body Mechanics   Body mechanics are a very important consideration in the application of FS. To prevent strain, avoid leaning over the client, and hold the limb close to your body (see Figure 8.12 ■). One hand should be placed close to the joint to help stabilize the joint. The second hand should be placed at the distal end of the bone. The distal hand provides the majority of the movement for the stretch. When moving the client's limb, your whole body should move so that you stay under the limb, making sure it is properly supported. Keep your back straight, and use your legs to lift heavy body parts (Figure 8.13 ■).

Work to Promote Ease of Movement   When moving a joint, use a slight *traction* (decompression) to prevent the joint from being "jammed." Traction decompresses the joint, which allows for greater mobility and prevents damage to the bones.

The main goal of FS is to promote ease of movement. Although an increase of ROM is a secondary goal, one should not stress it as the desired outcome. This will help to prevent a tendency to push the muscle too far or too fast. This technique emphasizes tuning into the client's ability to move and also working with small intervals of change. Facilitated

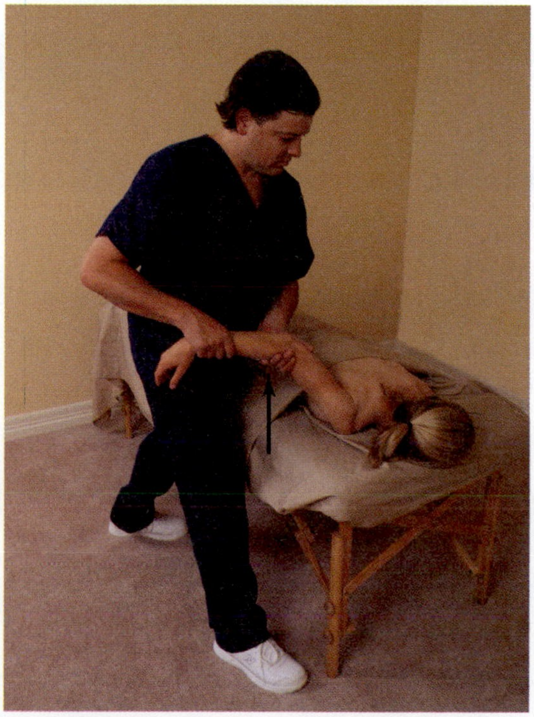

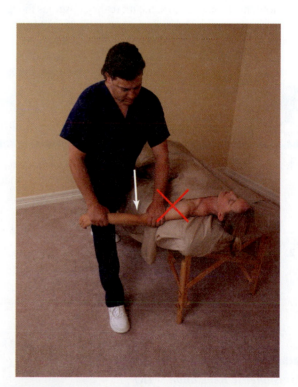

FIGURE 8.11

The Incorrect Positioning of the Client to Stretch the Chest and Anterior Shoulder. The Arrow Indicates the Direction the Arm Must Be Moved in Order to Stretch the Chest. The Position of the Client on the Table Prevents the Proper Movement for the Stretch.

FIGURE 8.10

The Proper Positioning of the Client to Stretch the Chest and Anterior Shoulder. The Arrow Shows That the Therapist Is Able to Lift the Limb to Produce the Desired Stretch.

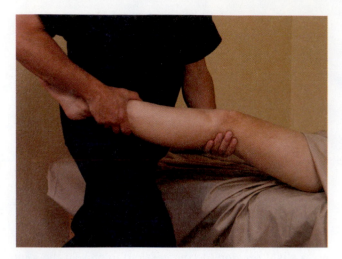

FIGURE 8.12

The Correct Hand Placement for Supporting the Leg While Performing the Adductor Stretch. Note That One Hand Is Close to the Joint and the Other Hand Is at the Distal End of the Limb.

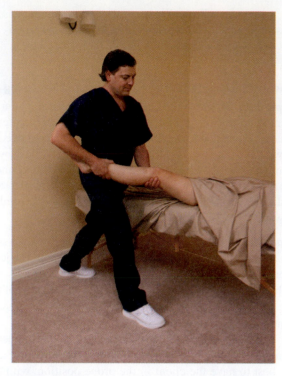

FIGURE 8.13

The Correct Posture of the Therapist During the Performance of the Adductor Stretch. Note That the Back Is Straight and the Legs Are Used to Support the Weight of the Client's Leg.

stretching works with the client's mind-muscle connection. The more the muscle relaxes, the more the conscious thoughts will let go of tension. The more the conscious thoughts release tension, the more each muscle will relax and lengthen.

QUICK QUIZ #15

1. When applying methods of trigger point pressure release, it is important to apply the greatest amount of pressure that the client can tolerate.
   a. True
   b. False

2. During a _____ contraction, there is movement at the joint. (Circle all that apply)
   a. isotonic
   b. eccentric
   c. concentric

   d. All of the above
   e. None of the above

3. Typically, when the end of the range is pathological, there is no feeling of residual springiness.
   a. True
   b. False

4. The main goal of facilitated stretching is to increase the range of motion of the joint.
   a. True
   b. False

Techniques of Facilitated Stretching

Postisometric Relaxation (PIR)

• **Physiology behind the technique:**   A strong, prolonged isometric contraction (no joint movement) loads the Golgi tendon organs and causes them to inhibit contraction of the muscle for a brief period. During this brief period, the muscle is said to be in a *refractory state*. Since the muscle is inhibited from contracting during this time, there is a 5 to 10 second window in which the muscle is

more receptive to lengthening. At this point, the target muscle (the muscle that is being treated) can often be moved slightly beyond the original pathological barrier.

• **Purpose:**   This method is used to re-educate a muscle to its best resting state. It is ideal for treating muscles that are chronically shortened. An important benefit of this technique is that it can be used when an area is either too painful or too tense to palpate or massage deeply. PIR can be used in the beginning stages of any treatment to release enough muscle tension to allow for deeper work. Once the muscles have been released through PIR, they are often more receptive to massage. This technique is also very effective when used in the re-education stage since it works by resetting the neural structures.

- **Procedure (Figures 8.14 to 8.17):**
  1. Use a passive stretch to lengthen the target muscle to the pathologic barrier. Figure 8.14 ■ shows the position for stretching the hamstrings.
  2. Ease off of the barrier slightly to find the comfort barrier. This will take the stress off of the tendons and fascia.
  3. Position your hands to provide resistance while the client presses against you to contract the target muscle. Instruct the client to gently contract the target muscle (push against you) at about 20 percent of his or her strength. Figure 8.15 ■ shows the direction in which the client must push to contract the hamstrings.
  4. While the client is contracting, counteract that pressure by resisting the movement (causing an isometric contraction) for 10 to 15 seconds. *Note:* It is important to make sure this is an isometric contraction with no movement at the joint. Figure 8.16 ■ shows the direction in which the therapist must resist the contraction of the hamstrings.

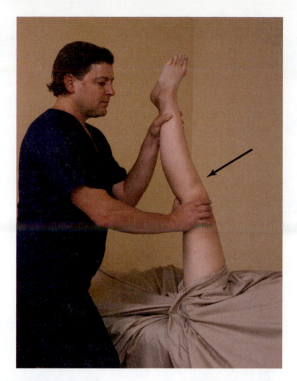

FIGURE 8.15

The Direction (as Indicated by the Arrow) in Which the Client Will Apply Pressure on the Hamstrings During the Contraction Phase of Postisometric Relaxation.

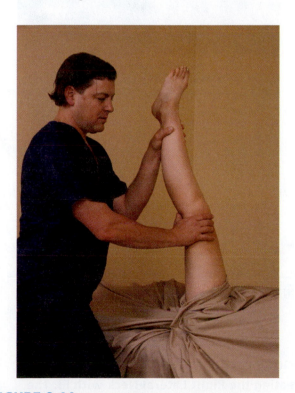

FIGURE 8.14

The Correct Position and Hand Placement to Stretch the Hamstrings During the Performance of Postisometric Relaxation.

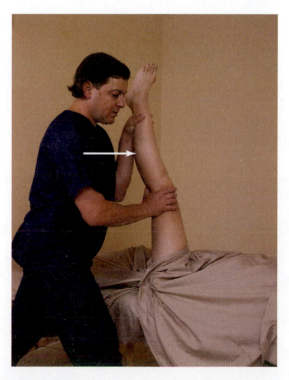

FIGURE 8.16

The Direction of Pressure Used by the Therapist to Resist the Client's Hamstring Contraction.

5. After 10 to 15 seconds, instruct the client to relax the contraction, and then perform one of two variations:
   a. Hold the limb in the same position (i.e., at the comfort barrier) for 3 seconds.
   b. Move the limb out of the stretch (i.e., relax the muscle) for 3 seconds.
   Figure 8.17 ■ shows the position the limb will be in when relaxing the hamstrings for 3 seconds.
6. After the 3 seconds, passively stretch the muscle to the next comfort barrier.
7. Repeat the procedure several times or until no further progress is achieved.

● **Special considerations:**
   ○ This technique is *not* good for muscles in spasm because it requires a contraction and a relaxation of the target muscle. In the case of a spasm, the target muscle is already in a state of severe contraction.
   ○ Pay heed to the general cautions and contraindications for all massage and stretching techniques (especially those that concern injury and joint conditions). A contraction under resistance can severely exacerbate an existing injury.
   ○ Don't use PIR on severely *atrophic* muscles. They may tear due to the resistance against the contraction.
   ○ This technique is best used on fairly healthy muscles that are hypertonic due to chronic overload or old injury.

Reciprocal Inhibition (RI)

● **Physiology behind the technique:** When a muscle isotonically contracts (with movement at the joint against resistance), its antagonist must relax to allow movement at the joint. This is due to an elaborate communication system between the muscle spindle cells, Golgi tendon organs, and the central nervous system. When the muscle opposing a tense muscle is contracted, it causes *reciprocal inhibition* in the tense target muscle (effectively relaxing it).

● **Purpose:** This is the best technique to use for a muscle currently in a spasm (a cramped muscle). It can also be used in place of PIR or more vigorous stretches for clients who cannot perform PIR due to pain or some other reason. Reciprocal inhibition is a good first-aid technique. Since the opposing muscle is doing all of the work, there is little risk of exacerbating problems in the target muscle.

● **Procedure (Figures 8.18 to 8.20):**
   1. Isolate the target muscle by putting it into passive contraction. This means that you move the insertion closer to the origin, effectively shortening the muscle. Figure 8.18 ■ shows the position for treating the right lateral neck. The neck is moved into right lateral flexion.

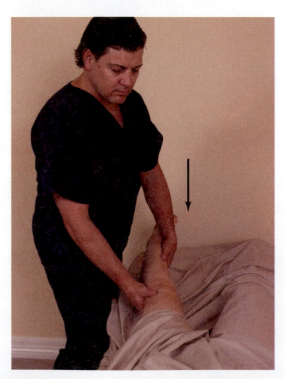

FIGURE 8.17
Following the Hamstring Contraction, the Leg Is Lowered and Relaxed for Three Seconds.

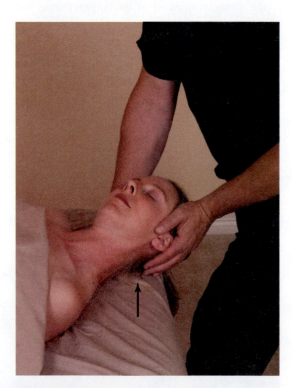

FIGURE 8.18
Treating the Right Lateral Neck with RI. The Therapist Begins by Moving the Target Muscles into Passive Contraction. The Origins of the Right Lateral Neck Muscles Have Been Moved Closer to Their Insertions.

2. Put pressure on the side opposite the target muscle (in this case the left side of the head), and instruct the client to resist your pressure and move the body part toward the opposite side. This will cause the client to contract the opposing muscle(s). Create just enough pressure to cause resistance, but not enough to hinder movement in the opposite direction. It is important to allow movement to occur slowly. Let the body part move as far in the opposite direction as it will go. This takes about 8 to 10 seconds. As the opposing muscle contracts, the the target muscle will relax and lengthen. Figure 8.19 ■ shows the direction of the movement for treating the right lateral neck. Figure 8.20 ■ shows the end of the movement.

3. Repeat the procedure three or four times or until the desired level of relaxation is achieved.

- **Special considerations:**
  - Make sure you allow the joint to move throughout the resistance.
  - RI is the first line of defense against a cramp (e.g., calf cramp, foot cramp) because contracting the antagonist muscle to the muscle in spasm causes the spastic muscle to relax.

- This is a gentle technique. It can be used in many cases where other techniques are unavailable or inapplicable due to pain or other restrictions.

Positional Release

- **Physiology behind the technique:**   In positional release, gentle pressure is applied to the pathology (trigger point, etc.), and then the body is repositioned in the "direction of ease" so the muscle tension can release on its own. The new position is held long enough to allow the pain receptors to stop sending pain signals. Through this process, the proprioceptors and pain receptors are essentially "reset" and the pain from the trigger point is diminished as well as its associated tension. The muscle incrementally achieves a longer resting length because of the systematic introduction to less painful positions before finally being reintroduced to the original positions that were uncomfortable.

- **Purpose:**   This technique is used directly on areas of tenderness and tension. Positional release treats all types of muscle tension as well as trigger points. It even works on nondescript spots of local pain called *tender points*. Positional release is a gentle way to re-educate the muscle and facilitate an increased ROM. It is one of the more effective ways of dealing with tender areas regardless of the pathology. It is especially good for releasing small areas of muscle spasm without inducing additional pain.

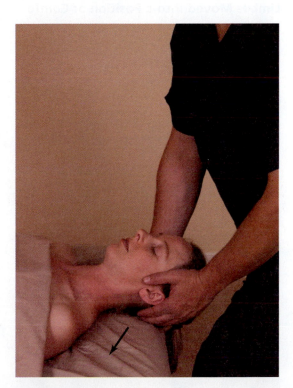

FIGURE 8.19

The Direction of Movement (as Indicated by the Arrow) Performed by the Client While Contracting the Opposing Muscles (the Left Lateral Neck Muscles), Which Allows the Target Muscles on the Right Side to Relax. The Client's Movement Is Met with a Slight Resistance by the Therapist.

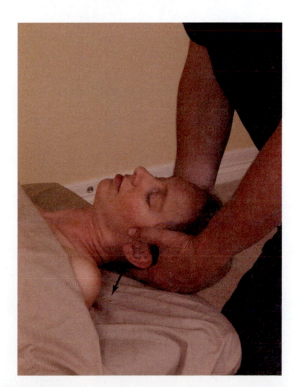

FIGURE 8.20

The Final Position of the Client's Neck and Head Once the Sequence for RI Has Been Applied to the Right Lateral Neck Muscles

- **Procedure (Figures 8.21 to 8.23):**

  1. Locate the site of pathology (e.g., tender point, trigger point).
  2. Using the thumbs, fingers, or elbows, press into the spot until the client feels a slight increase in tenderness (see Figure 8.21 ■).
  3. Using the sensation of tenderness as your guide, slowly reposition the client's body or limb until the pain subsides. This will often, but not always, mean moving the muscle in the direction of shortening it. It is most important to find a position where the pain is lessened or gone altogether (see Figure 8.22 ■).
  4. Hold the new position for at least 30 seconds and up to 90 seconds. Continue lightly holding the tender point while the new position is held.
  5. After 30 to 90 seconds at the new position, keep the pressure on the tender spot and slowly reposition the muscle toward the range where the client originally felt the pain (usually lengthening the muscle) (see Figure 8.23 ■).
  6. Once you have reached the position where the tenderness returns, pause, then slowly move back the body part to a new position where the pain diminishes, and hold for 30 to 90 seconds.
  7. Repeat the procedure until the original pain is gone, or the desired length of the muscle is obtained.

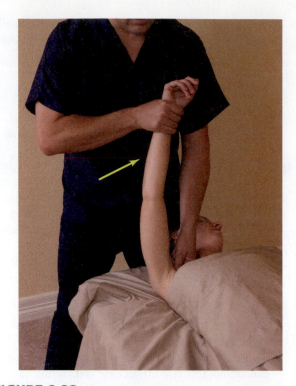

FIGURE 8.22

While Maintaining Pressure on the Tender Spot, the Limb Is Moved into a Position of Comfort.

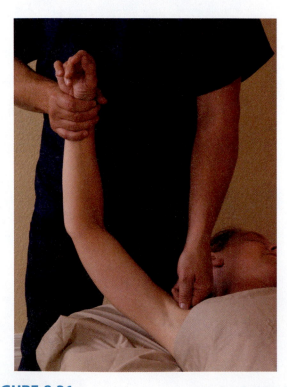

FIGURE 8.21

Possible Starting Position for Treating a Tender Spot in the Anterior Shoulder with the Positional Release Technique.

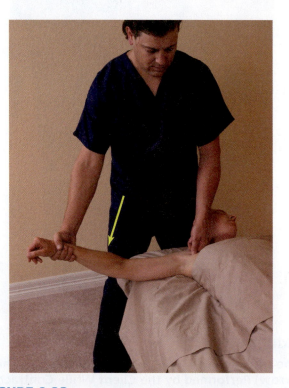

FIGURE 8.23

Pressure Is maintained as the Therapist Moves the Limb Gradually Back toward the Original Position, Which Had Been Uncomfortable.

- **Special considerations:**
  - ❍ Positional release is important because it helps to stimulate communication to the proprioceptors and allows the body to restore better balance.
  - ❍ Remember to hold the tender spot/trigger point through the entire procedure from step 1 through step 8. Keep pressure on the point while moving the limb and while holding it in place.
  - ❍ Use just enough pressure on the tender spot to illicit a slight tenderness at the spot. The pain is meant to be your guide, not the treating force.
  - ❍ It is important to remember that injury will affect the whole body, and thus positional release is a full-body process. For this reason, areas distant from the tender point must be considered during the positioning process. For example, when treating a tender point in the low back, you may need to consider the positioning of the client's legs, knees, and even the feet to arrive at a position where the pain is alleviated.

The Basic Neuromuscular Treatment Protocol

Even though the direct methods and indirect methods can be used independently of each other, they work best when combined into a five-stage treatment protocol. This ensures that the muscle is properly prepared and that all trigger points are located and treated. Once treated, the tissues are revitalized, which prepares them for the final goal of re-education.

STAGE 1. PREPARE THE TISSUES AND LOCATE THE TAUT BANDS

During this stage, techniques borrowed from Swedish massage, such as effleurage and petrissage, are used to warm up and loosen the tissues. Other relaxation techniques, such as jostling and compression, are also effective initial techniques. The goal is to warm up the muscle and connective tissue by stimulating circulation. This will prepare the tissues for the work to follow.

While warming up the tissues, it is important to assess the muscle looking for taut bands and knots.

STAGE 2. IDENTIFY THE TRIGGER POINTS

After locating the taut bands, it is important to narrow the focus and find the areas along the band that are the most tender. Often this is where there is a mass or knot in the muscle. These trigger points and tender spots are where the therapy will be focused. As discussed in Chapter 6, trigger points often give rise to referred pain. This phenomenon can be used to isolate the location of trigger points. Press the thumbs or fingertips along the taut band, looking for areas that cause a referred pain pattern. These will be the areas to focus on.

STAGE 3. TREAT THE TRIGGER POINTS

Use the direct method or methods indicated to treat the presenting trigger points. The number of trigger points treated in any single session depends on many factors. Healthier tissues and more robust clients may be able to handle more therapy. Generally speaking, keep communicating with the client. Continuously assess the client's responses and watch the tissues for responses, such as swelling and inflammation. This indicates the tissues are being overworked. Remember, sometimes less is more, and it is better to give the client space to heal than it is to push too fast or too far.

STAGE 4. REVITALIZE AND CLOSE THE TISSUES

This stage focuses on encouraging circulation to help heal the muscle. Swedish techniques, such as compression, petrissage, and *tapotement,* are used to invigorate and loosen the tissues. Then, effleurage strokes towards the heart are used to encourage movement of blood and lymph to the eliminatory organs, such as the kidneys.

STAGE 5. STRETCH THE TISSUES AND RE-EDUCATE THE NERVOUS SYSTEM

The objective of this stage is to restore flexibility and proper biomechanics through stretching.

Essentially, there are three ways to stretch a body: active, passive, and facilitated stretching. Each technique has its own benefits. In active stretching, clients are instructed how to perform the stretch. Then they perform the stretch on their own. This is good because clients can perform the stretch daily. The more often the stretch is performed, the better the results will be. During passive stretching, clients relax while the therapists move them through the stretches. This technique is effective because the muscles can be stretched further when they are relaxed. Both types of stretching are very effective for increasing length in the muscle. However, the indirect techniques of facilitated stretching are some of the most powerful ways to relax muscle and increase length. During the therapy session, use facilitated stretching to teach the muscle new resting lengths, effectively teaching it a new resting position.

GENERAL CAUTIONS FOR NEUROMUSCULAR THERAPY

In general, use common sense when performing neuromuscular techniques. There are no specific contraindications for trigger point pressure release and stripping strokes except those that are true for all forms of massage. These may include:

- Rashes
- Open wounds
- Recent injuries
- Infections

Always listen to your client and your client's body, and then adjust your pressure, number of repetitions, and other aspects of your treatment accordingly. This will ensure that you are always working in a therapeutic manner. Overall, in the application of facilitated stretching, when in doubt, take it *slower* and *easier* and move the client's body in *smaller* increments.

Contraindications for Facilitated Stretching

- **Pain**—These techniques should not be painful! They are designed to treat painful conditions by gently encouraging an increase in ROM. Furthermore, pain almost always induces a muscle contraction. It will be difficult to manipulate the neurology of the muscle if you are causing pain. Whenever there is pain during the technique, *stop immediately* and reassess the situation.

- **Hypermobility**—This is the state of extremely flexibility in the joint. Some clients already stretch to the end of the full range of motion (i.e., the physiologic barrier). These techniques are meant to extend the range of motion from the *pathologic* barrier to the *physiologic* barrier. It is never a good idea to take the body past this point. In addition, the muscle contractions used in some forms of FS, such as PIR, may in fact damage the joint if used at this extreme end range.

- **Inflammation**—When inflammation is present, continuous pain signals will be sent from the area being stretched. The pain signals cause the muscle to contract, thereby canceling out the stretch. Inflammation may also be an indication of injury, which could be further exacerbated by the stretch. Stripping strokes can increase the severity of inflammation because the technique often creates irritation as part of the healing process.

- **Acute injury (especially sprains and strains)**—Sprain is damage to the joint and its ligaments, often with lesions (tears) in those structures. Strain is damage to the muscle and its connective tissue, often including lesions. Stretching techniques, including FS, should not be used in acute injuries. They will often exacerbate the injury and may increase the size of the tears in the tissues.

- **Joint instability**—Facilitated stretching can place minor shearing forces on the joints because some techniques use contractions during the stretch. If a joint is unstable due to injury or disease, using FS may cause further damage.

QUICK QUIZ #16

1. Because postisometric relaxation (PIR) uses an isometric contraction, you should resist the client's contraction to ensure that there is no movement at the joint.
   a. True
   b. False

2. During reciprocal inhibition (RI), you should provide resistance but not stop movement at the joint as the client contracts the antagonist of the target muscle.
   a. True
   b. False

3. When applying the positional release technique: (Circle all that apply)
   a. move the limb just beyond the physiologic barrier so that the proprioceptors can reset.
   b. you will use trigger point pressure release on tender points to release tension.

   c. press on a tender point and then slowly reposition the client's body until the pain subsides.
   d. you will re-educate the muscle and facilitate an increased ROM.
   e. All of the above
   f. None of the above

4. Facilitated stretching techniques should never be used if any of these conditions exist: (Circle all that apply)
   a. Muscle spasm or cramp
   b. Inflammation
   c. Acute muscle sprains
   d. Joint instability
   e. All of the above
   f. None of the above

SUMMARY

There are a number of signs and symptoms a therapist can use to detect the presence of trigger points, including restricted movement and referred pain. There are also a variety of neuromuscular techniques designed to manipulate the neurology of the muscle in order to reduce pain and pathology or to lengthen a muscle. NMT combines techniques such as trigger point pressure release and facilitated stretching to release trigger points, lengthen muscles, and re-educate the nervous system. The trigger point pressure release method is used to treat trigger points directly. The trigger point may also be treated directly with either the intermittent pressure release method or by using deep stripping strokes.

Facilitated stretching techniques are used to treat TrPs indirectly as well as to re-educate muscles to a healthier resting length. It is important to understand the differences between isometric and isotonic contractions to effectively use FS techniques. Anatomic, physiologic, or pathologic barriers may limit joint movement, and it is also important to understand the difference between these.

Recognizing different types of joint end feel will help in assessing barriers to joint movement and how to work with range of motion. The main goal of FS is to improve ease of movement. While an increased ROM is desirable, and is often achieved, it is not the main goal. It is important to move slowly and easily at all times. Facilitated stretching should never be painful.

The basic NMT protocol follows a five-stage format. Stage one serves to warm up and investigate the tissues. Stage two helps locate and focus on the trigger points. Stage three is the treatment phase. Trigger points are treated with trigger point pressure release or facilitated stretching techniques. Stage four revitalizes the tissues. Stage five is designed to re-educate the muscles to new resting lengths. Re-educating muscles may include passive, active, and/or facilitated stretching.

Finally, there are some general cautions to keep in mind when performing facilitated stretching. In general it is best to move slowly, and adjust the client's body in small increments.

DISCUSSION QUESTIONS

1. Explain the physiology behind trigger point pressure release.
2. Explain the difference between the three variations of trigger point pressure release.
3. Explain the difference between isometric and isotonic contractions.
4. Describe the barriers to joint movement.
5. Explain the role that Golgi tendon organs play in the PIR technique.
6. Explain the roles that the target muscle and its opposing muscle play in the RI technique.

9 Sample Protocols for Neuromuscular Therapy

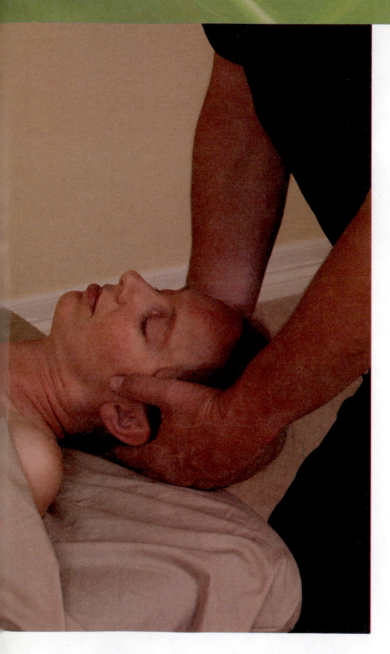

 CHAPTER HIGHLIGHTS

Chapter Objectives

Key Terms

Application of the Techniques

Sample Protocols

Summary

Discussion Questions

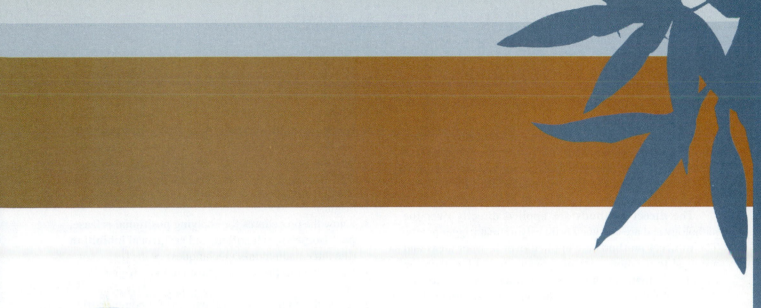

 CHAPTER OBJECTIVES

- Understand how to combine the techniques of neuromuscular therapy

- Explore sample neuromuscular therapy protocols for various body parts

- Rehearse assessment skills and practice neuromuscular techniques

 KEY TERMS

APPLICATION OF THE TECHNIQUES

The cornerstone of neuromuscular therapy is that the techniques are designed to treat myoskeletal pathology by manipulating the nerves and **neural structures.** When combined, the techniques of NMT will successfully relax hypertonic tissues, release trigger points, and then facilitate lengthening and relaxation by re-educating the muscles and nervous system.

The **direct methods** are applied directly over the pathology and are designed primarily to treat trigger points. The **indirect methods** are applied over broader areas and are used to promote ease of movement and lengthen the muscles. Remember that it is very important to warm up the tissues before applying neuromuscular techniques.

Here are a few key concepts to consider when formulating your NMT protocol.

1. Know all the muscles in the area that will be treated.
2. Know the origins, insertions, and actions of each muscle. Pay particular attention to the direction in which each muscle contracts and stretches. (When a muscle contracts the insertion moves towards the origin. When it stretches the insertion moves away from the origin.)
3. Know the procedures for applying **positional release, post-isometric relaxation,** and **reciprocal inhibition** (the three main indirect techniques)
4. Know the locations of the most common trigger points.
5. Know the common referral patterns for common trigger points.

A suitable protocol will be easy to prepare if you match your understanding of the muscles and pathologies being treated with the relative benefits of the various techniques. As discussed in Chapter 8, certain NMT techniques are better suited for each particular stage of treatment. Use Table 9.1 ■ as a guide to the appropriate techniques for each stage.

As discussed in Chapter 8, some techniques are better suited for certain areas and types of pathology. Table 9.2 ■ provides a quick reference to the common uses for each of the direct and indirect neuromuscular techniques.

 DID YOU KNOW

Before Every Massage

Remember to obtain a proper client history and perform a thorough assessment. This is important in order to develop a good plan and to rule out any techniques that may be contraindicated.

TABLE 9.1	Guide to Techniques for the Various Stages of NMT		
Warm-Up Phase	Treat the Trigger Points	Revitalize and Close	Stretch and Re-educate the Muscles
Swedish Massage Techniques	Direct Methods	Swedish Massage Techniques	Indirect Methods
Rocking, effleurage, light petrissage, light compression	Progressive pressure, barrier release, intermittent pressure, stripping strokes	Rocking, effleurage, light petrissage, light compression	Facilitated stretches—PIR, RI; positional release

TABLE 9.2	Guide to Common Uses of Neuromuscular Techniques	
	Description	Common Uses
Direct Methods		
Progressive pressure	Provides a moderate pressure without easing up.	Treats TrPs: This is best for robust muscles and deep-seated trigger points.
Barrier release	Same as progressive.	Same as progressive.
Intermittent pressure	Provides a moderate pressure, but eases up after a short time.	Treats TrPs: This is best for less robust muscles or when there is more pain involved in the trigger points.
Stripping strokes	Provides a grinding pressure to the trigger point.	Treats TrPs: This is for the most robust muscles or the most myogelotic (hardened) trigger points.

TABLE 9.2	*(Continued)*	
	Description	Common Uses
Indirect Methods		
Post-isometric relaxation (PIR)	A stretch is applied after of period of isometric contraction of the target muscle.	This is good for all muscular tension except muscles in spasm. It is best for chronic muscle tension.
Reciprocal inhibition (RI)	An isotonic contraction is applied to the opposing muscle to facilitate relaxation of the target muscle.	This is good for all muscular tension. It is best for acute tension, especially for muscles in spasm.
Positional release	Pressure is applied to a tender area or trigger point. Then the limb containing the target muscles is moved to a position of comfort.	Good for all focused areas of tenderness. Especially good for very sensitive pathology.

SAMPLE PROTOCOLS

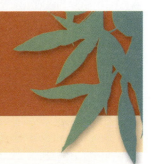

The Muscles of the Posterior Neck

☑ Review the muscles of the posterior neck (see Figure 9.1 ■).

• These muscles are responsible for moving the head and scapula.

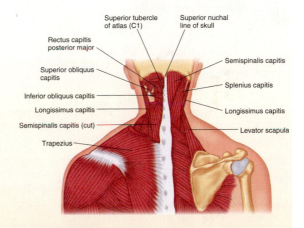

FIGURE 9.1

The Major Muscles of the Posterior Neck

WARM-UP AND ASSESS THE TISSUES

Using a selection of appropriate warm-up techniques, begin to warm and encourage circulation to the posterior neck. Make sure to work the entire area, including the upper back and shoulder. This is because the neck muscles extend well into these areas.

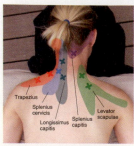

Trapezius
Splenius cervicis
Longissimus capitis
Splenius capitis
Levator scapulae

FIGURE 9.2

The Common Trigger Points and Referral Areas in the Posterior Neck

IDENTIFY THE TRIGGER POINTS

☑ Table 9.3 ■ lists the common locations of trigger points in the muscles of the posterior neck. In my experience, there are certain areas that are most likely to contain trigger points. Figure 9.2 ■ shows the locations of these areas and their referral zones. Palpate these areas and note any active trigger points. You may also find trigger points in any of the secondary referral zones. The client may present with trigger points that are not included here. It is important to address those as well.

TABLE 9.3	Common Trigger Points and Referral Zones of the Posterior Neck		
Muscle Group	Name of Muscle	Common Trigger Points	Common Secondary Referral Zones
Attaching to vertebra, scapula, and clavicle	*Trapezius*	Two in belly of muscle on top of shoulder near nape of neck Two at inferior angle of scapula One lateral to T1	Lateral head around the ear The temples
Cervical vertebrae	*Splenius capitus*	One or two in attachment, at base of skull	Top of head
	Splenius cervicis	One close to base of skull One in belly close to superior edge of scapula	Top of shoulders Behind eyes
Erector spinae	*Iliocostalis cervicis*	Two to three in belly and/or close to origins and insertions	Local over the muscle
	Longissimus capitis	Two to three in belly and/or close to origins and insertions	Local over the muscle
	Longissimus cervicis	Two to three in belly and/or close to origins and insertions	Local over the muscle
	Spinalis capitis	Two to three in belly and/or close to origins and insertions	Local over the muscle
	Spinalis cervicis	Two to three in belly and/or close to origins and insertions	Local over the muscle
Transversospinalis	*Semispinalis capitis*	One close to attachment at base of skull One at base of neck	Band around head at level of temples Back of head
	Semispinalis capitis	One or two in belly of muscle close to superior angle of scapula	Top of the shoulder
Suboccipital neck muscles	*Rectus capitis posterior major*	One or two in belly of muscle	Lateral head around the ear
	Rectus capitis posterior minor	One or two in belly of muscle	Local over the muscle
	Obliquus capitis inferior	One or two in belly of muscle	Local over the muscle
	Obliquus capitis superior	One or two in belly of muscle	Local over the muscle
Vertebral muscles	*Multifidis*	One or two in belly of muscle	Local over the muscle
	Rotatores	One or two in belly of muscle	Local over the muscle
	Interspinalis	Variable	Local over the muscle
Intertranversarii	*Intertransversarii posteriores*	Variable	Local over the muscle

TREAT THE TRIGGER POINTS

☑ Select the direct method(s) (Table 9.2) best suited to treat the trigger points discovered during assessment. Treat as many trigger points as is practical during your session.

REVITALIZE AND CLOSE

Use a selection of appropriate closing techniques to encourage circulation to the posterior neck. Also include some strokes to the shoulders and upper back to integrate those areas with the neck. Then finish with effleurage strokes towards the core to encourage movement of blood and lymph through the area.

STRETCH AND RE-EDUCATE

Consider your treatment plan and the client's needs to select one or more of the following indirect methods (also see Table 9.2).

☑ **Positional release**—The positioning will be unique for each client and each session. Generally the position of comfort will be found when the target muscle is shortened (in this case when the neck is moved into extension).

☑ **Post-isometric relaxation**—Place the neck into flexion to stretch the posterior muscles. Have the client resist your pressure, and continue with PIR protocol (Chapter 8). Figure 9.3 ■ shows the hand positions for the direction of pressure and stretch for applying post-isometric relaxation to the posterior neck.

☑ **Reciprocal inhibition**—Have the client actively move his or her neck into flexion while you slowly resist the movement. Continue with RI protocol (Chapter 8) until a full stretch is reached. Figure 9.4 ■ shows the hand positions as well as the direction of movement and resistance for applying reciprocal inhibition to the posterior neck.

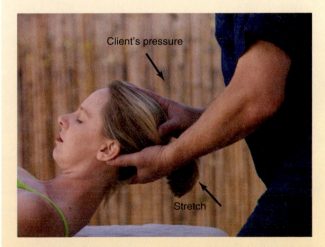

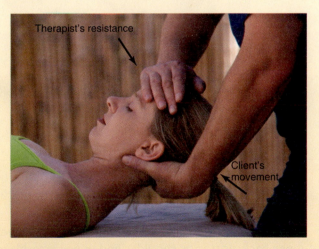

FIGURE 9.3

The Best Position for Applying PIR to the Posterior Neck. One Arrow Indicates the Direction the Therapist Uses to Passively Stretch the Muscles to the Comfort Barrier. Another Arrow Shows the Direction of Pressure Used by the Client to Resist the Stretch at the Comfort Barrier.

FIGURE 9.4

The Best Position for Applying RI to the Posterior Neck. One Arrow Indicates the Direction in Which the Client Is Moving to Stretch the Target Muscles. Another Arrow Shows the Direction of Pressure Used as the Therapist Resists the Client's Movement.

The Upper Back, Posterior Shoulder, and Upper Arm

☑ Review the muscles of the upper back, posterior shoulder, and upper arm (see Figure 9.5 ▪).

• These muscles are responsible for moving the scapula and upper arm.

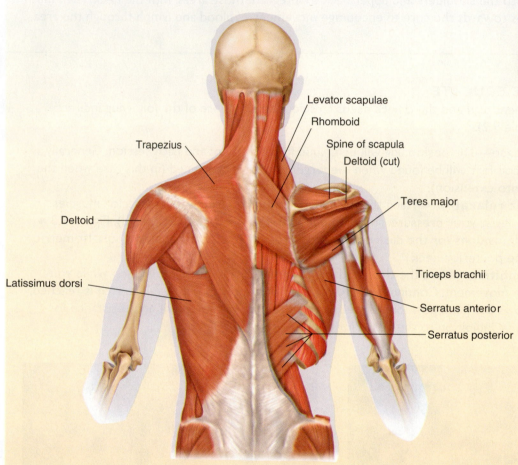

FIGURE 9.5

The Major Muscles of the Upper Back, Posterior Shoulder, and Upper Arm

Levator scapulae

Rhomboid

Spine of scapula

Deltoid (cut)

Trapezius

Teres major

Deltoid

Triceps brachii

Latissimus dorsi

Serratus anterior

Serratus posterior

WARM-UP AND ASSESS THE TISSUES

Using a selection of appropriate warm-up techniques, begin to warm and encourage circulation to the upper back, posterior shoulder, and upper arm. Make sure to work the entire area, including the neck and middle back. This is because these muscles extend well into those areas.

IDENTIFY THE TRIGGER POINTS

☑ Table 9.4 ■ lists the common locations of trigger points in the muscles of the upper back, posterior shoulder, and upper arm. In my experience, there are certain areas that are most likely to contain trigger points. Figure 9.6 ■ shows the locations of these areas and their referral zones. Palpate these areas and note any active trigger points. You may also find trigger points in any of the secondary referral zones. The client may present with trigger points that are not included here. It is important to address those as well.

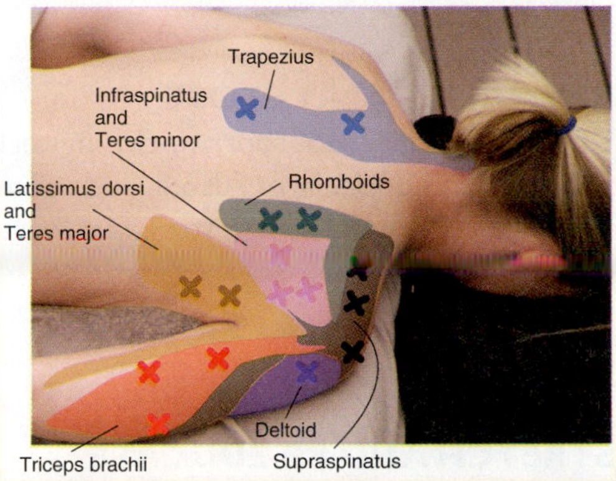

FIGURE 9.6

The Common Trigger Points and Referral Areas in the Upper Back, Posterior Shoulder, and Upper Arm

TABLE 9.4	Common Trigger Points and Referral Zones of the Upper Back, Posterior Shoulder, and Upper Arm		
Muscle Group	**Name of Muscle**	**Common Trigger Points**	**Common Secondary Referral Zones**
Attaching to trunk and arm	*Trapezius*	Two located in belly of muscle on top of the shoulder near the nape of the neck	Lateral head around ear and at the temples
		Two located at the inferior angle of the scapula	
		One located lateral to T1	
	Latissimus dorsi	Two located in belly of muscle along the lateral edge of muscle	Local over the muscle
Attaching to scapula and arm	*Deltoid*	Three to four located in belly of muscles	Local over the muscle
	Teres minor (shoulder rotator)	One located in belly of muscle close to axilla	Local over the muscle
	Teres major	Two located in belly of muscle	Local over the muscle
Attaching to scapula and trunk	*Levator scapulae*	Two located close to insertion at anterior superior angle of scapula	Local over the muscle
	Rhomboid major	Two or three located close to insertions along medial border of scapula	Local over the muscle
	Rhomboid minor	One or two located close to insertions along medial border of scapula	Local over the muscle
	Serratus anterior	One or two located close to origins below center of axilla	Medial lower border of scapula, lateral rib cage
Upper arm	*Triceps brachii*	One located in belly of muscle	Medal elbow and proximal forearm
		Two to three located at the elbow insertions of all three heads	
	Anconeus	One located in the belly of muscle over olecranon process	Lateral elbow
Rotators of the shoulder	*Supraspinatus*	One located close to origin	Lateral superior elbow
		One located close to acromioclavicular joint	
	Infraspinatus	Three located in the bellies of all three sections of muscle	Anterior shoulder and upper arm
	Subscapularis	Three or four located along inferior border and belly of the muscle	Posterior wrist

TREAT THE TRIGGER POINTS

☑ Select the direct method(s) best suited to treat the trigger points discovered during assessment (Table 9.2). Treat as many trigger points as is practical during your session.

REVITALIZE AND CLOSE

Use a selection of appropriate closing techniques to encourage circulation to the upper back, posterior shoulder, and upper arm. Also include some strokes to the middle back to integrate it with the shoulder. Then finish with effleurage strokes towards the core to encourage movement of blood and lymph through the area.

STRETCH AND RE-EDUCATE

Consider your treatment plan and the client's needs to select one or more of the following indirect methods (also see Table 9.2).

☑ **Positional release**—The positioning used will be unique for each client and each session. Generally the position of comfort will be found when the target muscle is shortened (in this case when the arm is moved into extension or the scapula is retracted).

☑ **Post-isometric relaxation**—Place the shoulder into flexion and slight adduction to stretch the posterior shoulder muscles. Have the client resist your pressure, and continue with PIR protocol (Chapter 8). Figure 9.7 ■ shows the hand positions for the direction of pressure and stretch for applying post-isometric relaxation to the upper back and shoulder.

☑ **Reciprocal inhibition**—Have the client actively move her or his shoulder into flexion and slight adduction while you slowly resist the movement. Continue with RI protocol (Chapter 8) until a full stretch is reached. Figure 9.8 ■ shows the hand positions as well as the direction of movement and resistance for applying reciprocal inhibition to the upper back and shoulder.

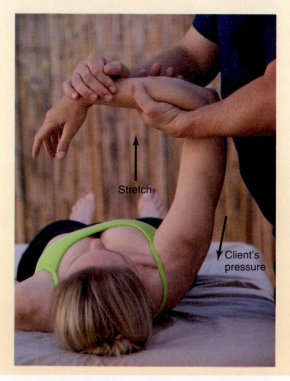

Stretch

Client's pressure

FIGURE 9.7

The Best Position for Applying PIR to the Upper Back, Posterior Shoulder, and Upper Arm. One Arrow Indicates the Direction the Therapist Uses to Passively Stretch the Muscles to the Comfort Barrier. Another Arrow Shows the Direction of Pressure Used by the Client to Resist the Stretch at the Comfort Barrier.

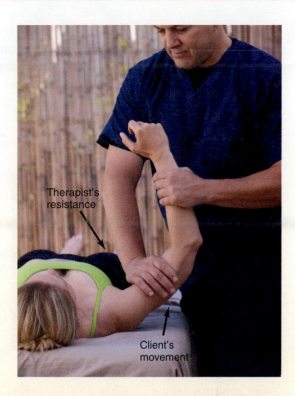

Therapist's resistance

Client's movement

FIGURE 9.8

The Best Position for Applying RI to the Upper Back, Posterior Shoulder, and Upper Arm. One Arrow Indicates the Direction in Which the Client Is Moving to Stretch the Target Muscles. Another Arrow Shows the Direction of Pressure Used as the Therapist Resists the Client's Movement.

The Posterior Forearm and Hand

☑ Review the muscles of the posterior forearm and hand (see Figure 9.9 ▪).

- These muscles are responsible for moving the wrist, hand, and fingers.

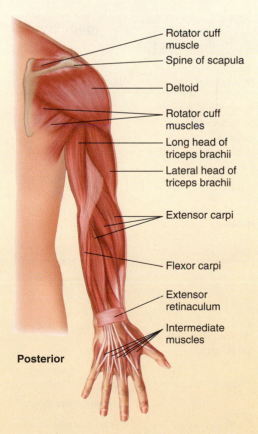

Rotator cuff muscle

Spine of scapula

Deltoid

Rotator cuff muscles

Long head of triceps brachii

Lateral head of triceps brachii

Extensor carpi

Flexor carpi

Extensor retinaculum

Intermediate muscles

Posterior

FIGURE 9.9

The Major Muscles of the Posterior Forearm and Hand

WARM-UP AND ASSESS THE TISSUES

Using a selection of appropriate warm-up techniques, begin to warm and encourage circulation to the posterior forearm and hand. Make sure to work the entire area, including the upper arm. This is because the forearm muscles extend well into this area.

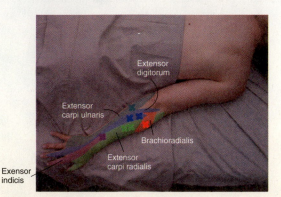

FIGURE 9.10

The Common Trigger Points and Referral Areas in the Posterior Forearm and Hand

IDENTIFY THE TRIGGER POINTS

☑ Table 9.5 ■ lists the common locations of trigger points in the muscles of the posterior forearm and hand. In my experience, there are certain areas that are most likely to contain trigger points.

Figure 9.10 ■ shows the locations of these areas and their referral zones. Palpate these areas and note any active trigger points. You may also find trigger points in any of the secondary referral zones. The client may present with trigger points that are not included here. It is important to address those as well.

TABLE 9.5	Common Trigger Points and Referral Zones of the Posterior and Lateral Forearm and Hand		
Muscle Group	Name of Muscle	Common Trigger Points	Common Secondary Referral Zones
Muscles of forearm	*Brachioradialis*	One to two located in belly of the muscle	Base of the thumb
	Supinator	One located in belly of the muscle	Base of the thumb
	Anconeus	One located in belly of the muscle	Local over the muscle
Muscles that move the wrist	*Extensor carpi radialis longus*	One to two located in belly of the muscle just distel to the elbow	Base of the thumb
	Extensor carpi radialis brevis	One to two located in belly of the muscle	Back of the hand
	Extensor carpi ulnaris	One to two located in belly of the muscle	Medial hand and wrist
Muscles that move the fingers	*Abductor pollicis longus*	One located in belly of the muscle	Anterior thumb and thenar
	Extensor pollicis brevis	One located in belly of the muscle	Posterior thumb and thenar
	Extensor pollicis longus	One located in belly of the muscle	Posterior thumb and thenar
	Extensor indicis	One located in belly of the muscle	Posterior aspect of index finger
	Extensor digitorum communis	One to two located in belly of the muscle just distal to the elbow	Posterior aspect of middle two fingers
	Extensor digiti minimi	One to two in belly of the muscle	Posterior little finger
Hand	*Dorsal interossei*	One located in belly of the each of the hands, between each finger	Local over the muscle

TREAT THE TRIGGER POINTS

☑ Select the direct method(s) best suited to treat the trigger points discovered during assessment (Table 9.2). Treat as many trigger points as is practical during your session.

REVITALIZE AND CLOSE

Use a selection of appropriate closing techniques to encourage circulation to the posterior forearm and hand. Also include some strokes to the upper arm to integrate those areas with the forearm. Then finish with effleurage strokes towards the core to encourage movement of blood and lymph through the area.

STRETCH AND RE-EDUCATE

Consider your treatment plan and the client's needs to select one or more of the following indirect methods (also see Table 9.2).

☑ **Positional release**—The positioning used will be unique for each client and each session. Generally the position of comfort will be found when the target muscle is shortened (in this case when the wrist and fingers are moved into extension).

☑ **Post-isometric relaxation**—Place the wrist into flexion to stretch the posterior hand and forearm muscles. Have the client resist your pressure, and continue with PIR protocol (Chapter 8). Figure 9.11 ■ shows the hand positions for the direction of pressure and stretch for applying post-isometric relaxation to the posterior forearm and hand.

☑ **Reciprocal inhibition**—Have the client actively move his or her wrist into flexion while you slowly resist the movement. Continue with RI protocol (Chapter 8) until a full stretch is reached. Figure 9.12 ■ shows the hand positions as well as the direction of movement and resistance for applying reciprocal inhibition to the posterior forearm and hand.

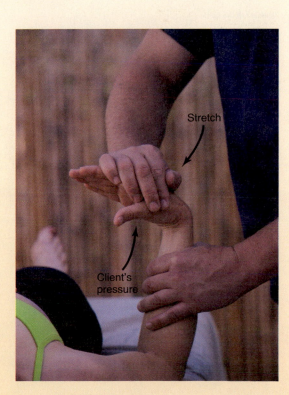

Stretch

Client's pressure

FIGURE 9.11

The Best Position for Applying PIR to the Posterior Forearm and Hand. One Arrow Indicates the Direction the Therapist Uses to Passively Stretch the Muscles to the Comfort Barrier. Another Arrow Shows the Direction of Pressure Used by the Client to Resist the Stretch at the Comfort Barrier.

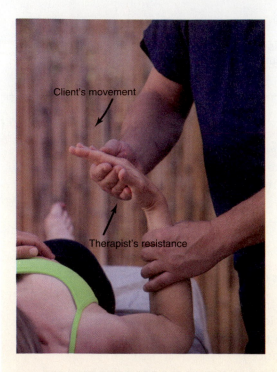

Client's movement

Therapist's resistance

FIGURE 9.12

The Best Position for Applying RI to the Posterior Forearm and Hand. One Arrow Indicates the Direction in Which the Client Is Moving to Stretch the Target Muscles. Another Arrow Shows the Direction of Pressure Used as the Therapist Resists the Client's Movement.

The Posterior Torso (Back and Sacrum)

☑ Review the muscles of the posterior torso (see Figure 9.13 ■).

   • These muscles are responsible for moving the vertebral column and the rib cage.

Muscles of the back

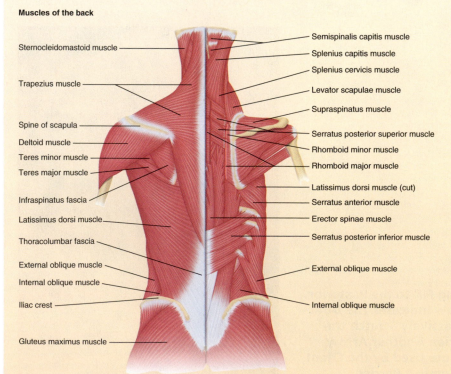

Sternocleidomastoid muscle

Trapezius muscle

Spine of scapula

Deltoid muscle

Teres minor muscle

Teres major muscle

Infraspinatus fascia

Latissimus dorsi muscle

Thoracolumbar fascia

External oblique muscle

Internal oblique muscle

Iliac crest

Gluteus maximus muscle

Semispinalis capitis muscle

Splenius capitis muscle

Splenius cervicis muscle

Levator scapulae muscle

Supraspinatus muscle

Serratus posterior superior muscle

Rhomboid minor muscle

Rhomboid major muscle

Latissimus dorsi muscle (cut)

Serratus anterior muscle

Erector spinae muscle

Serratus posterior inferior muscle

External oblique muscle

Internal oblique muscle

FIGURE 9.13

The Major Muscles of the Posterior Torso (Back and Sacrum)

ʾ

WARM-UP AND ASSESS THE TISSUES

Using a selection of appropriate warm-up techniques, begin to warm and encourage circulation to the posterior torso (back). Make sure to work the entire area, including the neck and hips. This is because the back muscles extend well into these areas.

IDENTIFY THE TRIGGER POINTS

☑ Table 9.6 ■ lists the common locations of trigger points in the muscles of the posterior torso. In my experience, there are certain areas that are most likely to contain trigger points. Figure 9.14 ■ shows the locations of these areas and their referral zones. Palpate these areas and note any active trigger points. You may also find trigger points in any of the secondary referral zones. The client may present with trigger points that are not included here. It is important to address those as well.

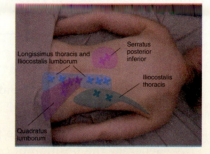

FIGURE 9.14

The Common Trigger Points and Referral Areas in the Posterior Torso (Back and Sacrum)

TABLE 9.6	Common Trigger Points and Referral Zones of the Posterior Torso (Back and Sacrum)		
Muscle Group	Name of Muscle	Common Trigger Points	Common Secondary Referral Zones
Attaching to trunk and arm	Trapezius	Two located in belly of muscle on top of the shoulder near the nape of the neck	Lateral head around ear and at the temples
		Two located at the inferior angle of the scapula	
		One located lateral to T1	
	Latissimus dorsi	Two located in belly of muscle along the lateral edge of muscle	Local over the muscle
Erector spinae	Iliocostalis thoracis	Four to six located in belly of each muscle	Lateral shoulder, side and lower buttocks
	Iliocostalis lumborum	Four to six located in belly of each muscle	Lateral shoulder, side and lower buttocks
	Longissimus thoracis	Four to six located in belly of each muscle	Lateral shoulder, side and lower buttocks
	Spinalis thoracis	Variable	Local over the muscle
Transverso-spinalis	Semispinalis thoracis	Three to four located in belly of each muscle	Local over the muscle
Muscles of inspiration	Serratus posterior inferior	One to two located in belly closer to ribs	Local over the muscle
	Serratus posterior superior	One to two located close to insertion and medial border of scapula	Lateral shoulder, elbow, and lateral wrist and hand
Vertebral muscles	Multifidis	One to two located in belly of each muscle	Local over the muscle
	Rotatores	One to two located in belly of each muscle	Local over the muscle
	Interspinalis	Variable	Local over the muscle
Intertransversarii	Intertransversarii posteriores	Variable	Local over the muscle
	Intertransversarii laterales	Variable	Local over the muscle
	Intertransversarii mediales	Variable	Local over the muscle
Prime mover	Quadratus lumborum	Two to four located in belly and at both attachments	Sacrum, lateral hip, and lower buttocks

TREAT THE TRIGGER POINTS

☑ Select the direct method(s) best suited to treat the trigger points discovered during assessment (Table 9.2). Treat as many trigger points as is practical during your session.

REVITALIZE AND CLOSE

Use a selection of appropriate closing techniques to encourage circulation to the posterior torso. Also include some strokes to the shoulders, neck, and hips to integrate those areas with the back. Then finish with effleurage strokes to encourage movement of blood and lymph through the area.

STRETCH AND RE-EDUCATE

Consider your treatment plan and the client's needs to select one or more of the following indirect methods (also see Table 9.2).

☑ **Positional release**—The positioning used will be unique for each client and each session. Generally the position of comfort will be when the target muscle is shortened (in this case when the back is moved into extension). When performing positional release on the torso it is often helpful or necessary to use bolsters or use a sitting or side-lying position.

☑ **Post-isometric relaxation**—Place the back into flexion to stretch the posterior back muscles. Have the client resist your pressure, and continue with PIR protocol (Chapter 8). Figure 9.15 ■ shows the hand positions for the direction of pressure and stretch for applying post-isometric relaxation to the back and sacrum.

☑ **Reciprocal inhibition**—Have the client actively move her or his torso into flexion while you slowly resist the movement. Continue with RI protocol (Chapter 8) until a full stretch is reached. Figure 9.16 ■ shows the hand positions as well as the direction of movement and resistance for applying reciprocal inhibition to the lower back and sacrum.

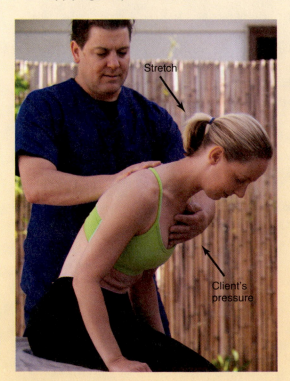

FIGURE 9.15

The Best Position for Applying PIR to the Posterior Torso (Back and Sacrum). One Arrow Indicates the Direction the Therapist Uses to Passively Stretch the Muscles to the Comfort Barrier. Another Arrow Shows the Direction of Pressure Used by the Client to Resist the Stretch at the Comfort Barrier.

FIGURE 9.16

The Best Position for Applying RI to the Posterior Torso (Back and Sacrum). One Arrow Indicates the Direction in Which the Client Is Moving to Stretch the Target Muscles. Another Arrow Shows the Direction of Pressure Used as the Therapist Resists the Client's Movement.

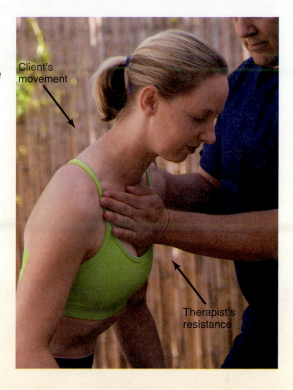

Client's movement

Therapist's resistance

The Posterior Hip and Thigh

☑ Review the muscles of the posterior hip and thigh (see Figure 9.17 ■).

- These muscles are responsible for moving the hip, knee and upper leg.

Muscles of the posterior left hip and thigh

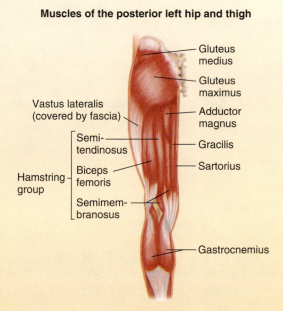

Gluteus medius

Gluteus maximus

Vastus lateralis (covered by fascia)

Adductor magnus

Semi-tendinosus

Gracilis

Hamstring group

Biceps femoris

Sartorius

Semimem-branosus

Gastrocnemius

FIGURE 9.17

The Major Muscles of the Posterior Hip and Thigh

WARM-UP AND ASSESS THE TISSUES

Using a selection of appropriate warm-up techniques, begin to warm and encourage circulation to the posterior hip and thigh. Make sure to work the entire area, including the lower back and lower leg. This is because these muscles extend well into those areas.

IDENTIFY THE TRIGGER POINTS

☑ Table 9.7 ■ lists the common locations of trigger points in the muscles of the posterior hip and thigh. In my experience, there are certain areas that are most likely to contain trigger points. Figure 9.18 ■ shows the locations of these areas and their referral zones. Palpate these areas and note any active trigger points. You may also find trigger points in any of the secondary referral zones. The client may present with trigger points that are not included here. It is important to address those as well.

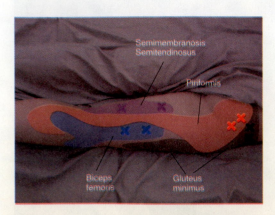

FIGURE 9.18

The Common Trigger Points and Referral Areas in the Posterior Hip and Thigh

TABLE 9.7	Common Trigger Points and Referral Zones of the Posterior Hip and Thigh		
Muscle Group	**Name of Muscle**	**Common Trigger Points**	**Common Secondary Referral Zones**
Gluteal muscles	*Gluteus maximus*	Three to four located in belly of muscle and along the sacral border	Sacrum and lower buttocks
	Gluteus medius	One located in belly of muscle Two located close to the iliac ridge	Sacrum
	Gluteus minimus	One located close to sacrum One located close to attachment at the trochanter	Lateral and posterior leg from thigh to foot
Posterior thigh muscles	*Biceps femoris*	One to two located in belly of muscle	Posterior knee
	Semitendinosis	Three to four located in belly of muscle	Lower buttocks
	Semimembranosis	Three to four located in belly of muscle	Lower buttocks
Lateral rotators	*Piriformis*	One located in belly of muscle One close to attachment at the sacrum	The posterior leg and foot
	Obturator internus	Variable	Hip
	Gemellus superior	Variable	Hip
	Gemellus inferior	Variable	Hip
	Obturator externus	Variable	Hip
	Quadratus femoris	Variable	Hip

TREAT THE TRIGGER POINTS

☑ Select the direct method(s) best suited to treat the trigger points discovered during assessment (Table 9.2). Treat as many trigger points as is practical during your session.

REVITALIZE AND CLOSE

Use a selection of appropriate closing techniques to encourage circulation to the posterior hip and thigh. Also include some strokes to the lower back to integrate those areas with the hip and thigh. Then finish with effleurage strokes towards the core to encourage movement of blood and lymph through the area.

STRETCH AND RE-EDUCATE

Consider your treatment plan and the client's needs to select one or more of the following indirect methods (also see Table 9.2).

☑ **Positional release**—The positioning used will be unique for each client and each session. Generally the position of comfort will be found when the target muscle is shortened (in this case when the hip is moved into extension and/or abduction or the thigh (knee) is moved into flexion).

☑ **Post-isometric relaxation**—Place the hip into flexion and the thigh into extension to stretch the posterior hip and thigh muscles. Have the client resist your pressure, and continue with PIR protocol (Chapter 8). Figure 9.19 ■ shows the hand positions for the direction of pressure and stretch for applying post-isometric relaxation to the hip and thigh.

☑ **Reciprocal inhibition**—Have the client actively move his or her hip into flexion with the thigh extended, while you slowly resist the movement. Continue with RI protocol (Chapter 8) until a full stretch is reached. Figure 9.20 ■ shows the hand positions as well as the direction of movement and resistance for applying reciprocal inhibition to the posterior hip and thigh.

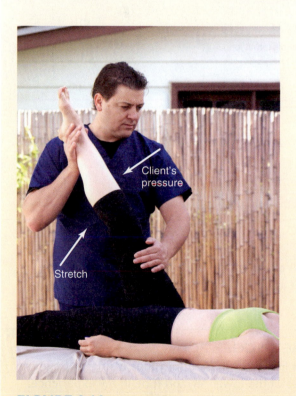

FIGURE 9.19

The Best Position for Applying PIR to the Posterior Hip and Thigh. One Arrow Indicates the Direction the Therapist Uses to Passively Stretch the Muscles to the Comfort Barrier. Another Arrow Shows the Direction of Pressure Used by the Client to Resist the Stretch at the Comfort Barrier.

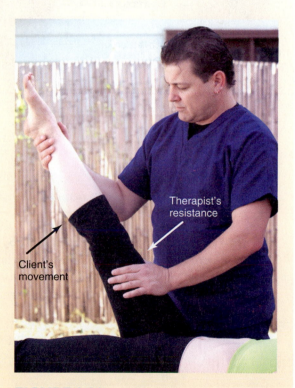

FIGURE 9.20

The Best Position for Applying RI to the Posterior Hip and Thigh. One Arrow Indicates the Direction in Which the Client Is Moving to Stretch the Target Muscles. Another Arrow Shows the Direction of Pressure Used as the Therapist Resists the Client's Movement.

The Posterior Lower Leg and Foot

☑ Review the muscles of the posterior lower leg and foot (see Figure 9.21 ■).

- These muscles are responsible for moving the ankle, foot, and toes.

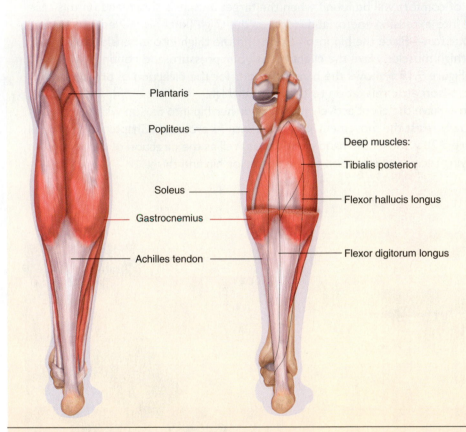

FIGURE 9.21

The Major Muscles of the Posterior Lower Leg and Foot

Plantaris

Popliteus

Soleus

Gastrocnemius

Achilles tendon

Deep muscles:

Tibialis posterior

Flexor hallucis longus

Flexor digitorum longus

WARM-UP AND ASSESS THE TISSUES

Using a selection of appropriate warm-up techniques, begin to warm and encourage circulation to the posterior lower leg and foot. Make sure to work the entire area, including the upper leg. This is because the lower leg muscles extend well into this area.

IDENTIFY THE TRIGGER POINTS

☑ Table 9.8 ■ lists the common locations of trigger points in the muscles of the lower leg and foot. In my experience, there are certain areas that are most likely to contain trigger points. Figure 9.22 ■ shows the locations of these areas and their referral zones. Palpate these areas and note any active trigger points. You may also find trigger points in any of the secondary referral zones. The client may present with trigger points that are not included here. It is important to address those as well.

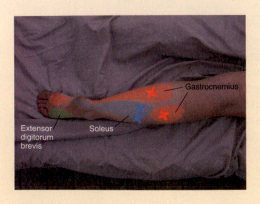

Gastrocnemius

Extensor digitorum brevis

Soleus

FIGURE 9.22

The Common Trigger Points and Referral Areas in the Posterior Lower Leg and Foot

TABLE 9.8	Common Trigger Points and Referral Zones of the Posterior Lower Leg and Foot		
Muscle Group	Name of Muscle	Common Trigger Points	Common Secondary Referral Zones
Lower leg	Gastrocnemius	One located in belly of the lateral head	Arch of foot
		One located close to the origin of both the medial and lateral heads	
	Soleus	Two located in belly of muscle on the lateral and/or medial side	Posterior ankle and bottom of heel
		One located close to origin	
		One located close to insertion	
	Plantaris	One located in belly of muscle	Local over the muscle
	Popliteus	One located in belly of muscle	Local over the muscle
	Tibialis posterior	One located in belly of muscle	Posterior ankle
Plantar surface of foot	Abductor hallucis	One to two located in belly of muscle	Medial ankle
	Abductor digiti minimi	One to two located in belly of muscle	Lateral ankle
	Quadratus plantae	One located in belly of muscle	Local over the muscle
	Lumbricales	Variable	Local over the muscle
	Flexor hallucis brevis	One to two located in belly of each head	Ball of foot at base of big toe
	Adductor hallucis	One to three located in belly of each of the three heads	Local over the muscle
	Flexor digiti minimi brevis	One located in belly of muscle	Lateral foot
	Dorsal interossei	Variable	Local over the muscle
	Plantar interossei	Variable	Local over the muscle
Lower leg and foot	Flexor hallucis longus	One located in belly of muscle	Bottom of the foot at the base of big toe
	Flexor digitorum longus	One located in belly of muscle	Ball of the foot
	Flexor digitorum brevis	One to two located in belly of muscle	Base of the toes

TREAT THE TRIGGER POINTS

☑ Select the direct method(s) best suited to treat the trigger points discovered during assessment (Table 9.2). Treat as many trigger points as is practical during your session.

REVITALIZE AND CLOSE

Use a selection of appropriate closing techniques to encourage circulation to the posterior lower leg and foot. Also include some strokes to the upper leg to integrate this area with the lower leg. Then finish with effleurage strokes towards the core to encourage movement of blood and lymph through the area.

STRETCH AND RE-EDUCATE

Consider your treatment plan and the client's needs to select one or more of the following indirect methods (also see Table 9.2).

- ☑ **Positional release**—The positioning used will be unique for each client and each session. Generally the position of comfort will be found when the target muscle is shortened (in this case when the foot is moved into plantar flexion).
- ☑ **Post-isometric relaxation**—Place the ankle into dorsiflexion to stretch the posterior lower leg muscles. Have the client resist your pressure, and continue with PIR protocol (Chapter 8). Figure 9.23 ■ shows the hand positions for the direction of pressure and stretch for applying post-isometric relaxation to the lower leg and foot.
- ☑ **Reciprocal inhibition**—Have the client actively move her or his foot into dorsiflexion while you slowly resist the movement. Continue with RI protocol (Chapter 8) until a full stretch is reached. Figure 9.24 ■ shows the hand positions as well as the direction of movement and resistance for applying reciprocal inhibition to the lower leg and foot.

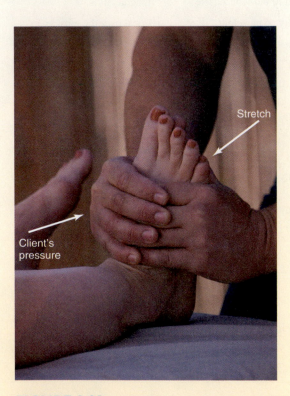

FIGURE 9.23

The Best Position for Applying PIR to the Posterior Lower Leg and Foot. One Arrow Indicates the Direction the Therapist Uses to Passively Stretch the Muscles to the Comfort Barrier. Another Arrow Shows the Direction of Pressure Used by the Client to Resist the Stretch at the Comfort Barrier.

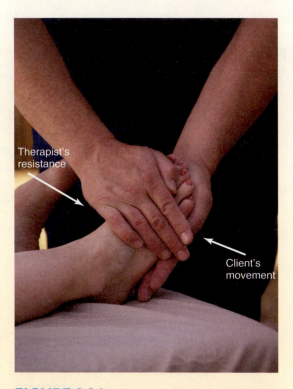

FIGURE 9.24

The Best Position for Applying RI to the Posterior Lower Leg and Foot. One Arrow Indicates the Direction in Which the Client Is Moving to Stretch the Target Muscles. Another Arrow Shows the Direction of Pressure Used as the Therapist Resists the Client's Movement.

QUICK QUIZ #17

1. It is best to use the indirect neuromuscular methods during the stretch and re-educate step of an NMT protocol.
   a. True
   b. False

2. Which of the following techniques are best suited for areas of sensitive pathology? (Circle all that apply)
   a. Progressive pressure
   b. Intermittent pressure
   c. Stripping strokes
   d. Positional release
   e. All of the above
   f. None of the above

3. The medial hand and wrist are the most common secondary referral zones for trigger points located in the: (Circle all that apply)
   a. brachioradialis.

   b. extensor carpi radialis longus.
   c. extensor carpi radialis brevis.
   d. extensor carpi ulnaris.
   e. All of the above
   f. None of the above

4. When applying PIR to the lower leg and foot, you should have the client resist your pressure as you place the ankle into dorsiflexion.
   a. True
   b. False

The Head and Face

☑ Review the muscles of the head and face (see Figure 9.25 ▪).

- These muscles are responsible for movement of the face and jaw.

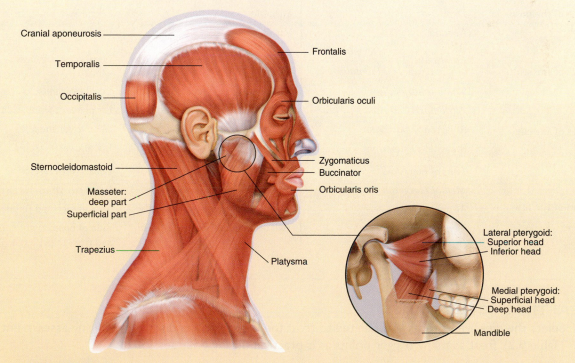

FIGURE 9.25

The Major Muscles of the Head and Face

WARM-UP AND ASSESS THE TISSUES

Using a selection of appropriate warm-up techniques, begin to warm and encourage circulation to the head and face. Make sure to work the entire area, including the anterior neck. This is because the face and head muscles have connections with this area.

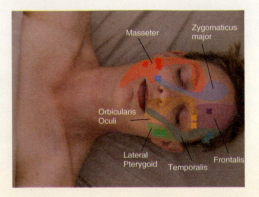

IDENTIFY THE TRIGGER POINTS

☑ Table 9.9 ■ lists the common locations of trigger points in the muscles of the head and face. In my experience, there are certain areas that are most likely to contain trigger points. Figure 9.26 ■ shows the locations of these areas and their referral zones. Palpate these areas and note any active trigger points. You may also find trigger points in any of the secondary referral zones. The client may present with trigger points that are not included here. It is important to address those as well.

FIGURE 9.26

The Common Trigger Points and Referral Areas in the Head and Face

TABLE 9.9	Common Trigger Points and Referral Zones of the Head and Face		
Muscle Group	Name of Muscle	Common Trigger Points	Common Secondary Referral Zones
Muscles of the eyelids	*Orbicularis oculi*	Two or three located in belly of the muscle	Over the bridge of the nose
	Levator palpebrae superioris	One or two in the muscle belly	Local over muscle
	Corrugator supercilii	Variable	Local over muscles
Muscles of the nose	*Procerus*	One or two in the muscle belly	Local over muscles
	Depressor septi	Variable	Local over muscles
	Nasalis	Variable	Local over muscles
Muscles of the scalp	*Epicranius* *Occipitalis* *Frontalis*	One or two in the muscle belly	Local over muscles
	Temporoparietalis	One or two in the muscle belly	Local over muscles
Muscles of the ear	*Auricularis anterior*	One or two in the muscle belly	Local over the muscles
	Auricularis posterior	Variable	Local over muscles
	Auricularis superior	Variable	Local over muscles
Muscles of the jaw	*Lateral pterygoid*	One or two in the muscle belly	Local over muscles
	Medial pterygoid	One or two in the muscle belly	Local over muscles
	Masseter	Two to three in the muscle belly	Side of face and forehead
	Temporalis	Two or three in the muscle belly	Side of head, zygomatic arch and front upper teeth

TREAT THE TRIGGER POINTS

☑ Select the direct method(s) best suited to treat the trigger points discovered during assessment (Table 9.2). Treat as many trigger points as is practical during your session.

REVITALIZE AND CLOSE

Use a selection of appropriate closing techniques to encourage circulation to the head and face. Also include some strokes to the neck to integrate the area with the head and face. Then finish with effleurage strokes towards the core to encourage movement of blood and lymph through the area.

STRETCH AND RE-EDUCATE

Consider your treatment plan and the client's needs to select one or more of the following indirect methods (also see Table 9.2).

☑ **Positional release**—The positioning used will be unique for each client and each session. Generally the position of comfort will be found when the target muscle is shortened (in this case when the jaw is closed).

☑ **Post-isometric relaxation**—Place the jaw into extension (open mouth) to stretch the jaw muscles. Have the client resist your pressure, and continue with PIR protocol (Chapter 8). Figure 9.27 ■ shows the hand positions for the direction of pressure and stretch for applying post-isometric relaxation to the jaw.

☑ **Reciprocal inhibition**—Have the client actively move his or her jaw into extension (open mouth) while you slowly resist the movement. Continue with RI protocol (Chapter 8) until a full stretch is reached. Figure 9.28 ■ shows the hand positions as well as the direction of movement and resistance for applying reciprocal inhibition to the jaw.

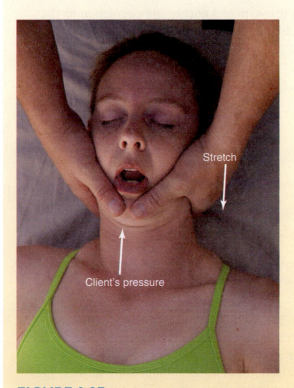

FIGURE 9.27

The Best Position for Applying PIR to the Jaw. One Arrow Indicates the Direction the Therapist Uses to Passively Stretch the Muscles to the Comfort Barrier. Another Arrow Shows the Direction of Pressure Used by the Client to Resist the Stretch at the Comfort Barrier.

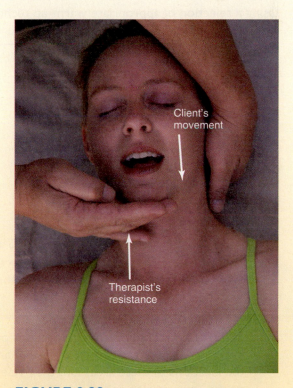

FIGURE 9.28

The Best Position for Applying RI to the Jaw. One Arrow Indicates the Direction in Which the Client Is Moving to Stretch the Target Muscles. Another Arrow Shows the Direction of Pressure Used as the Therapist Resists the Client's Movement.

The Anterior Neck

☑ Review the muscles of the anterior neck (see Figure 9.29 ■).

- These muscles are responsible for swallowing and moving the head.

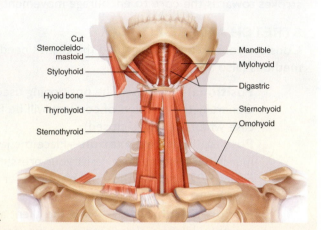

Cut Sternocleido-mastoid
Styloyhoid
Hyoid bone
Thyrohyoid
Sternothyroid
Mandible
Mylohyoid
Digastric
Sternohyoid
Omohyoid

FIGURE 9.29

The Major Muscles of the Anterior Neck

WARM-UP AND ASSESS THE TISSUES

Using a selection of appropriate warm-up techniques, begin to warm and encourage circulation to the anterior neck. Make sure to work the entire area, including the chest and shoulders. This is because the neck muscles extend well into this area.

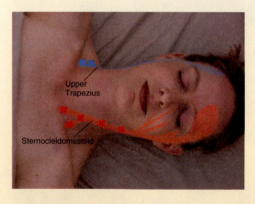

Upper Trapezius

Sternocleidomastoid

FIGURE 9.30

The Common Trigger Points and Referral Areas in the Anterior Neck

IDENTIFY THE TRIGGER POINTS

☑ Table 9.10 ■ lists the common locations of trigger points in the muscles of the anterior neck. In my experience, there are certain areas that are most likely to contain trigger points. Figure 9.30 ■ shows the locations of these areas and their referral zones. Palpate these areas and note any active trigger points. You may also find trigger points in any of the secondary referral zones. The client may present with trigger points that are not included here. It is important to address those as well.

TREAT THE TRIGGER POINTS

☑ Select the direct method(s) best suited to treat the trigger points discovered during assessment (Table 9.2). Treat as many trigger points as is practical during your session.

TABLE 9.10	Common Trigger Points and Referral Zones of the Anterior Neck		
Muscle Group	Name of Muscle	Common Trigger Points	Common Secondary Referral Zones
Superficial muscle	Platysma	Variable	Local over the muscle
Suprahyoid muscles	Digastricus	Variable	Local over the muscle
	Stylohyoid	Variable	Local over the muscle
	Mylohyoid	Variable	Local over the muscle
	Geniohyoid	Variable	Local over the muscle
Infrahyoid muscles	Sternohyoid	Variable	Local over the muscle
	Sternothyroid	Variable	Local over the muscle
	Thyrohyoid	Variable	Local over the muscle
	Omohyoid	Variable	Local over the muscle
Prime mover	Sternocleidomastoid	One to two located in belly of muscle	Lateral head around ear
Vertebral muscles	Longus colli	One to two located in belly of muscle	Local over the muscle
	Longus capitis	Variable	Local over the muscle
	Rectus capitus anterior	Variable	Local over the muscle
	Rectus capitus lateralis	Variable	Local over the muscle
	Intertransversarii anteriores	Variable	Local over the muscle
Lateral vertebral muscles	Scalenus anterior	Three to four located in belly and close to the origin and insertion of muscle	Lateral shoulder, arm, forearm, and hand / Anterior chest / Posterior medial border of scapula
	Scalenus medius	Three to four located in belly and close to the origin and insertion of muscle	Lateral shoulder, arm, forearm, and hand / Anterior chest / Posterior medial border of scapula
	Scalenus posterior	Three to four located in belly and close to the origin and insertion of muscle	Lateral shoulder, arm, forearm, and hand / Anterior chest / Posterior medial border of scapula

REVITALIZE AND CLOSE

Use a selection of appropriate closing techniques to encourage circulation to the anterior neck. Also include some strokes to the chest and shoulders to integrate those areas with the neck. Then finish with effleurage strokes towards the core to encourage movement of blood and lymph through the area.

STRETCH AND RE-EDUCATE

Consider your treatment plan and the client's needs to select one or more of the following indirect methods (also see Table 9.2).

☑ **Positional release**—The positioning used will be unique for each client and each session. Generally the position of comfort will be found when the target muscle is shortened (in this case, when the neck is moved into flexion).

☑ **Post-isometric relaxation**—Place the neck into extension to stretch the anterior neck muscles. Have the client resist your pressure, and continue with PIR protocol (Chapter 8). Figure 9.31 ■ shows the hand positions for the direction of pressure and stretch for applying post-isometric relaxation to the anterior neck.

☑ **Reciprocal inhibition**—Have the client actively move her or his neck into extension while you slowly resist the movement. Continue with RI protocol (Chapter 8) until a full stretch is reached. Figure 9.32 ■ shows the hand positions as well as the direction of movement and resistance for applying reciprocal inhibition to the anterior neck.

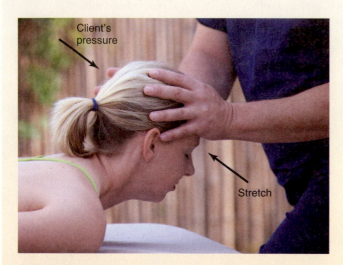

FIGURE 9.31

The Best Position for Applying PIR to the Anterior Neck. One Arrow Indicates the Direction the Therapist Uses to Passively Stretch the Muscles to the Comfort Barrier. Another Arrow Shows the Direction of Pressure Used by the Client to Resist the Stretch at the Comfort Barrier.

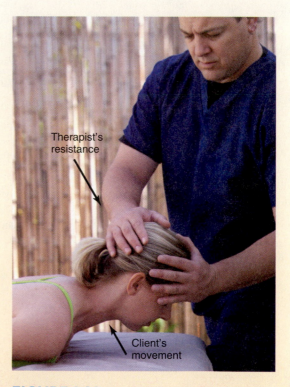

FIGURE 9.32

The Best Position for Applying RI to the Anterior Neck. One Arrow Indicates the Direction in Which the Client is Moving to Stretch the Target Muscles. Another Arrow Shows the Direction of Pressure Used as the Therapist Resists the Client's Movement.

The Chest, Anterior Shoulder, and Upper Arm

☑ Review the muscles of the chest, anterior shoulder, and upper arm (see Figures 9.33 ■ and 9.37).

• These muscles are responsible for moving the clavicle and upper arm.

FIGURE 9.33

The Major Muscles of the Chest, Anterior Shoulder, and Upper Arm

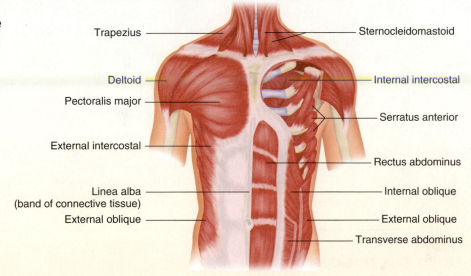

Trapezius — Sternocleidomastoid

Deltoid — Internal intercostal

Pectoralis major — Serratus anterior

External intercostal — Rectus abdominus

Linea alba (band of connective tissue) — Internal oblique

External oblique — External oblique

Transverse abdominus

WARM-UP AND ASSESS THE TISSUES

Using a selection of appropriate warm-up techniques, begin to warm and encourage circulation to the chest, anterior shoulder, and upper arm. Make sure to work the entire area, including the neck. This is because the anterior shoulder muscles have connections with this area.

IDENTIFY THE TRIGGER POINTS

☑ Table 9.11 ■ lists the common locations of trigger points in the muscles of the chest, anterior shoulder, and upper arm. In my experience, there are certain areas that are most likely to contain trigger points. Figure 9.34 ■ shows the locations of these areas and their referral zones. Palpate these areas and note any active trigger points. You may also find trigger points in any of the secondary referral zones. The client may present with trigger points that are not included here. It is important to address those as well.

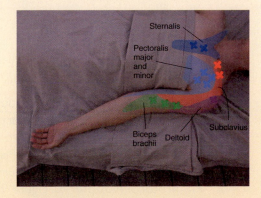

Sternalis

Pectoralis major and minor

Biceps brachii   Deltoid

Subclavius

FIGURE 9.34

The Common Trigger Points and Referral Areas in the Chest, Anterior Shoulder, and Upper Arm

TABLE 9.11	Common Trigger Points and Referral Zones of the Chest, Anterior Shoulder, and Upper Arm		
Muscle Group	Name of Muscle	Common Trigger Points	Common Secondary Referral Zones
Attaching to trunk and arm	*Pectoralis major*	Six to eight located in belly of muscle and on the superior and inferior edges	Lateral shoulder
Attaching clavicle to arm	*Deltoid*	Three to four located in belly of muscle	Local over the muscle
Attaching to arm and scapula	*Biceps brachii*	Two located in the belly of each of the two heads	Anterior upper shoulder and proximal forearm
	Coracobrachialis	One located in belly of the muscle close to the axilla	Posterior upper arm, forearm, and wrist
Attaching to scapula and trunk	*Pectoralis minor*	One located in the inferior belly of long section. One located close to axilla	Local over the muscle
	Subclavius	One located in the belly of the muscle inferior to the clavicle	Anterior arm and lateral elbow
Upper arm	*Brachialis*	One located in belly of muscle. One located distal end close to elbow	Anterior thumb

TREAT THE TRIGGER POINTS

☑ Select the direct method(s) best suited to treat the trigger points discovered during assessment (Table 9.2). Treat as many trigger points as is practical during your session.

REVITALIZE AND CLOSE

Use a selection of appropriate closing techniques to encourage circulation to the chest, anterior shoulder, and upper arm. Also include some strokes to the neck to integrate this area with the anterior shoulder and chest. Then finish with effleurage strokes towards the core to encourage movement of blood and lymph through the area.

STRETCH AND RE-EDUCATE

Consider your treatment plan and the client's needs to select one or more of the following indirect methods (also see Table 9.2).

☑ **Positional release**—The positioning used will be unique for each client and each session. Generally the position of comfort will be found when the target muscle is shortened (in this case when the arm is moved into flexion and/or horizontal adduction).

☑ **Post-isometric relaxation**—Place the shoulder into extension and horizontal abduction to stretch the anterior shoulder muscles. Have the client resist your pressure, and continue with PIR protocol (Chapter 8). Figure 9.35 ■ shows the hand positions for the direction of pressure and stretch for applying post-isometric relaxation to the anterior shoulder and upper arm.

☑ **Reciprocal inhibition**—Have the client actively move his or her shoulder into extension and horizontal abduction while you slowly resist the movement. Continue with RI protocol (Chapter 8) until a full stretch is reached. Figure 9.36 ■ shows the hand positions as well as the direction of movement and resistance for applying reciprocal inhibition to the chest and upper arm.

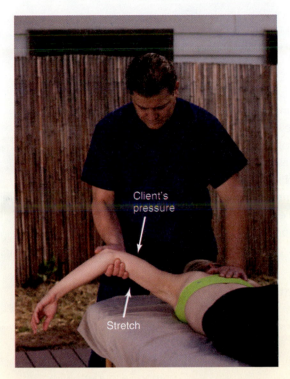

Client's pressure

Stretch

FIGURE 9.35

The Best Position for Applying PIR to the Chest, Anterior Shoulder, and Upper Arm. One Arrow Indicates the Direction the Therapist Uses to Passively Stretch the Muscles to the Comfort Barrier. Another Arrow Shows the Direction of Pressure Used by the Client to Resist the Stretch at the Comfort Barrier.

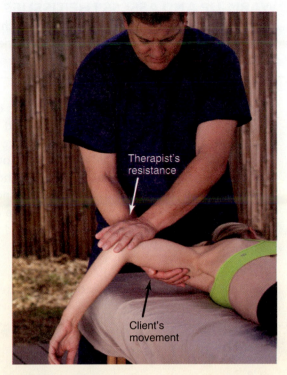

Therapist's resistance

Client's movement

FIGURE 9.36

The Best Position for Applying RI to the Chest, Anterior Shoulder, and Upper Arm. One Arrow Indicates the Direction in Which the Client Is Moving to Stretch the Target Muscles. Another Arrow Shows the Direction of Pressure Used as the Therapist Resists the Client's Movement.

The Anterior Forearm and Hand

☑ Review the muscles of the anterior forearm and hand (see Figure 9.37 ■).

- These muscles are responsible for moving the wrist, hand, and fingers.

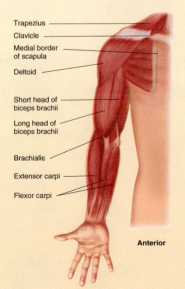

Trapezius
Clavicle
Medial border of scapula
Deltoid
Short head of biceps brachii
Long head of biceps brachii
Brachialis
Extensor carpi
Flexor carpi

Anterior

FIGURE 9.37

The Major Muscles of the Anterior Forearm and Hand

WARM-UP AND ASSESS THE TISSUES

Using a selection of appropriate warm-up techniques, begin to warm and encourage circulation to the anterior forearm and hand. Make sure to work the entire area, including the upper arm. This is because the shoulder muscles extend well into that area.

IDENTIFY THE TRIGGER POINTS

☑ Table 9.12 ■ lists the common locations of trigger points in the muscles of the anterior forearm and hand. In my experience, there are certain areas that are most likely to contain trigger points. Figure 9.38 ■ shows the locations of these areas and their referral zones. Palpate these areas and note any active trigger points. You may also find trigger points in any of the secondary referral zones. The client may present with trigger points that are not included here. It is important to address those as well.

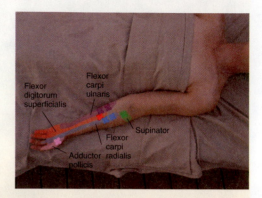

FIGURE 9.38

The Common Trigger Points and Referral Areas in the Anterior Forearm and Hand

TABLE 9.12	**Common Trigger points and Referral Zones of the Anterior and Medial Forearm and Hand**		
Muscle Group	**Name of Muscle**	**Common Trigger Points**	**Common Secondary Referral Zones**
Forearm/hand muscles	*Pronator teres*	One located in belly of the muscle	On palm side of the lateral wrist at the base of the thumb
	Flexor carpi radialis	One to two located in belly of the muscle	On palm at the base of the thumb
	Palmaris longus	One located in belly of the muscle	Center of the palm
	Flexor carpi ulnaris	One to two located in belly of the muscle	On palm at the base of the little finger
	Flexor digitorum superficialis	One to two located in belly of the muscle	On palm side of the third fourth and fifth fingers
	Flexor digitorum profundus	One to two located in belly of the muscle	On palm side of the third fourth and fifth fingers
	Flexor pollicis longus	One located in belly of the muscle	On palm side of the thumb
	Pronator quadratus	One located in belly of the muscle	On palm side of the lateral wrist at the base of the thumb
Hand	*Palmaris brevis*	One located in belly of the muscle	Local over the muscle
	Abductor pollicis	One located in belly of the muscle	Local over the muscle
	Flexor pollicis brevis	One located in belly of the muscle	Local over the muscle
	Opponens pollicis	One to two located in belly of the muscle	On palm side of the base of the thumb and along the thumb
	Adductor pollicis	One to two located in belly of the muscle	On palm side of the thumb
	Abductor digiti minimi	One located in belly of the muscle	Local over the muscle
	Flexor digiti minimi brevis	One located in belly of the muscle	Local over the muscle
	Opponens digiti minimi	One located in belly of the muscle	Local over the muscle
	Palmar interossei	One located in belly of the each of the heads, between each finger	No common area
	Lumbricales	One common TrP located in belly of the each of the heads, between each finger	Local over the muscle

TREAT THE TRIGGER POINTS

☑ Select the direct method(s) best suited to treat the trigger points discovered during assessment (Table 9.2). Treat as many trigger points as is practical during your session.

REVITALIZE AND CLOSE

Use a selection of appropriate closing techniques to encourage circulation to the anterior forearm and hand. Also include some strokes to the upper arm to integrate this area with the forearm. Then finish with effleurage strokes towards the core to encourage movement of blood and lymph through the area.

STRETCH AND RE-EDUCATE

Consider your treatment plan and the client's needs to select one or more of the following indirect methods (also see Table 9.2).

☑ **Positional release**—The positioning used will be unique for each client and each session. Generally the position of comfort will be found when the target muscle is shortened (in this case when the wrist and fingers are moved into flexion).

☑ **Post-isometric relaxation**—Place the wrist into extension to stretch the anterior forearm and hand muscles. Have the client resist your pressure, and continue with PIR protocol (Chapter 8). Figure 9.39 ■ shows the hand positions for the direction of pressure and stretch for applying post-isometric relaxation to the anterior hand and forearm.

☑ **Reciprocal inhibition**—Have the client actively move her or his wrist into extension while you slowly resist the movement. Continue with RI protocol (Chapter 8) until a full stretch is reached. Figure 9.40 ■ shows the hand positions as well as the direction of movement and resistance for applying reciprocal inhibition to the anterior forearm and hand.

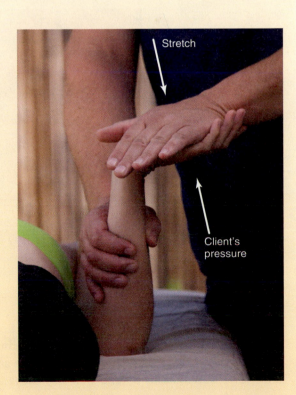

FIGURE 9.39

The Best Position for Applying PIR to the Anterior Forearm and Hand. One Arrow Indicates the Direction the Therapist Uses to Passively Stretch the Muscles to the Comfort Barrier. Another Arrow Shows the Direction of Pressure Used by the Client to Resist the Stretch at the Comfort Barrier.

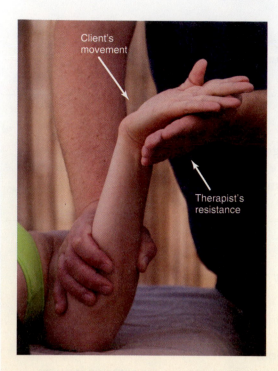

Client's movement

Therapist's resistance

FIGURE 9.40

The Best Position for Applying RI to the Anterior Forearm and Hand. One Arrow Indicates the Direction in Which the Client Is Moving to Stretch the Target Muscles. Another Arrow Shows the Direction of Pressure Used as the Therapist Resists the Client's Movement.

The Anterior Torso (Abdomen)

☑ Review the muscles of the anterior torso (see Figure 9.41 ■).

- These muscles are responsible for breathing and movement of the abdomen.

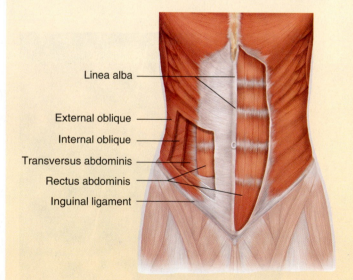

Linea alba

External oblique

Internal oblique

Transversus abdominis

Rectus abdominis

Inguinal ligament

FIGURE 9.41

The Major Muscles of the Anterior Torso (Abdomen)

WARM-UP AND ASSESS THE TISSUES

Using a selection of appropriate warm-up techniques, begin to warm and encourage circulation to the anterior torso. Make sure to work the entire area, including the *costal area* and hips. This is because the anterior torso muscles extend well into these areas.

IDENTIFY THE TRIGGER POINTS

☑ Table 9.13 ■ lists the common locations of trigger points in the muscles of the anterior torso. In my experience, there are certain areas that are most likely to contain trigger points. Figure 9.42 ■ shows the locations of these areas and their referral zones. Palpate these areas and note any active trigger points. You may also find trigger points in any of the secondary referral zones. The client may present with trigger points that are not included here. It is important to address those as well.

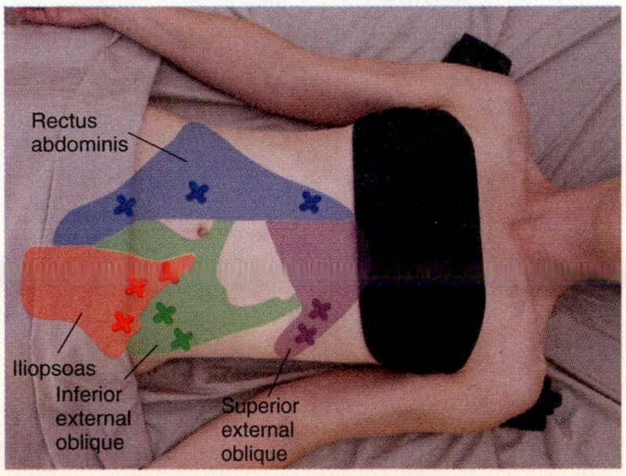

Rectus abdominis
Iliopsoas
Inferior external oblique
Superior external oblique

FIGURE 9.42

The Common Trigger Points and Referral Areas in the Anterior Torso (Abdomen)

TABLE 9.13	Common Trigger Points and Referral Zones of the Anterior Torso (Abdomen)		
Muscle Group	Name of Muscle	Common Trigger Points	Common Secondary Referral Zones
Abdominal muscles	*Obliquus externus abdominis*	Two to four located close to upper pelvis, lateral side, and upper border near ribs	Across the back in bands at level of trp
	Rectus abdominis	Two to four located at both attachments (i.e., close to pubis, and upper border near ribs and sternum)	Across the back in bands at level of trp
	Obliquus internus abdominis	Two to four located close to upper pelvis, lateral side, and upper border near ribs	Across the back in bands at level of trp
	Transverses abdominis	Variable	Local over the muscle
	Cremaster	None	Local over the muscle
Thoracic muscles	*Intercostales externi*	Variable	Local over the muscle
	Intercostales interni	Variable	Local over the muscle
	Subcostales	Variable	Local over the muscle
	Transverses thoracis	Variable	Local over the muscle
	Levatores costarum	Variable	Local over the muscle
	Diaphragm	Variable along anterior attachments	Local over the muscle

TREAT THE TRIGGER POINTS

☑ Select the direct method(s) best suited to treat the trigger points discovered during assessment (Table 9.2). Treat as many trigger points as is practical during your session.

REVITALIZE AND CLOSE

Use a selection of appropriate closing techniques to encourage circulation to the anterior torso. Also include some strokes to the costal area and hips to integrate those areas with the torso. Then finish with effleurage strokes towards the core to encourage movement of blood and lymph through the area.

STRETCH AND RE-EDUCATE

Consider your treatment plan and the client's needs to select one or more of the following indirect methods (also see Table 9.2).

☑ **Positional release**—The positioning used will be unique for each client and each session. Generally the position of comfort will be found when the target muscle is shortened (in this case when the torso is moved into flexion). When performing positional release on the abdomen, it is often helpful or necessary to use bolsters or use the side-lying position.

☑ **Post-isometric relaxation**—Place the torso into extension to stretch the anterior abdominal muscles. Have the client resist your pressure, and continue with PIR protocol (Chapter 8). Figure 9.43 ■ shows the hand positions for the direction of pressure and stretch for applying post-isometric relaxation to the anterior torso.

☑ **Reciprocal inhibition**—Have the client actively move his or her torso into extension while you slowly resist the movement. Continue with RI protocol (Chapter 8) until a full stretch is reached. Figure 9.44 ■ shows the hand positions as well as the direction of movement and resistance for applying reciprocal inhibition to the anterior torso.

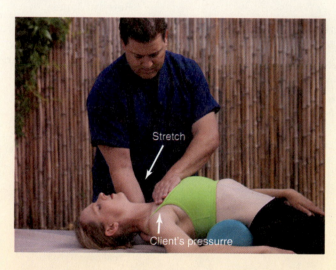

FIGURE 9.43

The Best Position for Applying PIR to the Anterior Torso (Abdomen). One Arrow Indicates the Direction the Therapist Uses to Passively Stretch the Muscles to the Comfort Barrier. Another Arrow Shows the Direction of Pressure Used by the Client to Resist the Stretch at the Comfort Barrier.

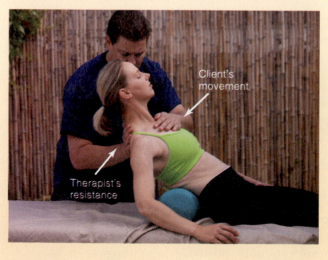

FIGURE 9.44

The Best Position for Applying RI to the Anterior Torso (Abdomen). One Arrow Indicates the Direction in Which the Client Is Moving to Stretch the Target Muscles. Another Arrow Shows the Direction of Pressure Used as the Therapist Resists the Client's Movement.

The Anterior Hip and Thigh

☑ Review the muscles of the anterior hip and thigh (see Figure 9.45 ■).

• These muscles are responsible for moving the hip, knee, and upper leg.

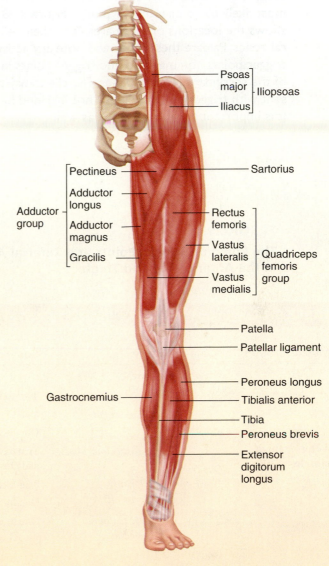

FIGURE 9.45

The Major Muscles of the Anterior Hip and Thigh

WARM-UP AND ASSESS THE TISSUES

Using a selection of appropriate warm-up techniques, begin to warm and encourage circulation to the anterior hip and thigh. Make sure to work the entire area, including the abdomen and knee. This is because the anterior hip and thigh muscles extend well into these areas.

IDENTIFY THE TRIGGER POINTS

☑ Table 9.14 ■ lists the common locations of trigger points in the muscles of the anterior hip and thigh. In my experience, there are certain areas that are most likely to contain trigger points. Figure 9.46 ■ shows the locations of these areas and their referral zones. Palpate these areas and note any active trigger points. You may also find trigger points in any of the secondary referral zones. The client may present with trigger points that are not included here. It is important to address those as well.

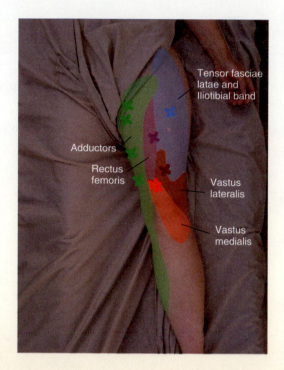

FIGURE 9.46

The Common Trigger Points and Referral Areas in the Anterior Hip and Thigh

TABLE 9.14	Common Trigger Points and Referral Zones of the Anterior and Medial Hip and Thigh		
Muscle Group	**Name of Muscle**		**Common Trigger Points**	**Common Secondary Referral Zones**
Anterior thigh muscles	Tensor fascia latae		One to two located in belly of muscle	Lateral hip
	Sartorius		Two to five located in belly of muscle	Medial knee
	Quadriceps femoris	Rectus femoris	One located in belly of muscle One located close to origin	Anterior knee
		Vastus lateralis	Two to seven located in belly of muscle and close to both attachments	Lateral knee and lateral buttocks
		Vastus medialis	One located in belly of muscle One located close to the knee	Medial lower knee
		Vastus intermedius	One to two located close to origin	Local over the muscle
Medial thigh muscles	Gracilis		Two to three located in belly of muscle	Medial knee
	Adductor longus		One to two located in belly of muscle	Medial superior knee
	Adductor magnus		Two located in belly of muscle Two close to origin at ischium	Pubis and sacrum
	Pectineus		One to two located in belly of muscle	Local over the muscle
	Adductor brevis		One to two located in belly of muscle	Medial superior knee
Hip muscles	Psoas major		One to two located in belly of muscle	Lower back
	Iliacus		One to two located in belly of muscle	Anterior thigh

TREAT THE TRIGGER POINTS

☑ Select the direct method(s) best suited to treat the trigger points discovered during assessment (Table 9.2). Treat as many trigger points as is practical during your session.

REVITALIZE AND CLOSE

Use a selection of appropriate closing techniques to encourage circulation to the anterior hip and thigh. Also include some strokes to the abdomen and knee. Then finish with effleurage strokes towards the core to encourage movement of blood and lymph through the area.

STRETCH AND RE-EDUCATE

Consider your treatment plan and the client's needs to select one or more of the following indirect methods (also see Table 9.2).

- ☑ **Positional release**—The positioning used will be unique for each client and each session. Generally the position of comfort will be found when the target muscle is shortened (in this case when the hip is moved into flexion or the thigh is moved into extension).
- ☑ **Post-isometric relaxation**—Place the hip into extension and the thigh into flexion to stretch the anterior hip and thigh muscles. Have the client resist your pressure, and continue with PIR protocol (Chapter 8). Figure 9.47 ■ shows the hand positions for the direction of pressure and stretch for applying post-isometric relaxation to the anterior hip and thigh.
- ☑ **Reciprocal inhibition**—Have the client actively move her or his hip into extension and the thigh into flexion while you slowly resist the movement. Continue with RI protocol (Chapter 8) until a full stretch is reached. Figure 9.48 ■ shows the hand positions as well as the direction of movement and resistance for applying reciprocal inhibition to the posterior hip and thigh.

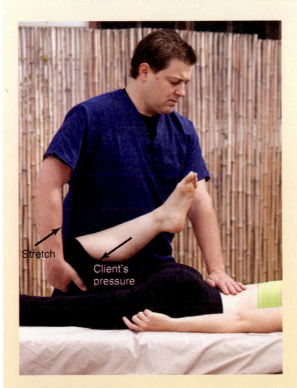

FIGURE 9.47

The Best Position for Applying PIR to the Anterior Hip and Thigh. One Arrow Indicates the Direction the Therapist Uses to Passively Stretch the Muscles to the Comfort Barrier. Another Arrow Shows the Direction of Pressure Used by the Client to Resist the Stretch at the Comfort Barrier.

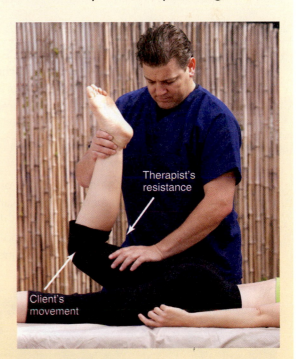

FIGURE 9.48

The Best Position for Applying RI to the Anterior Hip and Thigh. One Arrow Indicates the Direction in Which the Client Is Moving to Stretch the Target Muscles. Another Arrow Shows the Direction of Pressure Used as the Therapist Resists the Client's Movement.

The Anterior Lower Leg and Foot

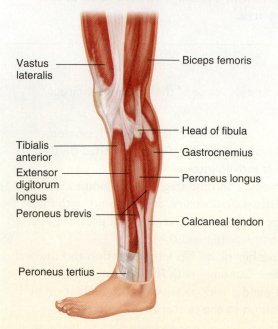

Vastus lateralis

Biceps femoris

Tibialis anterior

Head of fibula

Gastrocnemius

Extensor digitorum longus

Peroneus longus

Peroneus brevis

Calcaneal tendon

Peroneus tertius

☑ Review the muscles of the anterior lower leg and foot (see Figure 9.49 ■).

• These muscles are responsible for moving the ankle, foot, and toes.

FIGURE 9.49

The Major Muscles of the Anterior Lower Leg and Foot

WARM-UP AND ASSESS THE TISSUES

Using a selection of appropriate warm-up techniques, begin to warm and encourage circulation to the anterior lower leg and foot. Make sure to work the entire area, including the upper leg. This is because the lower leg muscles extend well into this area.

IDENTIFY THE TRIGGER POINTS

☑ Table 9.15 ■ lists the common locations of trigger points in the muscles of the anterior lower leg and foot. In my experience, there are certain areas that are most likely to contain trigger points. Figure 9.50 ■ shows the locations of these areas and their referral zones. Palpate these areas and note any active trigger points. You may also find trigger points in any of the secondary referral zones. The client may present with trigger points that are not included here. It is important to address those as well.

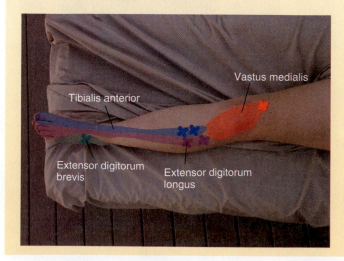

Vastus medialis

Tibialis anterior

Extensor digitorum brevis

Extensor digitorum longus

FIGURE 9.50

The Common Trigger Points and Referral Areas in the Anterior Lower Leg and Foot

TABLE 9.15	Common Trigger Points and Referral Zones of the Anterior Lower Leg and Foot		
Muscle Group	Name of Muscle	Common Trigger Points	Common Secondary Referral Zones
Lower leg	*Tibialis anterior*	One located in belly of muscle	Anterior ankle and big toe
Lateral lower leg and foot	*Peroneus longus*	One located in belly of muscle	Lateral ankle
	Peroneu brevis	One located in belly of muscle	Lateral ankle
	Peroneus tertius	One located in belly of muscle	Anterior ankle and lateral heel
Dorsal foot	*Extensor digitorum brevis*	One to two located in belly of the medial and lateral heads of muscle	Local over the muscle
Lower leg and foot	*Extensor hallicus longus*	One located in belly of muscle	Anterior big toe
	Extensor digitorum longus	One located in belly of muscle	Anterior foot

TREAT THE TRIGGER POINTS

☑ Select the direct method(s) best suited to treat the trigger points discovered during assessment (Table 9.2). Treat as many trigger points as is practical during your session.

REVITALIZE AND CLOSE

Use a selection of appropriate closing techniques to encourage circulation to the anterior lower leg and foot. Also include some strokes to the upper leg to integrate those areas with the lower leg. Then finish with effleurage strokes towards the core to encourage movement of blood and lymph through the area.

STRETCH AND RE-EDUCATE

Consider your treatment plan and the client's needs to select one or more of the following indirect methods (also see Table 9.2).

☑ **Positional release**—The positioning used will be unique for each client and each session. Generally the position of comfort will be found when the target muscle is shortened (in this case when the foot is moved into dorsiflexion).

☑ **Post-isometric relaxation**—Place the ankle into plantar-flexion to stretch the anterior lower leg and foot muscles. Have the client resist your pressure, and continue with PIR protocol (Chapter 8). Figure 9.51 ■ shows the hand positions for the direction of pressure and stretch for applying post-isometric relaxation to the anterior lower leg and foot.

☑ **Reciprocal inhibition**—Have the client actively move his or her foot into plantar-flexion while you slowly resist the movement. Continue with RI protocol (Chapter 8) until a full stretch is reached. Figure 9.52 ■ shows the hand positions as well as the direction of movement and resistance for applying reciprocal inhibition to the anterior lower leg and foot.

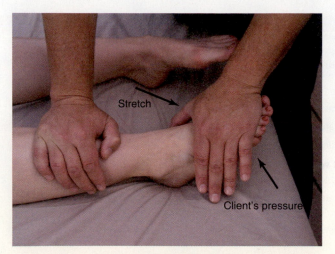

FIGURE 9.51

The Best Position for Applying PIR to the Anterior Lower Leg and Foot. One Arrow Indicates the Direction the Therapist Uses to Passively Stretch the Muscles to the Comfort Barrier. Another Arrow Shows the Direction of Pressure Used by the Client to Resist the Stretch at the Comfort Barrier.

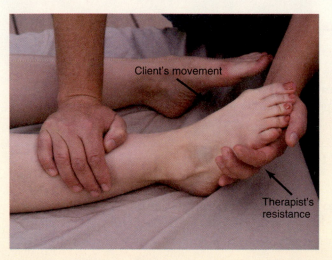

FIGURE 9.52

The Best Position for Applying RI to the Anterior Lower Leg and Foot. One Arrow Indicates the Direction in Which the Client Is Moving to Stretch the Target Muscles. Another Arrow Shows the Direction of Pressure Used as the Therapist Resists the Client's Movement.

QUICK QUIZ #18

1. Which of the following are common secondary referral zones for trigger points in the Scalenus anterior? (Circle all that apply)
   a. Anterior chest
   b. Lateral shoulder
   c. Lateral border of scapula
   d. Forearm and hand
   e. All of the above
   f. None of the above

2. When applying RI to the anterior forearm and hand, you should have the client resist your pressure as you place his or her wrist into extension.
   a. True
   b. False

3. Which of the following are common secondary referral zones for trigger points in the Pectineus? (Circle all that apply)
   a. Medial knee
   b. Medial superior knee
   c. Lower back
   d. Pubis and sacrum
   e. All of the above
   f. None of the above

4. When applying RI to the anterior lower leg and foot, you should slowly resist the client's movement as the client actively moves her or his foot into plantar-flexion.
   a. True
   b. False

HOLISTIC CONNECTION

Reflexology is a complementary treatment modality in which pressure is applied to specific areas of the feet, hands, and/or ears that correlate with other distant areas of the body. It is thought that reflexology may work by affecting energy flow within the body, releasing endorphins, stimulating nerve circuits, or by promoting lymphatic flow. Evidence suggests that reflexology is useful for relaxation. It may be effective for symptoms of multiple sclerosis and in edema of the legs and feet in pregnant women (Aetna InteliHealth Inc., 1996–2010).

Consider getting basic training in the use of reflexology. Adding this therapy to the beginning or end of your massage routines is a great way to broaden your focus and treat the whole client.

SUMMARY

When applying your neuromuscular therapy protocol, remember the basic principles of this approach. Keep in mind the physiology behind the techniques you are using. There are specific reasons for the use of the various techniques and for the order in which they are performed. If necessary, review the details of the techniques or the muscle areas you are working on. It can be helpful to keep handy some reference materials regarding referral zones, trigger point locations, etc.

Before starting your protocol, determine if you will need any additional tools or supplies, such as an extra blanket, bolsters, a heat source, etc. Adjust any furniture or objects in the room to accommodate for stretches you may be performing with the client.

With each massage, pay special attention to your body mechanics. Take care to use leverage to preserve your energy and posture.

Focus on the client and remember the mental and emotional connection to the pathology you are treating. Communicate regularly with the client to monitor the effects of your treatment.

As you become more practiced you will begin to develop more variable protocols. The NMT protocols for any specific body part or set of body parts can be combined with other methods, such as deep tissue massage, myofascial therapy, acupressure, and more.

DISCUSSION QUESTIONS

1. Why is it important to know the direction in which each muscle contracts when applying NMT?
2. Why is it useful to know the common referral patterns for common trigger points?
3. What factors should you consider when choosing to use positional release, post-isometric relaxation, and/or reciprocal inhibition?

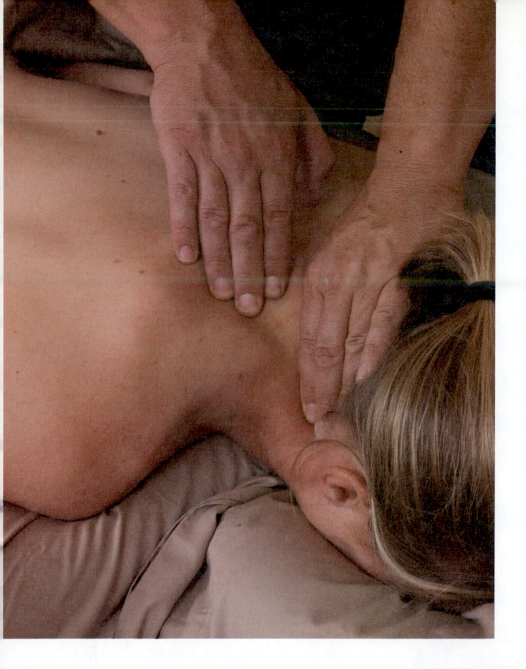

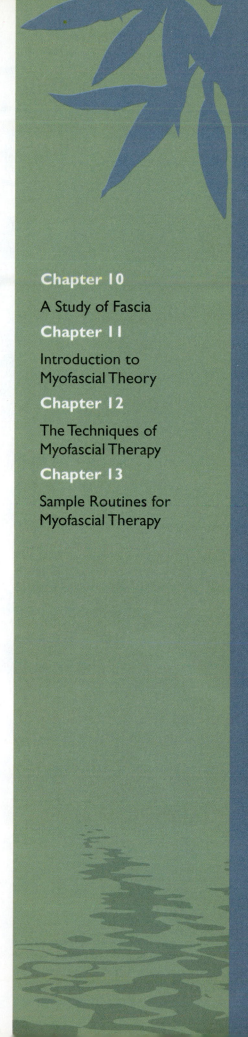

PART

4

The Myofascial Approach

10 A Study of Fascia

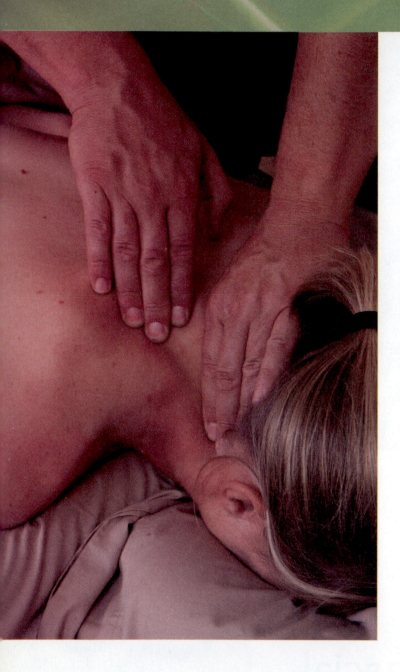

CHAPTER HIGHLIGHTS

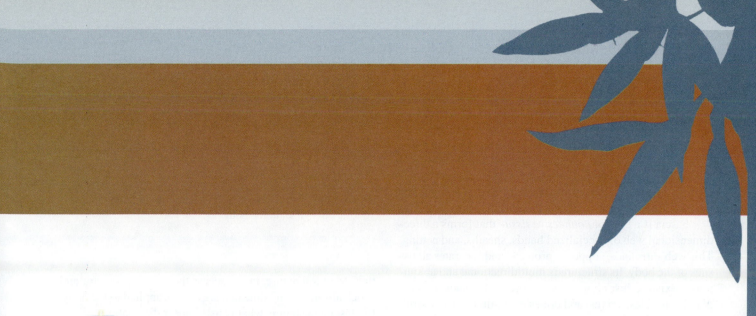

CHAPTER OBJECTIVES

- Examine the structure of fascia
- Consider the relationship between fascia and muscle tissue

- Understand the physiology of fascia
- Investigate pathology in the myofascia

KEY TERMS

THE INTERCONNECTED WEB

In anatomic studies, the body is often described in terms of its parts. Muscles, bones, and their supporting structures are individually categorized and explained in terms of their specific place in or on the body. Sometimes it can be helpful to view the body this way. However, it is very important to realize that all the muscles, bones, ligaments, and tendons are interconnected by a type of tissue called *fascia*.

Fascia is a type of *connective tissue* that forms a three-dimensional web of specialized bands, sheaths, and netting. This web surrounds, supports, protects, and separates all tissues of the body. Its structure is multidirectional and ubiquitous—existing just about everywhere. All tissues, organs, glands, muscles, nerves, and bones are built on a framework of fascia and are surrounded by it.

The framelike, or scaffoldlike, nature of fascia not only supports the tissues, organs, etc., but also creates the spaces between the tissues. These spaces serve as pathways for *interstitial fluid* movement, cellular exchange, and metabolic activity. Because of this, most of the tissue repair and rebuilding processes take place in the fascia.

Fascia not only provides the space and support for organs and tissues, but for all vessels in the body as well. Lymph vessels, blood vessels, and nerves are all constructed with layers of fascia that connect to and spread through the fascia in the other tissues. Therefore fascia can be highly sensitive. If you have ever bumped your shin on a coffee table, you have felt how sensitive the *periosteum* (fascia that wraps the bone) can be.

As mentioned, fascia not only forms and organizes the structures, but also connects them. This creates a continuous network that extends throughout the body from head to toe, from superficial to deep, and from front to back. Because of

DID YOU KNOW

Think of the construction of the body like the construction of a house. A house has a foundation (the concrete footers). Anchored into the foundation is a frame for the walls. The frame for the walls provides the space for the internal wiring, plumbing, and insulation. Over the frame is the roof that is anchored into the walls.

In the body, the bones are the foundation. Anchored into the bones (via the periosteum) is fascia, which is the frame for the muscles and other structures. The space between the fascia is filled with vessels, nerves, and cells. Then, anchored into the framework of the fascia is the subcutaneous fascia, which wraps and holds everything together.

In a house, the foundation, frame, and roof are made of different substances (e.g., wood, concrete). In the body these areas are made of fascia. Fascia is the internal structure, and, at the same time, it covers and protects the body.

DID YOU KNOW

The name *macrophage* means "big eater." I like to picture macrophages as little Pac-Man cells going around eating all the "ghosts" or "junk" in the body.

this structural nature, fascia acts as the body's protector and shock absorber. Any time that pressure is applied to the body, the fascial system is what resists and/or dissipates it.

The Components of Fascia

The structure of all connective tissue (including fascia) can be broken into two basic components: **cells** and a conglomerate of fibers and gels called the **extracellular matrix** (see Figure 10.1 ■).

CELLS

Many types of cells exist in the fascia. Cells called **fibroblasts** are one of the most important and predominant types. These cells secrete both the fibers and the ground substance that make up the extracellular matrix. Fibroblasts are very active and can be mobilized to an area of tissue that has been damaged. Once at the site of injury, the fibroblasts will fill the area in with fibers. Pressure, injury, and muscle growth in a particular area may all cause fibroblasts to move in and secrete fibers. Mature fibroblasts become **fibroclasts,** which are less active and help to maintain the health of the matrix. Interestingly, in the case of serious injury, fibroclasts can revert back to being fibroblasts to speed up the rebuilding process (Marieb, 2004).

Because fascia infuses and surrounds all structures of the body, it is uniquely positioned to provide an environment for immune function. **Plasma cells** produce *antibodies* and *white blood cells* and are found throughout fascia. These cells migrate freely from the bloodstream into the extracellular matrix to patrol for harmful foreign substances.

Another type of cell that is found in large numbers in fascia is the **macrophage.** Macrophages are cells that have the ability to break down foreign substances, such as viruses and bacteria. They also play an important role in the reabsorption of damaged or worn out tissues and cells. Macrophages clear the way for the rebuilding process. Some macrophages are fixed to fascial fibers, while others migrate freely throughout the matrix (Marieb, 2004).

Mast cells are plentiful in the fascia. They release histamine in response to inflammation and help maintain osmotic balance in the ground substance.

Another major function of fascia is to provide a reservoir for nutrients. This reservoir is maintained by fat cells. Fat cells are found all over fascia and are especially concentrated in the superficial layers, just under the skin.

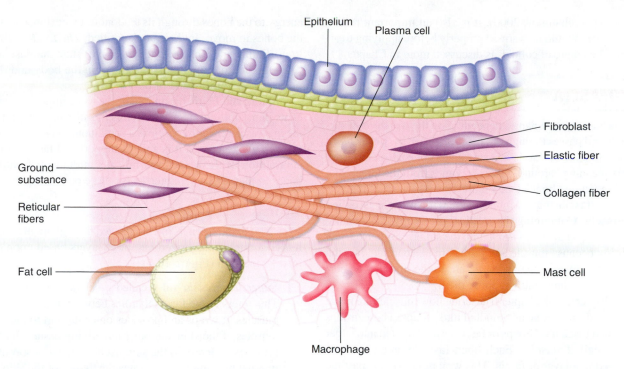

Epithelium
Plasma cell
Fibroblast
Elastic fiber
Collagen fiber
Ground substance
Reticular fibers
Fat cell
Mast cell
Macrophage

FIGURE 10.1

The Components of Fascia: Fibroblasts, Fat Cells, Plasma Cells, Macrophages, Fibers, Mast Cells, and Ground Substance

EXTRACELLULAR MATRIX

Extracellular matrix (ECM) is the primary structural component of fascia. It is composed of *fibers*, which give dimension to the matrix, and *ground substance*, which acts as a sort of mortar that supports and holds the fibers together as well as provides a lubricant for movement.

Fibers Three types of fibers make up the extracellular matrix:

- **Collagen** (Figure 10.1)—This is a strong, inelastic fiber. It provides stability to the fascial network. Collagen is made of a fibrous protein, which forms thick, ropelike structures with a white color. The ratio of collagen fibers in a given area of fascia depends on the general amount of stress applied to it. The fascia of structures such as muscles, which experience more stress, has a higher ratio of collagen fibers. In contrast, the fascia surrounding soft organs like the spleen has a much lower ratio of collagen fibers (Turchaninov, 2000).
- **Elastin** (Figure 10.1)—These are long, thin fibers that can stretch and recoil. They lend a flexible element to fascia. These fibers are found in branched networks throughout the matrix and have a yellow color. The fascia associated with tissues that need a higher degree of flexibility, such as those of the lungs, have a higher ratio of elastin.
- **Reticulin** (Figure 10.1)—This is an altered form of collagen fiber that is much smaller and finer. Reticulin forms a spongelike "mesh" that creates spaces in the

fascia. The mesh provides room for structures such as lymph and blood vessels and also connects the layers of fascia together.

Ground Substance **Ground substance** is a semigelatinous material that has the appearance of egg whites (Figure 10.1). It is made up of *interstitial fluid* and proteins. One of its components is hyaluronic acid, which is a *viscous* substance. Ground substance surrounds the cells, maintaining distance between the fibers while also lubricating them and acting as a shock absorber. Because of its gel-like consistency, it provides an environment for waste products and nutrients to move in and out of the cells. Ground substance also functions as a mechanical barrier against bacteria by surrounding each cell in a viscous envelope, thus protecting it (Marieb, 2004).

One of the unique features of ground substance is that it is a colloidal solution. **Colloids** are substances made up of particles which are evenly dispersed within another substance. Gelatin, shaving cream, and milk are all familiar colloidal substances. The ground substance of fascia is a colloid which contains proteins and other substances evenly dispersed in water. Colloids have some special properties which help to explain some of the important effects massage can have on the fascia.

The colloidal nature of ground substance means that it has the property of **thixotropy.** This is the tendency of colloids to change in *viscosity* from a liquid nature to a more solid, gel-like consistency, depending on the temperature. When cool, the ground substance can become sticky and thick. When it is warm, it is more fluid and flexible. This is an important concept to bodyworkers as it explains how a number of pathologies can develop (Turchaninov, 2000). It is also an important reason why tissues should be warmed properly before applying treatment. The nature of colloids is discussed more in Chapter 11.

MYOFASCIA

Fascia has different names depending on the structures it surrounds and passes through. As mentioned earlier, **periosteum** is the name for the fascia that surrounds bone. *Peri* is a Greek prefix meaning "around." *Osteum* comes from the Greek root word meaning "bone" (see Figure 10.2 ■).

The fascia that is interwoven with muscle is called **myofascia.** Combining the medical prefix *myo* (indicating "muscle") and the word *fascia* into the single word *myofascia* is fitting because muscle and fascia are inseparable. It is the fascia that gives shape and structure to the muscles by permeating, dividing, and wrapping them.

Chapter 2 and Chapter 6 describe how muscles are made up of small fibers that are bundled into groups. These groups are called **fascicles.** Groups of fascicles are bundled into larger groups called *muscles*. Each fiber, fascicle, and muscle is wrapped in a layer of fascia. This wrapping extends past the muscle tissue to become the tendon, which attaches the muscle to the periosteum around the bone (see Figure 10.3 ■). Furthermore, groups of muscles are wrapped together, as are larger groupings of groups of muscles. Finally the whole body part is wrapped in a superficial layer of fascia.

Examine the upper arm, for example. It has three muscles, which divide into six distinct heads. In the anterior compartment, the two heads of the biceps and the coracobrachialis are each individually wrapped. The two heads of the biceps are then wrapped together in a layer. Then another layer wraps them with the coracobrachialis. In the posterior compartment, the three heads of the triceps are individually wrapped. They are all then wrapped together. Finally, both the anterior and the posterior compartment are wrapped in a layer called the superficial or *subcutaneous* layer. Figure 10.4 ■ shows a cross-section of the upper arm and the individual muscles and compartments that are divided by fascial wrappings.

Due to the intricate interweaving of muscle and fascia, myofascia is involved in all aspects of motion. Muscle tissue pulls on its surrounding fascia. The fascia then transmits the

energy to the bones through its tendonous extension, causing the bones to move. In their book entitled, *The Endless Web*, Louis Shultz and Rosemary Feitis (1996) state that fascia is "The 'organ' that transmits movement in the body and that makes a structural whole of us" (p. 27).

Shultz and Feitis hit on one of the most important concepts in myofascial theory, which is the structural aspect of the myofascia. Because fascia is a continuous net that extends through all structures, it is able to support and facilitate the contraction of the muscles, while it simultaneously holds bones in place. (See Chapter 11 for more on this topic.)

Myofascial Layers

Even though the fascia is interconnected throughout the body, it is commonly categorized into three layers based upon the relative location (Figure 10.4).

1. *Superficial fascia* (also called *subcutaneous* fascia)— This refers to the fascia that lies between the skin and muscles. It wraps and provides outer support to the muscles of the skin and other underlying tissues. It also provides structure to the skin itself, acting as a sort of internal backing that separates the tissues of the skin from the muscle below.

DID YOU KNOW

Using the house analogy, the roof of the house would be like the superficial layer of fascia (skin, etc.). The frame of the house is like the middle layer that supports the muscles. The foundation of the house is like the deep layer of fascia around the bones and joints.

All of these layers are interconnected just like the structure of a house. If you were a giant and you grabbed and shook the roof of a house, you would not only affect the roof, but the frame and foundation as well. The same thing happens in the body. During bodywork, when you move the skin, the muscles and the deeper fascial layers will move as well.

FIGURE 10.2

The Meanings and Origins of the Words "Periosteum" and "Myofascia"

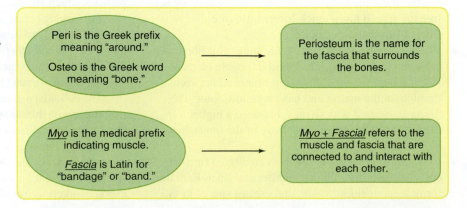

Peri is the Greek prefix meaning "around."

Osteo is the Greek word meaning "bone."

→ Periosteum is the name for the fascia that surrounds the bones.

Myo is the medical prefix indicating muscle.

Fascia is Latin for "bandage" or "band."

→ *Myo + Fascial* refers to the muscle and fascia that are connected to and interact with each other.

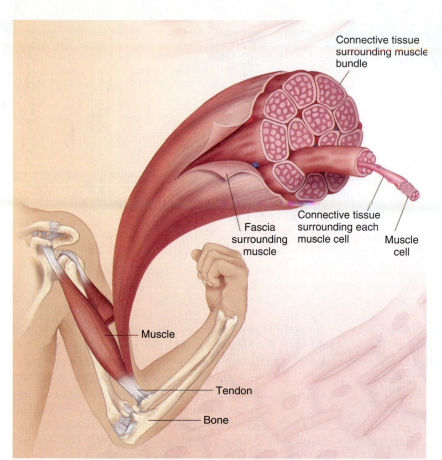

FIGURE 10.3

A Tendon Is an Extension of the Fascia That Wraps the Muscle and of the Fascia That Becomes the Periosteum.

Connective tissue surrounding muscle bundle

Fascia surrounding muscle

Connective tissue surrounding each muscle cell

Muscle cell

Muscle

Tendon

Bone

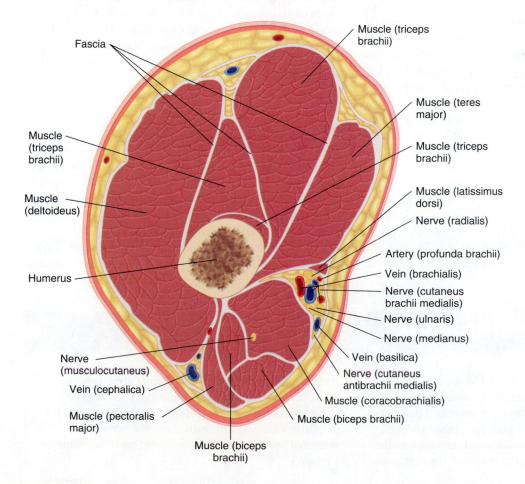

FIGURE 10.4

A Cross-Section View of the Arm Illustrates How the Wrapping of Fascia Creates Compartments for Various Structures.

Fascia

Muscle (triceps brachii)

Muscle (teres major)

Muscle (triceps brachii)

Muscle (triceps brachii)

Muscle (deltoideus)

Muscle (latissimus dorsi)

Nerve (radialis)

Artery (profunda brachii)

Vein (brachialis)

Nerve (cutaneus brachii medialis)

Nerve (ulnaris)

Humerus

Nerve (medianus)

Vein (basilica)

Nerve (musculocutaneus)

Nerve (cutaneus antibrachii medialis)

Vein (cephalica)

Muscle (coracobrachialis)

Muscle (pectoralis major)

Muscle (biceps brachii)

Muscle (biceps brachii)

FIGURE 10.5

Fascia Can Be Classified as Superficial, Middle, or Deep Depending on Where It Is Located.

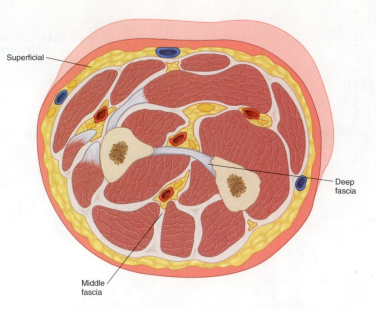

2. *Middle fascia*—This fascia is located in, around, and between the muscle fibers. It provides shape and support to muscles by wrapping the individual fibers and groups of fibers. This is the fascia that extends out from the ends of the muscles to form tendons.

3. *Deep fascia*—This fascia is located around the bones and joints. It provides stability to joints and blends with joint capsules, tendons, and ligaments.

Figure 10.5 ■ shows a cross-cut of the forearm. The white areas represent fascia and the red color represents muscle tissue. In the center you can see the radius and ulna. The deep layer includes the fascia around the radius and ulna including the fascial membrane between them. All of the fascia around the muscles is the middle layer, and the layer around the outside is the superficial layer.

Although it can be helpful to categorize fascia in different levels, the fact is the layers of fascia are all interconnected and multidirectional. Essentially, fascia forms layers of netting that create an elaborate web. The web of fascia connects all parts of the body together and holds everything in place. Dr. Jean-Claude Guimberteau in his groundbreaking video entitled, *Strolling Under the Skin: Images of Living Fascia* (2005), reveals the nature of this weblike connectedness. Upon careful observation, Dr. Guimberteau discovered a microsystem of tiny reticular fibers that connect and run through all the myofascial layers and all other structures of the body. He called this system the "multimicrovacuolar collagenic dynamic absorbing system." The fibers are arranged in geometric patterns that extend through all tissues and fill all of the spaces of the body. This network simultaneously supports, stretches, and maintains the shape of all tissues. It is capable of absorbing, resisting, and transmitting both pressure and movement throughout the body.

According to Dr. Guimberteau, this network uses the principles of *tensegrity* to allow the fibers to both maintain shape as well as transmit movement. (See Chapter 11 for more about tensegrity.) This helps to explain how bodywork which treats the superficial layers always affects the deeper layers. This is important because it means one doesn't always have to work deep into the tissues to create profound changes in all the layers.

FASCIA AND PIEZOELECTRICITY

A unique feature of fascia is that it has piezoelectric properties (Myers, 2001; Turchaninov, 2000). **Piezoelectricity** is the tendency of some materials to produce an electric charge when stress is applied to them. Quartz crystal has this property and so do the collagen fibers in fascia.

When stress such as pressure or a stretch is applied to the fascial structures, the collagen fibers release a piezoelectric

HOLISTIC CONNECTION

A holistic view of the body means looking at the body and its tissues from different perspectives. Layers of fascia are integrated with layers of muscle. The layers of myofascia are connected with each other and are integrated with other important structures, such as the bones and internal organs. Furthermore, the myofascia itself also includes important vascular structures (such as capillaries, veins, and arteries) and neural tissue (such as motor neurons, proprioceptors, and more). It is helpful to examine and learn about the parts of the body, but it is essential to remember that it functions as a whole.

QUICK QUIZ #19

1. Fibroblasts: (Circle all that apply)
   a. secrete the fibers and the ground substance that make up the extracellular matrix.
   b. revert back to being fibroclasts in case of serious injury.
   c. produce antibodies and white blood cells.
   d. break down foreign substances such as bacteria and viruses.

2. The extracellular matrix: (Circle all that apply)
   a. is the primary structural component of fascia.
   b. contains collagen.
   c. contains ground substance.

   d. is composed of fibers and ground substance.
   e. All of the above
   f. None of the above

3. Ground substance is a semigelatenous substance made up of fluid and proteins.
   a. True
   b. False

4. Fascia is arranged into three distinct layers that are separated from each other by clear boundaries.
   a. True
   b. False

DID YOU KNOW

Interestingly, as massage therapists, we are in a unique position of being able to encourage the fibers to align in a healthier position. Massage strokes apply mechanical forces such as pressure, pulling, and stretching on the collagen fibers. This stimulates the piezoelectric charge, which enhances the effectiveness of our work by helping the fibers align.

charge. This charge has two effects. It causes the fibers to align and also stimulates the laying down of more fibers in the area. This helps the tissue to respond by strengthening and aligning the fibers in such a way that the structure becomes thicker and able to withstand the new stress (Myers, 2001).

A common example of this process is exercising or working out a muscle. The increased pulling of the muscle fibers will cause an increase of piezoelectric charge. The electric charge stimulates the fascia to lay down more fibers, so that it becomes stronger to resist the pull. This process also occurs during postural distortions or injury. When the body is held in a chronic fixed position, the increased stress caused by the position will create an increased piezoelectric charge. The fibers will be stimulated to grow and align along that stress line to help the muscle withstand that force. The laying down of more fibers also causes the area to become more rigid and resistant to movement.

PATHOLOGIES OF FASCIA

Because of the dynamic role that fascia plays in supporting all of the body's structures, it is often an area where pathology develops and is harbored. Fascia can become rigid, dehydrated, *fibrotic*, and "glued down" due to stresses, injury, degenerative processes, or anything that causes lack of movement.

Pathologies in the fascia can be categorized as either **adhesions** or **restrictions.**

Adhesions

Adhesions can take on two basic forms.

1. *Adhesions in the ground substance (see Figure 10.6 ■):* When the ground substance is hydrated and healthy, the fibers are able to move independently of each other. The free movement of fibers is essential to the health of a muscle. When the ground substance is free flowing, it can provide the proper medium for nutrient and waste exchange. Also, a more liquid ground substance provides freedom of movement to the fibers which it surrounds (i.e., muscle fibers, collagen, elastin, etc.).

   If a muscle or joint is damaged or unused, the ground substance can become sticky. This is due to dehydration and temperature changes resulting from lack of circulation. When the ground substance becomes sticky, it binds the fibers together. Now, as each fiber tries to move independently, it pulls on the surrounding resting fibers,

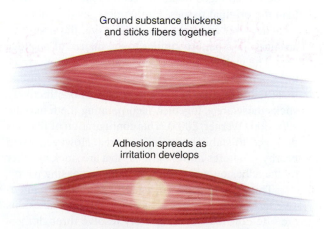

Ground substance thickens and sticks fibers together

Adhesion spreads as irritation develops

FIGURE 10.6

The Formation of a Ground Substance Adhesion

Damaged muscle

Collagen fibers fill in the space

The fibers spread and attach to the surrounding tissues

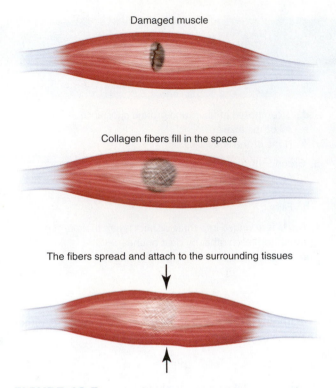

FIGURE 10.7

The Formation of a Fibrous Adhesion

which often causes pain. These types of adhesions often surround trigger points, because the chronic tension of the TrP will restrict the fascia and its blood supply. Adhesions at this stage respond well to bodywork. It is relatively easy to release the ground substance.

2. *Fibrous adhesions (see Figure 10.7 ■):* This type of adhesion is often called a *scar*. As mentioned, when muscle is damaged, fibroblasts deposit fibers into the lesion to fill in the space and reconnect the tissues. The predominant fibers secreted are collagen fibers. This is because collagen is the strongest fiber and therefore better able to resist pull on the damaged tissues.

   However, since the newly patched area is primarily formed of collagen fibers, it becomes much more rigid than the original tissues. Furthermore, as the adhesion stretches over and across the injury site, the fibers are arranged in a pattern similar to the matrix of a spider web. The weblike fibers extend into surrounding structures, such as other muscle fibers, surrounding fascia, local tendons, ligaments, and bones. This effectively sticks these areas together, incorporating them into the adhesion (Werner, 2005). This configuration of fibers is designed to stabilize the injured area. However, when nearby structures move, the areas that are stuck together by the adhesion will pull on each other, causing pain.

   This type of adhesion usually needs a more intensive technique to promote healing. Fibrous adhesions are often difficult to completely resolve through therapy. The scar will always be a part of that structure, as one cannot completely eliminate the fibers that form it.

However, proper therapy can be effective in reducing the rigidity of the scar. The fibers can be softened and the adhesions loosened so that the scar is more flexible and functional. A functional scar is less painful.

Restrictions

Restrictions are often called **chronic holding patterns.** Whenever the muscles become stiff or the joints lose their range of motion, this is considered a restriction. Restrictions can be localized, affecting only one or two joints. They can also be systemic, affecting multiple joints, even the entire body.

When a body part is held still for extended periods due to pain or injury, the blood supply will diminish and the area will cool considerably. This has an effect on the viscosity and elasticity of the fascia. It will become rigid and inflexible. Due to influences such as piezoelectricity, the rigid fascia perpetuates the holding pattern by laying down fibers and forming adhesions, which causes more pain. More pain results in more holding. Over time, adjacent areas are affected as they take on the extra stress and the restriction is perpetuated.

Injury is one of the most common causes of restrictions. Certain types of injuries can cause lesions (tears) in the myofascial tissues. As discussed, the repair process often binds the injury site to other local tissues. It is precisely this binding that causes pain. As the pain from the adhesion increases, the person will limit movement of the injured area. As the area is used less, the circulation to and from the area becomes impaired. The lack of circulation affects everything: from nutrient content to hydration of the fascia. This may then cause more adhesions, and as the cycle repeats itself, the condition may develop into a **contracture.**

A contracture is a severe form of restriction. The tissues (especially the joint capsule) become immovable to the degree that they will *atrophy* from the loss of movement. In cases of contracture, the nerves as well as the blood and lymph vessels may also become adhered and restricted. Because fascia is multilayered and continuous throughout the entire body, adhesions in one area will affect other areas through the network of fascia.

Acute injury is not the only reason for the development of restrictions. Often, the habitual way we carry our bodies during work, sports, etc. impacts our posture and causes restrictions. People tend to move about life and engage in the same activities, day in and day out. These habitual movement patterns wear on the posture. In fact, any activity that we engage in on a regular basis has the potential to create a holding pattern. When the activity requires us to hold our bodies in a specific position for an extended time (e.g., working on an assembly line) or when the activity focuses on just a few muscle groups, it can lead to fixation in those positions or movements.

Even the way we sleep can be a cause of restrictions. Since sleeping takes up roughly one-third of our lives, sleep positions have a profound effect on posture. Any restrictions developed during the hours we are awake are compounded by long hours lying still. Further complicating the issue is sleeping on old mattresses or using too many pillows. These can add new restricted patterns and/or aggravate postural holding patterns that are already present.

QUICK QUIZ #20

1. When stress is applied to fascia through exercise or by fixed chronic tension: (Circle all that apply)
   a. the tissue is stimulated to lay down more fibers.
   b. the collagen fibers release an electrical charge.
   c. the fibers tend to come out of alignment.
   d. All of the above
   e. None of the above

2. A contracture:
   a. is a written agreement signed by the therapist and the client prior to treatment.
   b. is a severe form of adhesion in which the ground substance becomes sticky and dehydrated.
   c. is a severe form of restriction in which blood and lymph vessels may become restricted.

3. It is generally easier to release fibrous adhesions than it is to release adhesions of the ground substance.
   a. True
   b. False

4. Any time the muscles become stiff or the joints lose their range of motion, this is considered an adhesion.
   a. True
   b. False

Finally, emotions are a common contributor to postural holding patterns. The body is the subconscious expression of the mind. How we feel is directly expressed through our posture and other body positions. If a great deal of time is spent in certain emotional states (sadness, for example), a person will spend a proportionate amount of time in the physical expression of sadness. Their shoulders, perhaps their neck and back, will be slumped and rounded, causing stress to the spine and the ligaments of the vertebrae. This position may become fixed in the fascia.

SUMMARY

Fascia is a connective tissue that is found in all structures of the body. It makes up the foundation and scaffolding of all organs, tissues, and glands. Fascia also connects the body, holding all structures in dynamic balance with the others. Fascia is made up of cells, fibers, and ground substance. Each component has a unique role in the form and function of fascia. Fascia has a thixotropic nature. It is flexible when it is warm and rigid when cool.

Myofascia is the term for the fascia that wraps and infuses muscle. All muscle fibers, muscles, and groups of muscles are wrapped in myofascia. Myofascia then extends to form the tendons, which attach the muscle to the bone.

Myofascia can be divided into three layers: superficial, middle, and deep. These categories are good to keep in mind when assessing and treating pathology, but it is also important to remember that fascia is connected and continuous throughout the body.

Fascia has a piezoelectric property that causes the fibers to release an electric charge when stress or pressure is applied to them.

There are two major pathologies that occur in the fascial network: adhesions and restrictions. Adhesions are local areas where the fascia is bound together. Tissues may be bound together by ground substance that has become sticky or by fibers that are laid down in the injury repair process.

Restrictions occur when the body gets locked into a particular position or a limb is immobile for an extended time. They can be caused by injury and a host of other causes including work, recreation, sleep habits, and emotional states.

DISCUSSION QUESTIONS

1. Explain the function of three types of cells found in fascia.
2. Compare and contrast the three types of fibers found in the extracellular matrix.
3. Why is the thixotropic nature of the ground substance important in massage therapy?
4. Explain how piezoelectricity in the fascia can be helpful and how it can contribute to pathology.
5. Explain the differences between adhesions in the ground substance and fibrous adhesions.

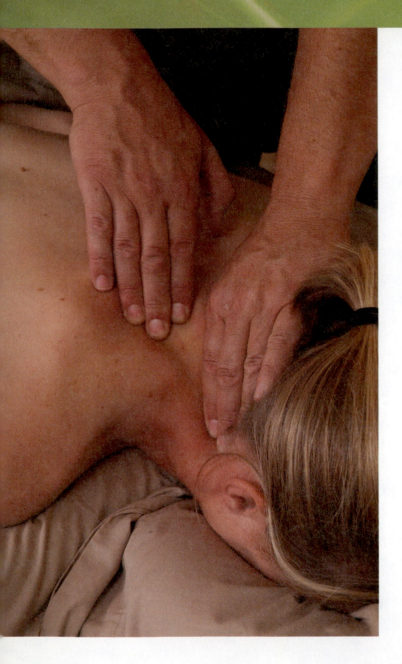

11 An Introduction to Myofascial Theory

CHAPTER HIGHLIGHTS

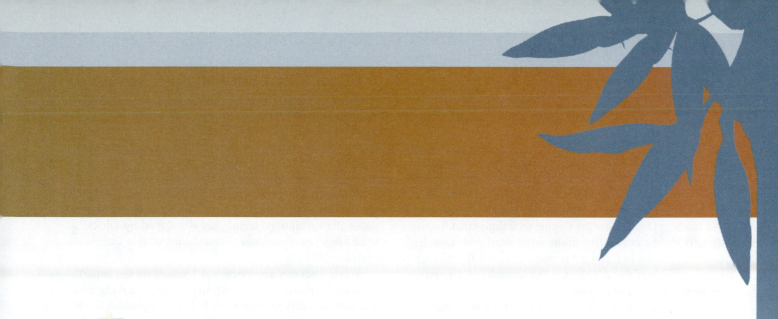

CHAPTER OBJECTIVES

- Survey the history and development of the myofascial approach
- Investigate the contributors to myofascial theories

- Explore tensegrity and its relationship to myofascial theory
- Consider the myofascial approach to resolving adhesions and restrictions

KEY TERMS

THE FUNDAMENTALS OF MYOFASCIAL THEORY

The Roots of Myofascial Treatment

The term *myofascial therapy* was not popularized until Simons, Travell, and Simons used it in their textbook, *Myofascial Pain and Dysfunction: The Trigger Point Manual* (1999). However, as early as the 1920s, physiotherapists such as Elizabeth Dickie were developing techniques that focused directly on the connective tissue associated with muscles, bones, and skin. In fact, Dickie was one of the first to focus on the pathology that develops in the specialized connective tissue we have come to know as fascia.

Dickie recognized the continuous nature of connective tissue and saw a relationship between the superficial layers and the deep layers. She was aware that internal pathology (in an organ, for example) could affect the connective tissue in the structures that surround and envelop the area. This pathology can then spread through the connective tissue web, eventually affecting the skin and muscles. Dickie and her colleagues were able to observe and map onto the body areas that they called "connective tissue zones." These zones consistently reflect pathologies of specific inner organ systems (Turchaninov, 2006; see Figure 11.1 ■).

Dickie and others went on to theorize that if internal pathology can be reflected in the superficial tissues, then treatment of the superficial tissues could work in the opposite direction. A system was developed in which the affected organ could be treated by releasing the restrictions in the superficial layers. This system came to be known as **connective tissue massage (CTM).** CTM has a complete protocol, including how to perform the strokes and in which direction the strokes must be applied for maximum results. One of the specialized techniques developed by Dickie is called *bindegewebmassage*. Some forms of this technique are still used today.

While Dickie's approach was focused on the superficial fascial structures, other physicians were looking a little deeper for this reflective pathology. Beginning in the 1930s and continuing to the 1950s, physicians such as Dr. P. Vogler and Dr. H. Krauss were researching the effects of pathology on the *periosteum* (the fascia that wraps the bone). They reached similar conclusions as Dickie. Pathology originating in an organ or other tissue can, over time, affect its surrounding connective tissue and spread along the fascial web, causing damage to other structures. They noted that the pathology spreads not only to the superficial tissues, but to the underlying connective tissue structures as well.

FIGURE 11.1

The Diagram Shows Some Examples of the Connective Tissue Zones.

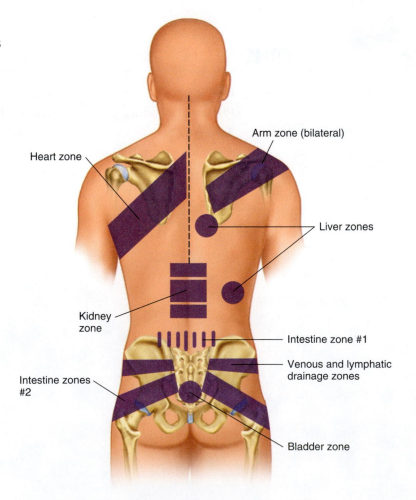

Vogler and Krauss focused on the periosteum and how it is affected through reflective pathology. Periosteum is responsible for the nutritional support and healing of bone. Treatment focused directly on it can be very powerful in the health of bone and related tissues. This is important because the periosteum is the anchor for the tendons and ligaments and can be disrupted through injury. Therefore it must be addressed during the treatment of any local injury to muscle or associated fascia. Vogler and Krauss developed a method called **periostal massage (PM).** This system applies ischemic pressure and friction techniques directly over the periosteum. The goal was to smooth out rough, bumpy areas, to realign the fibers, and promote flexibility. They theorized that treating the deepest layers of fascia would have a reflective effect on the entire system, including the internal organs (Turchaninov, 2006).

THE INFLUENCE OF SEGMENT-REFLEX MASSAGE

These earlier researchers focused on healing a variety of pathologies, but mostly on treating diseases of the internal organs. Their focus was limited to the signs of pathology as it is reflected in the fascia. Other practitioners, such as Dr. I. Z. Zabludovsky and the Russian physiotherapist Dr. A. Sherbak, recognized that *all* tissues have the capacity to reflect pathology originating in other tissues. Therefore, therapists must take into account that disease can unfold in this way. They found that the health of the entire body is both dictated by and reflected in the entire myoskeletal system (joints, bones, muscles, fascia). In fact, they argued that in order for internal structures to function efficiently, the superficial structure (i.e., myoskeletal system and skin) must be healthy, flowing, and aligned. They developed a system called segment-reflex massage that incorporated connective tissue massage, periostal massage, and other neurological concepts into a comprehensive system that attempts to address all aspects of health by aligning the body's muscles bones and joints. This system was based on the discovery of the segmented nature of nerve distribution in the body discussed in Chapter 6.

MODERN ARCHITECTS OF MYOFASCIAL THEORY

One modern researcher, Dr. John Upledger, D.O., O.M.M., was looking into how posture and the myofascial system affect the health of the central nervous system (the brain and spinal cord). In 1975, Dr. Upledger investigated an osteopathic approach called *craniosacral therapy*. Originally developed around the turn of the century by William Sutherland, D.O., this therapy focuses on gently aligning the fascia around the bones of the cranium and vertebral column (axial skeleton). Upledger theorized that when the axial skeleton is balanced, the cerebrospinal fluid flows evenly. He felt that the health of the brain and spinal cord is reliant upon healthy flow of the cerebrospinal fluid.

Upledger was also concerned with keeping the lymph system flowing. Healthy lymphatic movement is essential to the health of the tissues as well as to systems such as the immune system. Freeing the myofascial system opens the pathways for lymphatic flow (Turchaninov, 2006). John Upledger went on to found the Upledger Institute, which continues to develop and teach this unique perspective on the myofascial system.

During the 60s and 70s, other therapists, such as John Barnes, P.T., developed their own styles of myofascial therapy. John Barnes developed a very comprehensive approach to addressing the myofascial system. He combined physical therapy techniques with craniosacral therapies and traditional massage to form a technique he calls *myofascial unwinding*. Barnes' technique employs slow sustained pressure for 90 to 120 seconds to completely soften the ground substance and get full movement in the fascia.

Barnes' approach underlines the need to focus on the structure, movement, and posture of the whole body. In order to affect change in one area, therapy must address all restrictions, even those far away from the original site of injury. This is due to the continuous nature of fascia throughout the body.

Building upon the work done before him, Barnes' method is mindful of the concept that restriction in one area will almost always affect other areas. Barnes recommends doing a thorough analysis of the body, taking into account all restrictions, no matter how small and insignificant they may seem.

THE INFLUENCE OF ROLFING AND STRUCTURAL INTEGRATION

One system of body analysis and therapy called **Rolfing** has had a profound impact on the field of myofascial therapy. Originally called *structural integration*, this approach was developed by Dr. Ida Rolf in the 1950s and 60s. She was one of the first to use a holistic integrated view of the myoskeletal system. She saw posture as a dynamic interaction between the muscles, bones, and connective tissue.

Rolf used the analogy of the body as a series of blocks stacked on top of each other with myofascial "bags" holding them all together. When the blocks are out of balance, they put pressure on the myofascial bags that wrap and hold it all together. This causes tension, adhesions, and a host of other pathological responses in the myofascia. The pathology over time becomes fixed in the system. Therefore Ida Rolf emphasized assessing then working the entire myoskeletal system using a holistic method of soft tissue manipulation and movement education. Her technique involves positioning the body and using a variety of myofascial techniques designed to address all fascial structures. Rolfing realigns the body through a series of preset treatments. The primary goal is to balance the body as it resists the pull of gravity upon it. Since her death in 1979, other schools using the name *structural integration* have been formed, each one building upon Dr. Rolf's ideas. Rolfing and these other forms of structural integration are still taught in associated schools and have many enthusiastic proponents.

Recent Developments in Myofascial Theory

One of Dr. Rolf's students, Thomas Myers, has developed one of the most accessible contributions to myofascial theory. His system, described in the book, *Anatomy Trains: Myofascial*

QUICK QUIZ #21

1. Connective tissue massage was developed based on the idea that releasing pathology in the superficial layers could affect pathology of the internal organs.
   a. True
   b. False

2. Periostal massage is intended to: (Circle all that apply)
   a. affect conditions of the internal organs.
   b. align the fascia around the bones of the cranium.
   c. realign the fibers and promote the flexibility of the periosteum.
   d. All of the above
   e. None of the above

3. Craniosacral therapy is intended to: (Circle all that apply)
   a. promote the healthy flow of lymph.

   b. realign the fibers and promote the flexibility of the periosteum.
   c. promote healthy flow of the cerebrospinal fluid.
   d. align the fascia around the bones of the cranium.
   e. All of the above
   f. None of the above

4. Rolfing is mainly intended to: (Circle all that apply)
   a. align the fascia around the bones of the cranium.
   b. affect conditions of the internal organs.
   c. promote the healthy flow of lymph.
   d. realign the fibers and promote the flexibility of the periosteum.
   e. All of the above
   f. None of the above

Meridians for Manual and Movement Therapists (2001), defines an alignment of the myofascia, as it exists, functions, and moves together through the whole body.

According to conventional thinking, the body and its movements are discussed and analyzed in terms of individual *myotatic units*. The focus is only on specific movements of individual joints. This viewpoint neglects the fact that in order for one joint to move, the rest of the body must also adjust to assist that movement. Thomas Myers points out that the body moves as a whole and that almost every motion requires the participation of the entire body in order to achieve it.

For example, the simple act of lifting an arm up over the head requires the rest of the body to either stabilize or assist this movement. It's not just the muscles of the arm working. The shoulder muscles must contract to stabilize the scapula to allow the arm muscles to pull upon it. The back muscles must contract to resist the increased tension on that side of the body. In fact, if a person is standing, the legs must also be involved to help hold the body still while the arm moves. Some of these adjustments may go unnoticed because they can be quite subtle, especially those that are far away from the intended movement. They are nevertheless all critical to the proper function of lifting the arm.

Myers mapped general patterns of muscle coordination as they exist and interact from head to toe. He came up with a series of muscular interconnections, or **myofascial meridians** (see Figure 11.2 ■). These meridians show how muscles are connected as "lines of pull" through the body. The lines of pull demonstrate the way that muscles and fascia integrate with each other. Myers' ideas illustrate that myofascial structures throughout the body work together to create every movement and postural pattern.

For example, the flexors of the forearm commonly work in conjunction with the biceps of the upper arm and the pectoralis of the anterior shoulder. Anytime you bring something

to your mouth, you are using these muscle groups together. Therefore, any injury or compensation pattern in one of these muscles will often affect the others. The myofascial meridian can be seen as a line through all of these groups. Myers used this same concept and formulated meridians for groups of muscles throughout the entire body.

Myers' theory is best appreciated through understanding the concept of **tensegrity.** Tensegrity refers to the way that structures can have integrity through the combined forces of tension and compression. The term *tensegrity* was coined by Buckminster Fuller, an American architect. Fuller is famous for developing the geodesic dome and used the term *tensegrity* to describe the type of forces and pressures present in its construction. Fuller drew upon models developed by Kenneth Snelson, a popular American artist (Myers, 2001).

Snelson's models are formed by rods suspended between ropes of material, such as rubber. What is intriguing about these models is that the rods do not touch each other. The rods float in the forces of tension of the rubber bands (see Figure 11.3 ■). Fuller and Snelson unwittingly discovered one of the most important concepts in myofascial theory.

Modern researchers analyzing the structure of the body discovered that it demonstrates a geometry similar to Snelson's models. Donald E. Ingber M.D., Ph.D., a professor at Harvard University, proposed that tensegrity is the basic model for every aspect of our bodies. He states:

The principles of tensegrity apply at essentially every detectable size scale in the body. At the macroscopic level, the 206 bones that constitute our skeleton are pulled up against the force of gravity and stabilized in a vertical form by the pull of tensile muscles, tendons, and ligaments (similar to the cables in Snelson's sculptures). In other words, in the complex tensegrity structure inside

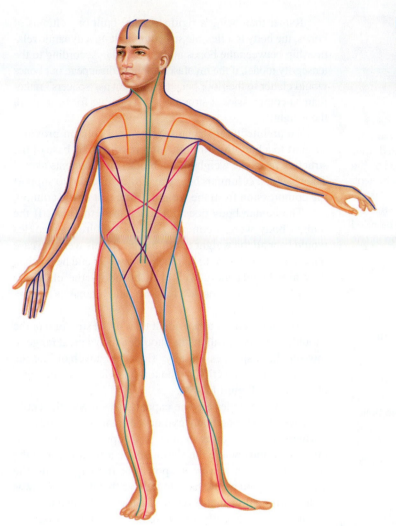

FIGURE 11.2

Myofascial Meridians Can Be Represented by Lines Running Through Interconnected Muscles.

FIGURE 11.3

One of Kenneth Snelson's Models, in Which the Rods Seem to Float Between the Tension of the Bands.

every one of us, bones are the compression struts, and muscles, tendons, and ligaments are the tension-bearing members. (Ingber, 1998, p. 50)

Essentially, the muscles and fascial structures hold the bones in place by a balanced tension between them. This is similar to Snelson's models except, in this case, the bones are the rods and the myofascia are the rubber bands. This concept contrasts with the old idea that the bones are columns that hold up the body and that the tissues simply rest and act upon them.

Rather than being a rigid structure built on columns of bones, the body is a flexible structure built on a dynamic relationship between the bones and myofascia. According to the tensegrity model, if the myofascia were to disappear, our bones would clatter to the floor because they act as "spacers" rather than as compressional structures responsible for bearing all the weight.

An architectural structure such as a column provides support to a building through compression. The base of the structure bears the weight of the blocks and elements above. The base of a column is heavy and thick in order to support the compression from the weight of the rest of the column.

The human body does not function in this way. If the human body were a compressional structure, our ankles would bear all the weight of our bodies. If this were the case our ankles would have to be much more solid and heavy than they are. In fact more weight is borne by the elaborate dynamic system of muscles, tendons, and ligaments than by the bones.

Nowhere is this more evident than in the structure of the shoulder. In order to allow the shoulder such a great range of motion, the scapula essentially "floats" in a web of muscle. Its only bony connection to the torso is via the small clavicle bone (see Figure 11.4 ■).

Yet the shoulder has the capacity to support the entire body weight. During many gymnastics maneuvers, and even during simple exercises such as push-ups, there are a variety of positions where the shoulders bear the weight of the body. If the bones were responsible for supporting the weight, then you would have to believe that the clavicle was transmitting all of that force to the torso. The clavicle is a small bone which really acts more like a strut than a weight-bearing structure. The force of the body weight is carried through the shoulder via the complex muscular arrangement that surrounds and supports the scapula. In order for the scapula to be stabilized and support the body's weight, the muscles that surround it must contract to hold it in place. The scapula, like the hub of a wheel on a mountain bike, is held in place by the tension on all sides. The weight is carried to the torso not through the bones but along the muscles and fascia.

This model of muscular reinforcement and support is repeated throughout our skeletal system. It allows our body

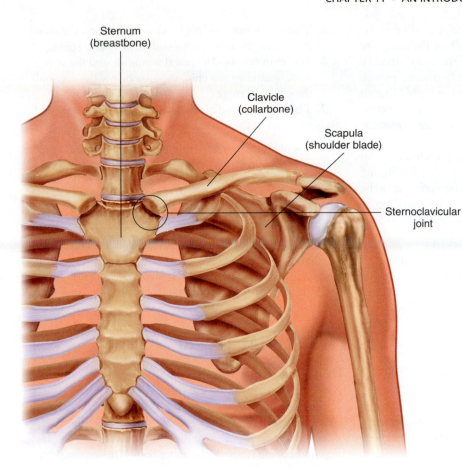

Sternum
(breastbone)

Clavicle
(collarbone)

Scapula
(shoulder blade)

Sternoclavicular
joint

FIGURE 11.4

The Articulation of the Clavicle with the Sternum Is the Only Bony Joint Connecting the Entire Shoulder Girdle to the Axial Skeleton. The Rest of the Shoulder Is Supported by Muscles.

to be flexible and adaptive. This flexibility allows the structures of the body to act like a spring—absorbing pressure and releasing it when needed. This process is seen in our ability to perform amazing physical feats as in gymnastics and martial arts.

For example, in karate, trained artists are able to break a stack of bricks with their bare hands. The flexible body is able to compress and load, then release like a spring. This generates many times the power of the muscle alone. The flexible nature of the body allows it to withstand larger impacts.

The body is occasionally subject to heavy focused blows. These may occur during accidents or during sports. If our bodies were rigid structures, those focused blows could be quite harmful. However, the body is able to absorb the impact and dissipate the energy of the blow along the flexible myofascial net. This is similar to the way a trampoline responds to the impact of a jumping person. The trampoline fabric is attached by springs on all sides. When the jumping person falls into the fabric, it stretches in all directions, therefore minimizing the focused impact of the person.

ADDITIONAL MYOFASCIAL DISCOVERIES

Another discovery about myofascial anatomy is the existence of a number of bands, or **retinacula,** that wrap the body. In their book, *The Endless Web: Fascial Anatomy and Physical Reality*, R. Louis Schultz and Rosemary Feitis describe the retinacula as "bands that we see running horizontally

---

HOLISTIC CONNECTION

The holistic tensegrity model clarifies important concepts in deep tissue massage. The principle of balanced tension and support helps explain the layering of muscles and their arrangement in reinforcing patterns. The connections between muscle layers and myotatic units are not just structural; they have to do with motion and energy. For more about the layering of myofascia, see Chapters 2–5.

around the body, almost like retaining belts holding in the soft tissue" (p. 53). They go on to discuss how the bands are "independent of the muscle anatomy of the body" (p. 53), yet seemingly run through the body like horizontal planes. These planes almost appear to segment the body "like an armadillo" (p. 53). These bands seem to perform the function of holding the muscles, viscera, and other tissues in place as the body bends and moves about.

In most individuals, there are seven major retinacula that are located in strategic areas where the body folds during forward and lateral flexion. There is some variation in the exact position of the retinacula between individuals, but in most people they are found in the following locations (see Figure 11.5 ■):

1. **The pubic band**—This band wraps the body at the level of the pubis and the lower gluteals.
2. **The inguinal band**—This band wraps the hips at the level of the anterior superior iliac spine. It wraps around the iliac crest and then runs through the back in the area of the sacroiliac joints.
3. **The umbilical band**—This band wraps around the lower torso at the level of the navel. The umbilical band may also be located superior to the navel at the level of the *costal arch*.
4. **The chest band**—This band wraps around the upper torso just below the level of nipples and the lower border of the pectoralis muscles.

5. **The collar band**—This band wraps around the shoulders along the collar bone and the scapular spine.
6. **The chin band**—This band wraps around the upper neck, including the chin, the area below the ear, and the occipital ridge.
7. **The eye band**—This band wraps around the head at the level of the eyes and the bridge of the nose.

It is important to remember the location of these bands, as they are common areas where the fascial net can become restricted. Because these bands incorporate large portions of the body, focusing therapy on them will help to release the entire net.

In addition to the larger retinacula described by Schultz and Feitus, it is important to note that there are smaller bands that wrap the elbows, knees, wrists, and ankles. These smaller retinacula are significant myofascial structures, and it is essential to investigate them any time you are addressing pathology in the limbs (see Figure 11.6 ■).

MYOFASCIAL THERAPY

Myofascial therapy seeks to achieve balance in the myoskeletal system by realigning the entire fascial net. Releasing the fascial net has both a local and a systemic effect. Locally, it releases the joint and associated myotatic unit. Because the fascia is continuous throughout the body, releasing the myofascia in any local area impacts the entire body. The tensional forces

FIGURE 11.5

The Seven Major Bands, or Retinacula

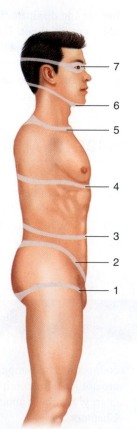
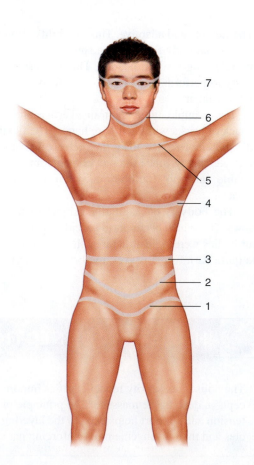

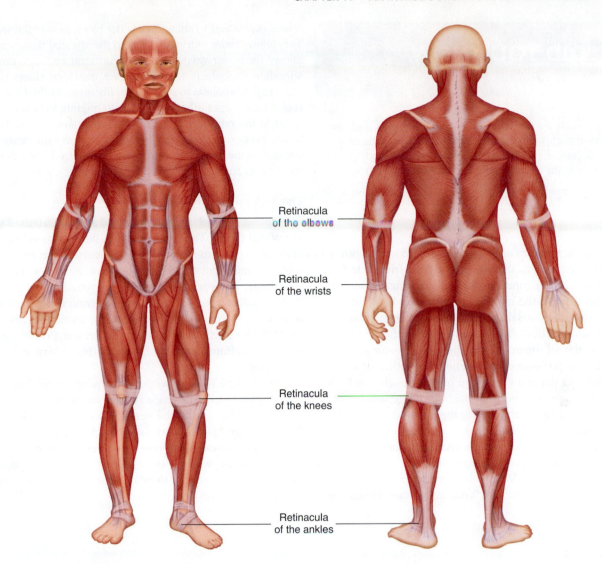

Retinacula of the elbows

Retinacula of the wrists

Retinacula of the knees

Retinacula of the ankles

FIGURE 11.6

The Smaller Retinacula That Wrap the Wrists, Elbows, Knees, and Ankles

are transmitted along the general lines of pull mapped by Myers. Understanding the myofascial meridians and the retinacula is invaluable to understanding how injury in one area can have a profound effect on another seemingly unrelated area.

Myofascial therapy (MFT) is a term used for a collection of bodywork techniques that stretch the fascial net. The focus is on releasing adhesions and restrictions in the myofascial system. The techniques have had other names such a bingewebmassage, soft tissue mobilization, and connective tissue massage. Some of these names are still used today. For the purpose of simplicity, they will all be included under the heading of "myofascial therapy" in this text. The techniques range from gentle pressure to vigorous rubbing. The type used depends on the pathology that is present.

As mentioned, MFT addresses local pathologies as well as systemic dysfunctions. To address both of these, MFT has a direct method, which includes techniques that manipulate

the fascia directly over the pathology and an indirect method that works indirectly over broader areas. Each technique allows the practitioner to address the major pathologies in the fascia. The type and scope of pathology determines which techniques are used.

The Direct Method

The direct method is focused specifically on the localized adhesions. The techniques focus on directly stretching the tissue over the adhesion or mobilizing adhesions by working directly into them. These techniques work well for fibrous adhesions as well as for adhesions in the ground substance. The main goal is to directly break down the adhesion, allowing the fibers to move more independently of each other.

One of the primary *direct methods* is called **deep fiber friction.** This technique originated in the field of osteopathy and physical therapy in the 30s and 40s. Dr. James Cyriax

DID YOU KNOW

Just like shaking the roof of a house would disturb its walls and foundation, manipulating the superficial fascia affects the deeper layers. The superficial, middle, and deep layers are connected in much the same way as the important structural components of a house.

was one of the pioneers of this technique. He was an orthopedist who emphasized the use of deep fiber friction to free the tissue and restore function. His method primarily worked across the grain of the majority of the fascial and muscle fibers. His assertion was that working across the grain exerted a greater healing effect. Interestingly, tests on the piezoelectric stimulation of the myofascia showed a greater stimulation when the pressure of the friction is applied almost at right angles to the main direction of the muscle fibers. A greater stimulation of piezoelectric discharge will have a greater effect on the fibers, causing them to align more completely (Turchaninov, 2006).

Deep fiber friction also encourages an increase in metabolism and tissue rebuilding. It does this by causing a local inflammatory response. When tissues are irritated, *histamine* is released to speed up the body's healing process. Histamine

dilates *capillaries* to encourage better blood flow to the area. This allows more nutrients to get to the affected tissues and allows for better waste removal. Furthermore, histamines stimulate fibroclasts to break down damaged fibers and encourage fibroblasts to secrete new fibers to rebuild the area. It also encourages other fibroblasts to migrate to the area to assist in the rebuilding process (Turchaninov, 2006). This whole process speeds the healing and allows the body to strengthen the weak, overstretched tissues by laying down more fibers for support (Myers, 2001).

The Indirect Method

The indirect method involves the use of a gentle stretch of the superficial fascia. The idea is to work the superficial layers of fascia in order to indirectly affect the deeper layers. Usually, the contact covers a larger area than just the local adhesive tissue. By working the larger surrounding areas, the therapy addresses any compensations spreading out from the adhesion. Indirect methods work well for restrictions involving multiple structures and postural distortions. Practitioners, such as John Barnes, make wide use of this style of myofascial therapy.

Myofascial therapy works by moving layers over the top of other layers to release restrictions between them. It treats the entire myofascial net, not just the myotatic unit. Release of myofascial restrictions can even affect the health of the organs through a release of tension in the whole fascial system. So, while it is important to treat local adhesions, it is also important to treat the net as a whole through indirect myofascial therapy.

QUICK QUIZ #22

1. Thomas Myers' concept of "anatomy trains": (Circle all that apply)
   a. focuses on specific movements of individual joints.
   b. analyzes the body and its movements in terms of individual myotatic units.
   c. recognizes that almost any movement of the body causes a response of the entire body.
   d. All of the above
   e. None of the above

2. The "myofascial meridians" demonstrate how myofascial structures operate through lines of pull within the body.
   a. True
   b. False

3. According to the tensegrity model, the bones hold the muscles and fascial structures in place within the body.
   a. True
   b. False

4. Myofascial therapy is intended to: (Circle all that apply)
   a. help the layers of fascia move independently of one another.
   b. mobilize the ground substance.
   c. increase range of motion of specific joints.
   d. change unhealthy postural patterns by releasing the fascial net.
   e. All of the above
   f. None of the above

SUMMARY

Myofascial therapy has its roots in the 1920s and 30s with a system of connective tissue massage developed by Elizabeth Dickie. Her system focused on how the connective tissue reflects disease from all over, including the internal organs. Others such as Vogler and Krauss looked at how the periosteum is affected by reflected disease from other organs and tissues. The segment-reflex massage system incorporated these ideas and combined them into a comprehensive approach that addresses pathology reflected in the entire myoskeletal system. Modern practitioners, such as John Upledger, developed myofascial approaches that focused on the flow of lymph and cerebral spinal fluid. Later practitioners, such as Ida Rolf, took up the treatment of the myofascia and developed a very comprehensive postural analysis and system of therapy called *Rolfing*. Thomas Myers, a student of Ida Rolf, developed the concept of anatomy trains. His idea describes the lines of pull called *myofascial meridians*.

Myofascial meridians are based on the concept of tensegrity. The tensegrity model proposes the importance of a dynamic constant tension of the muscles on the bones. The tension is what holds the body together and can be distorted by injury or postural distortions. Myofascial therapy attempts to correct imbalances in the myoskeletal system by addressing pathology that falls under two categories: local and systemic. It does this by using a direct method and an indirect method. The direct methods involve working the local site of injury. It stimulates an inflammatory response that encourages metabolism of the tissues. Direct friction stimulates the piezoelectric stimulation of the fibers, which enhances healing. The indirect methods focus on gently stretching larger areas of fascia to release postural distortions.

DISCUSSION QUESTIONS

1. How does myofascial theory explain that treatment of connective tissues can influence the organs and other systems?
2. Explain how the concept of *tensegrity* works within the myoskeletal system.
3. Explain the relationship between myofascial meridians and principles of movement in the body.
4. How does a local inflammatory response encourage healing?

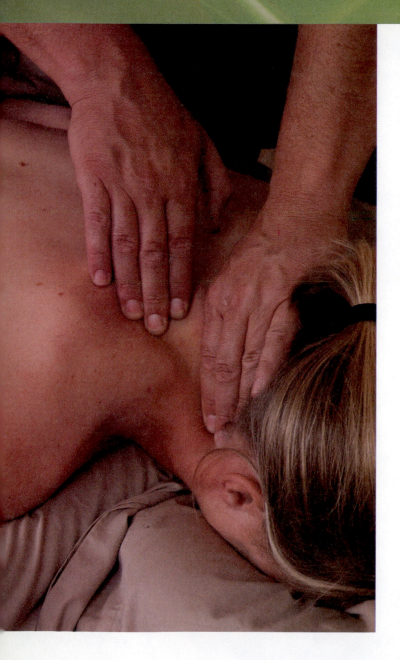

12 The Techniques of Myofascial Therapy

CHAPTER HIGHLIGHTS

Chapter Objectives
Key Terms
General Guidelines for Myofascial Therapy
The Techniques of Myofascial Therapy
Contraindications for Myofascial Therapy
Summary
Discussion Questions

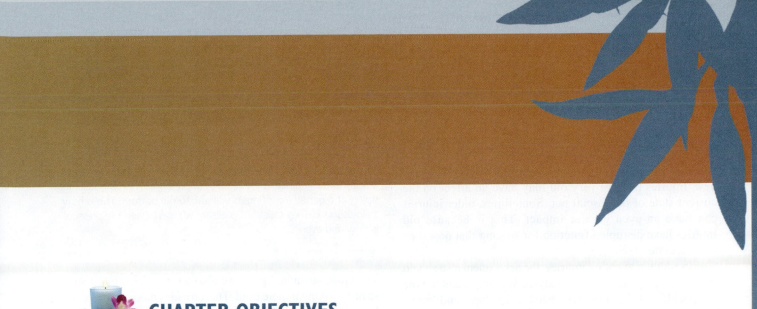

CHAPTER OBJECTIVES

- Understand general guidelines for applying myofascial therapy techniques
- Learn to apply the direct methods

- Learn to apply the indirect methods
- Recognize the contraindications to myofascial therapy

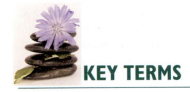

KEY TERMS

GENERAL GUIDELINES FOR MYOFASCIAL THERAPY

Assessment

Myofascial therapy, like all forms of massage, requires that a comprehensive history and assessment be taken prior to performing the techniques. The history should note all damage or disturbances to the myofascial net, both old and new. Injuries that are very old may have an affect on the current state of the fascial net. Sometimes, older injuries can have an even greater impact. This is because old injuries have disrupted function for so long that now they have become fixed.

In addition to noting injuries, the assessment also should include a complete postural analysis. It is important to note the position of the shoulders, head, neck, hips, and knees. Perform postural analysis while keeping in mind myofascial theories, such as myofascial meridians and the locations of retinacula.

Observation is only part of the analysis. It is important to palpate the tissues looking for any restrictions in the muscles as well as between the muscles and other structures (such as the skin and joint capsule). Areas of restriction may be cooler than the surrounding tissue. This is due to lack of circulation. It is also a good idea to look at the health of the skin, as it may point to pathology below the skin affecting its health. The history and assessment will help focus the therapy and will also highlight any contraindications.

No Lubricant

The goal of myofascial therapy is to stretch and free the layers of fascia. In order to do this, you must move the skin. Moving the skin pulls on the deeper layers of fascia due to the continuity of the fascial net. Unlike many forms of massage where the contact point glides over the skin, in myofascial therapy you must have a good grip on the skin's surface in order to move it. To create and maintain the grip, do not use lubricant before or during the application of the techniques. If the skin is moist and slippery, or lubricant was already used, you can put a cloth between your hands and the client. This is kind of like using a towel to improve your grip on the tight lid of a jar. The cloth will grip the skin of your hands as well as the client's skin. The sheet used for draping may also be used to create the proper grip.

Be Patient

Myofascial work requires patience. The fascia responds better to slow sustained pressure and tends to resist fast, forceful movements. One reason for this is the nature of the colloids found in the ground substance. A unique property of colloids is that they will resist abrupt pressure. However, when the pressure is slow and sustained, they will yield and move, allowing the therapy to work deeper into the tissues.

DID YOU KNOW

Explore the nature of colloids. Fill one-half of a small bowl with cornstarch, and add water to make a thin paste. Push your fingers quickly into the paste. It will resist your pressure. Then try pushing slowly and gently. Your fingers will sink to the bottom. This is how colloids work. They resist fast pressure yet yield when the pressure is slow and even.

The slow, sustained pressure also warms the ground substance, making it more fluid. This provides more room for the fascial fibers to stretch and move.

Fascial restrictions, especially scars, can be very painful. Moving into these tissues too quickly will increase the incidence of guarding during therapy. Use slow, sustained pressure to help prevent guarding. When you ease into the tissues and move slowly, the client will be able to relax and allow the pressure. Instruct the client to breathe out on the pressure, because breathing out relaxes the rib cage which helps the whole body relax. Breathing can also act as a simple distraction. When clients are paying attention to their breathing, they are less attentive to their soreness and/or pathology.

Maintain Focus

Myofascial work requires focus. Focusing your complete attention on the tissues is extremely important, as changes in the fascial layers can be very subtle. This is because of the netlike structure of fascia. Think about stretching out a fishing net that has shrunk up a little. When stretching a net, the movement happens in many directions. Some fibers may release before some of the others. Often it will stretch in multiple directions at once. The fascial net responds the same way. When pressure is applied, the net will begin to release. The fibers that are less adhered will release first. Pay close attention to the directions in which the fascia is releasing, and follow those movements with your pressure. Then come back and work in opposite directions and at right angles to get at the more restricted areas.

Work in Many Directions

Remember that, unlike muscles—which run from origin to insertion—fascia's fibers run in many different directions. Therefore, it is important to apply each technique in multiple directions. This helps stretch the entire fabric and to create space between all of the fibers. Think of a shirt that may be too tight. The shirt squeezes your body in all directions. In order to loosen the shirt, you must stretch it in all directions.

Warm the Tissues Thoroughly

All myofascial therapy techniques require a thorough warm-up. The thixotropic nature of the ground substance in fascia means that it will be much more pliable when it is warm. Warming up the tissues before applying heavier pressure also helps to minimize discomfort to the client. Some techniques, such as skin rolling (described below) can be somewhat uncomfortable. When the tissues are warmer, there will be less resistance in the fibers and the client will not be inclined to resist the therapy.

Use Proper Body Mechanics

Finally, it is important to maintain proper body mechanics throughout the application of myofascial techniques. Weight and leverage should be used to apply pressure. This will save wear and tear on your body and uses energy more efficiently. Refer to Chapter 4 for more on proper body mechanics.

THE TECHNIQUES OF MYOFASCIAL THERAPY

The Direct Methods

The **direct methods** are applied right over the pathology. They are designed to break apart fibrous adhesions as well as adhesions in the ground substance. This is done by mechanically separating the fibers and by causing inflammation in the area of the adhesion. Remember it is the local inflammation that stimulates the body's natural breakdown and rebuilding response. Because of the local inflammatory response, it is important to keep the therapy focused directly over the adhesion. This will limit any potential irritation to the surrounding healthy tissues. If too much of the area is irritated, it will be harder for the body to heal the original injured area.

There are two direct methods presented here. The first technique, called the *direct stretch technique,* is designed to slowly sink into the restricted fascia, then push the fibers in multiple directions. The second technique, called *deep fiber friction*, employs a grinding motion that slowly works down through the layers of the fascia. This can be an invasive technique and causes the most local inflammation. In either technique, the pressure is placed right over the adhesion with the intention of separating the fibers and breaking apart the glued tissues.

DIRECT STRETCH TECHNIQUE

- **Direction of stroke:** Multiple directions
- **Contact point:** Palms, knuckles, elbows
- **Physical description:** Using the palms, knuckles, or elbow, sink into the tissues until the restricted layer is contacted (see Figures 12.1 ■ through 12.3 ■). Without gliding over the surface, push into the tissue so that the skin and the superficial fascia slightly move in the direction of your choice. It is important that you stay "glued" to the skin's surface, essentially pushing a fold in a particular direction, but not sliding in the surface at

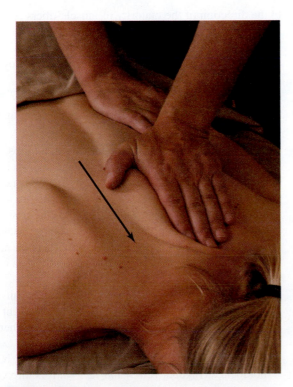

FIGURE 12.1

The Position of the Hand and the Direction of Movement for Applying the Direct Stretch Technique with the Palm

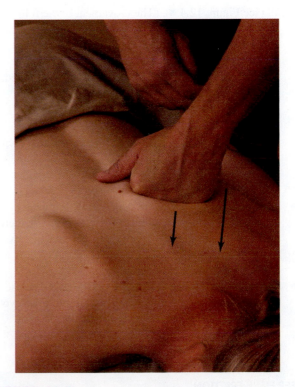

FIGURE 12.2

The Position of the Hand and the Direction of Movement for Applying the Direct Stretch Technique with the Knuckles

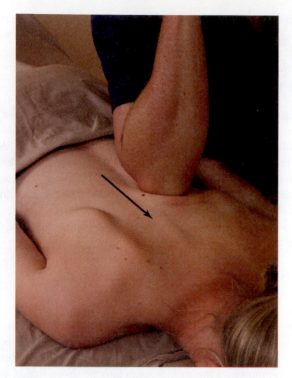

FIGURE 12.3

The Position of the Arm and the Direction of Movement for Applying the Direct Stretch Technique with the Elbow

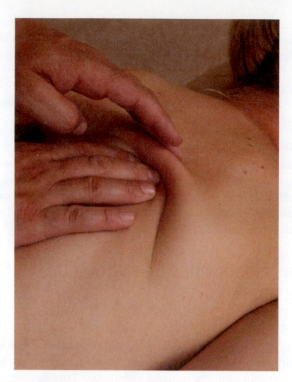

FIGURE 12.4

The Fingers Must Engage the Skin to Push a Fold in the Direction of the Stroke.

all (see Figure 12.4 ■). (The movement of the fold will be minimal.) Hold the position for 3 to 5 seconds, then release the tissues. Repeat in multiple directions.

○ When using the palms or knuckles, you should hold the elbows relatively straight but not locked. It is important that the arms stay rigid enough to transfer the weight of your body into the client (Figures 12.1 and 12.2).

○ When using the elbows as the contact point, keep the shoulder firm and lowered to transfer your weight into the client (Figure 12.3). Avoid raising your shoulders toward your ears.

● **Common areas of use:** This is a relatively gentle technique, therefore it can be applied anywhere there are local restrictions. It is good for sensitive clients and sensitive skin areas, such as the inside of the upper arms and upper legs.

● **Special considerations:** In less muscular areas, use your palms for contact. You can even use one or two fingers in small shallow areas such as the face. In thicker, more muscular areas, use the elbows and knuckles.

DEEP FIBER FRICTION

● **Direction of stroke:** Deep fiber friction can be applied using the familiar cross-fiber and lengthwise strokes. Cross-fiber strokes are applied at right angles

to the direction of the majority of muscle fibers (see Figure 12.5 ■), and lengthwise strokes are applied along the grain with the majority of muscle fibers (see Figure 12.6 ■). You may also choose to employ **circular strokes,** where the stroke is applied in a circular motion over the adhesion (see Figure 12.7 ■).

● **Contact point:** The fingertips, knuckles, elbows, and thumbs (see Figures 12.8 through 12.11 ■)

● **Physical description:** Using the fingertips, thumbs, knuckles, or elbows, press down to engage the fascia, and move back and forth in the desired direction (i.e., cross-fiber, lengthwise, circular) several times (up to a minute in duration). This essentially grinds the tissue between your contact point and the bone below. Make sure the contact point is glued to the skin's surface and that the skin moves with you. Repeat several times in multiple directions.

○ Using the fingertips and knuckles, it is important that the bones of the fingers are relatively straight (the finger bones should be in line with each other). The wrist should be in a relatively straight line with the fingers. The elbows should be straight, but not locked (Figures 12.8 ■ and 12.9 ■). It is important that the arms stay rigid enough to transfer the weight of your body into the client.

○ When using the thumb it is best to hold it tight to your fist for support (Figure 12.10 ■).

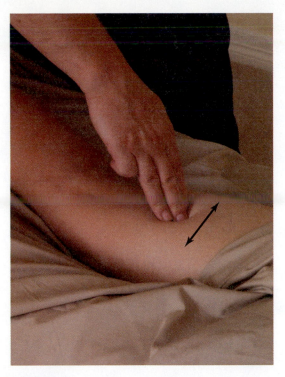

FIGURE 12.5

The Arrow Indicates the Direction of Movement for Applying Deep Fiber Friction Across the Grain of the Majority of Muscle Fibers on the Posterior Leg.

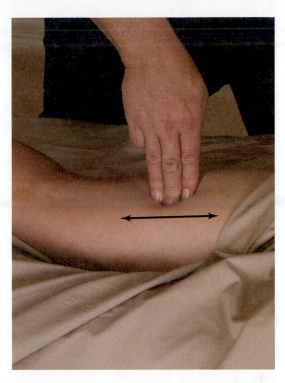

FIGURE 12.6

The Arrow Indicates the Direction of Movement for Applying Deep Fiber Friction with the Grain of the Majority of Muscle Fibers on the Posterior Leg.

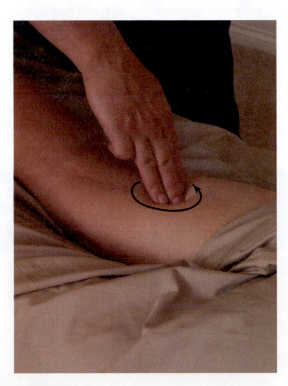

FIGURE 12.7

The Arrow Indicates the Direction of Movement for Applying Deep Fiber Friction in a Circular Motion on the Posterior Leg.

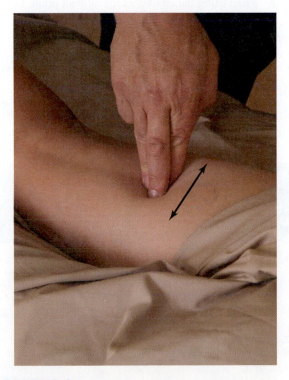

FIGURE 12.8

The Arrow Indicates the Direction of Stroke and the Application of Deep Fiber Friction Using the Finger Tips.

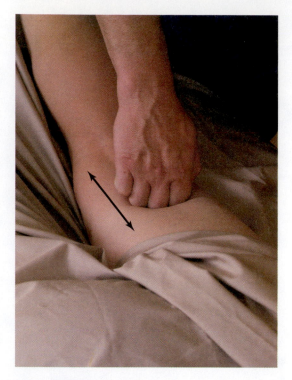

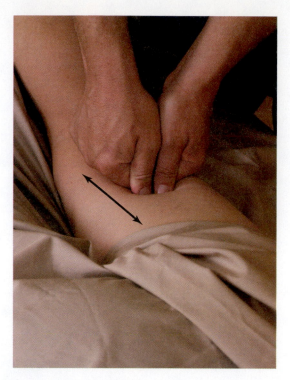

FIGURE 12.9

The Arrow Indicates the Direction of Stroke for the Application of Deep Fiber Friction Using the Knuckles.

FIGURE 12.10

The Arrow Indicates the Direction of Stroke for the Application of Deep Fiber Friction Using the Thumbs.

○ When using the elbows as the contact point, keep the shoulder firm and low to transfer your weight into the client (Figure 12.10). Avoid raising your shoulders toward your ears.

● **Common areas of use:** This technique is used for all adhesions and is especially effective on entrenched fibrous adhesions (scars). It can be used anywhere these are found. The pressure should be varied depending on the area being treated and the

depth of the adhesion. Thinner, less muscular areas require less pressure than thicker areas with more muscle.

● **Special considerations:** This technique causes the most inflammation and should be focused on the site of adhesions only. Use friction judiciously because of the level of inflammation it can cause. The body can only manage so much before the inflammation becomes problematic in and of itself.

QUICK QUIZ #23

1. In order to have a good grip on the skin, plenty of lubrication should be used when performing myofascial therapy techniques.
   a. True
   b. False

2. Just like muscle fibers, the fibers of the fascia run from origin to insertion.
   a. True
   b. False

3. Deep fiber friction: (Circle all that apply)
   a. is a relatively gentle technique.

   b. is good for sensitive areas such as the inside of the arms.
   c. is especially effective on scars.
   d. All of the above
   e. None of the above

4. The direct stretch technique:
   a. can cause significant inflammation as part of the healing effect.
   b. is especially effective on scars.
   c. is designed to push the fascial fibers in multiple directions.

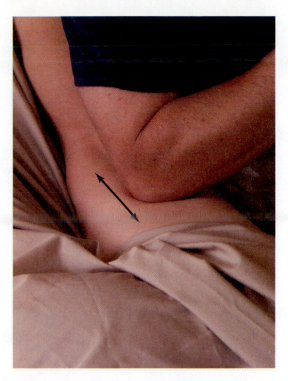

FIGURE 12.11

The Arrow Indicates the Direction of Stroke for the Application of Deep Fiber Friction Using the Elbows.

The Indirect Methods

The **indirect methods** work the superficial layers of fascia in order to indirectly affect the deeper layers. Usually the contact covers a larger area than just the local adhesive tissue. By working the larger surrounding areas, you will be sure to address any compensations spreading out from the adhesion. This technique works well for restrictions involving multiple structures and for systemic postural distortions.

The technique is to engage the superficial layer and slowly apply pressure in opposite directions. This will effectively stretch the tissues underneath. The hands are allowed to gently travel with the fascia letting it "unwind" itself. It can be especially difficult to feel the fascial release when performing the indirect methods because these methods use

pressure applied over a larger distance, which can make it harder to feel the movement. The gentle traction stretches the fibers and also increases blood flow in the tissues.

When treating indirectly, work on as large an area as possible. Remember that the fascia is a continuous structure, and restrictions in one area affect other adjacent areas. So, in addition to working the affected tissues:

- Work above the pathology
- Work below the pathology
- Work to the left of the pathology
- Work to the right of the pathology

Using this simple strategy will ensure that the net is released sufficiently around the pathology and that associated compensations are also addressed. Because the indirect methods are designed to treat a broader area, the strokes are often applied in many different directions.

Whenever possible, it is important to treat the entire body, as compensation can spread throughout. If the rest of the body is overlooked, the untreated compensations will, over time, cause their own restrictions and new patterns of pathology.

STANDARD RELEASE

- **Direction of stroke:** Multiple directions
- **Contact point:** Palms, knuckles, fingers, and forearms (see Figures 12.12 ■ through 12.15 ■)
- **Physical description:** Position yourself so you are ready to push in opposite directions. Make contact with the client using the palms, knuckles, fingers, or forearms. Apply a slight pressure down into the client to engage the fascia, while simultaneously applying a greater pressure to push the skin in opposite directions (see Figures 12.12 through 12.15 to see the direction of pressure and position for various body parts). Like most myofascial techniques, the contact point is glued to the surface of the skin. As the fascia releases, there may be some movement. It will feel as though your hands are slowly sliding. When this occurs, allow your hands to move with the stretching of the skin. Resist the urge to let your hands glide over the skin's surface by staying engaged with the skin and subcutaneous fascia. Like a

 HOLISTIC CONNECTION

Tellington-touch (T-touch) is a subtle form of bodywork which incorporates the idea of working broad areas of the body. Linda Tellington-Jones originally developed the system for work with sensitive animals, but it is now widely used with people as well. The hallmark of the method is its use of very light, circular touches that are usually applied in a variable and random pattern on the skin's surface. T-touch engages the nervous system through working skin and myofascia. It activates an awareness of the interconnectedness of the whole body. Explore T-touch as a tool for awakening whole-body awareness in your clients.

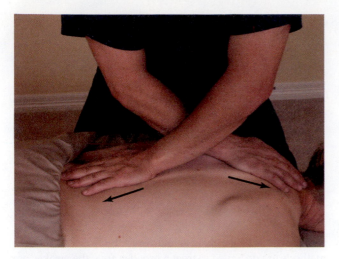

FIGURE 12.12

The Hands Are Crossed to Apply Pressure in Opposite Directions While Performing the Standard Release Technique with the Palms.

net, the superficial layers may stretch in many directions, as the patterns of fascia will vary. Follow the stretch for 2 to 10 minutes, allowing your hands to move in the direction that the fascia releases. Repeat the entire procedure in as many directions as possible.

○ When using the palms and knuckles, it is easier to cross your hands to apply the pressure (Figures 12.12 and 12.13). Your elbows should be slightly bent but held firmly when using the hands to make contact. It is important that the arms and shoulders stay rigid enough to transfer the weight of your body into the client. (When using forearms, keep the shoulders down and the wrists and hands relaxed.)

● **Common areas of use:** This is a gentle technique, so it can be applied to any area where there is a restriction.

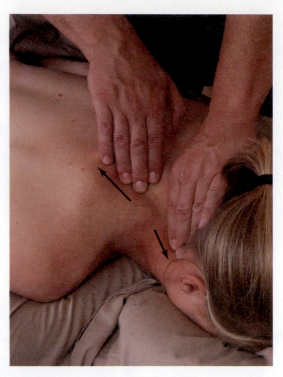

FIGURE 12.14

The Arrows Indicate the Opposite Directions of Pressure Used While Applying the Standard Release Technique with the Fingers.

It works very well across joints to release contracture and in large areas such as the back and legs.

● **Special considerations:** In addition to being very gentle, this technique is very versatile. It can be applied virtually anywhere. In small areas such as the face, the technique can be applied with one or two fingers. Large areas can be treated with the forearms and palms.

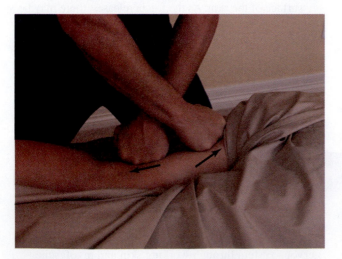

FIGURE 12.13

The Hands Are Crossed to Apply Pressure in Opposite Directions While Performing the Standard Release Technique with the Knuckles.

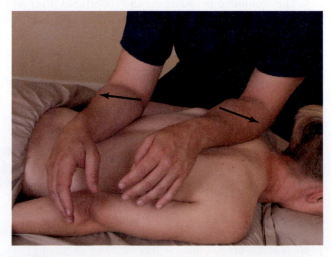

FIGURE 12.15

The Arrows Indicate the Opposite Directions of Pressure Used While Applying the Standard Release Technique with the Forearms.

TORQUING

- **Direction of stroke:** Multiple directions
- **Contact point:** Palms, knuckles, and forearms (see Figures 12.17 ■ through 12.19 ■)
- **Physical description:** Apply a slight downward and opposite pressure to engage the fascia. Then proceed to torque the fascia by twisting both hands in opposite directions (see Figures 12.16 ■ through 12.18 to see the direction of pressure and the hand positions on various body parts). You will see a twisting effect on the surface of the skin. Hold the position for 30 seconds to 2 minutes. Repeat several times in multiple directions. This technique is similar to the standard release in that the contact point is used to apply pressure in opposite directions. However, a twist is added to the contact point to give something of a wringing action. This is helpful on more entrenched restrictions.
  - When using the knuckles, it is important to keep the bones of the hand relatively straight and the wrist in a relatively straight line with the hand. The elbows should be straight but not locked. It is important that the arms stay rigid enough to transfer the weight of your body into the client.
- **Common areas of use:** Like the standard release, this technique can be used most anywhere on the body. Torquing is particularly effective when working around curves, such as the sides of the body and limbs.

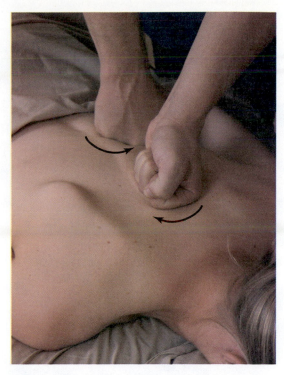

FIGURE 12.17

The Arrows Show the Opposite and Twisting Pressure Applied with the Knuckles to Perform the Torquing Technique.

- **Special considerations:** This technique is slightly more intense than the standard release. Therefore, areas with sensitive skin, such as the inner thighs, should be approached with care.

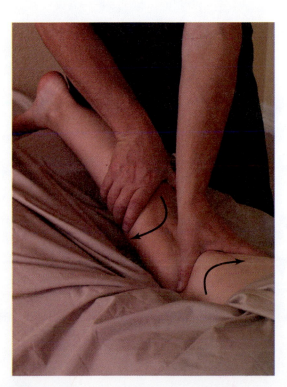

FIGURE 12.16

The Arrows Show the Opposite and Twisting Pressure Applied with the Palms to Perform the Torquing Technique.

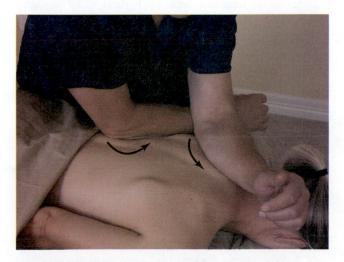

FIGURE 12.18

The Arrows Show the Opposite and Twisting Pressure Applied with the Forearms to Perform the Torquing Technique.

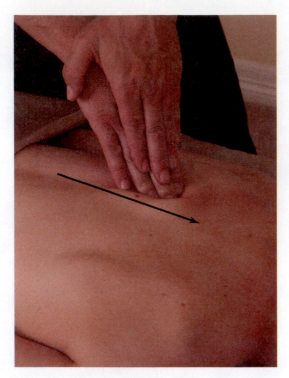

FIGURE 12.19

The Direction of Pressure and the Hand Positions for Using the Fingers During the Application of the Skin Pushing Technique

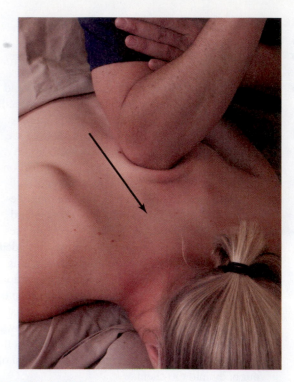

FIGURE 12.20

The Direction of Pressure and the Arm Position for Using the Elbow During the Application of the Skin Pushing Technique

SKIN PUSHING

- **Direction of stroke:** Multiple directions
- **Contact point:** The fingertips, elbows, and knuckles
- **Physical description:** Choose a contact point, and apply a slight downward and forward pressure to engage the fascia while pushing up a fold of tissue. Push the fold of tissue away from you like a "wave" across the treatment area (see Figures 12.19 through 12.21 ■ to see the direction of the stroke). The key is to move along the skin's surface, pushing up the fold as you go. Repeat in several directions.
  - ○ When using the fingertips, contact is made using the four fingers of one hand, while the four fingers of the other hand are placed on top of the first. This adds stability to the treating hand and decreases fatigue. It is important that the bones of the fingers are in a relatively straight line and the wrist is in line with the fingers. The elbows should be straight but not locked. It is important that the arms stay rigid enough to transfer the weight of your body into the client (Figure 12.19).
  - ○ When using the elbows to contact the client, keep the shoulders low and firm (Figure 12.20).
  - ○ When using the knuckles, keep them in a relatively straight line with the wrist. The elbows should be straight but not locked. It is important that the arms stay rigid enough to transfer the weight of your body into the client (Figure 12.21).

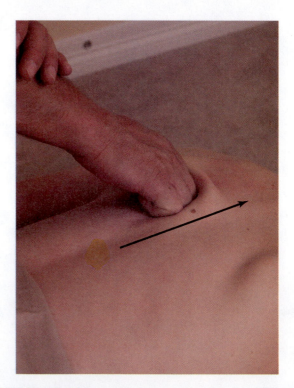

FIGURE 12.21

The Direction of Pressure and the Hand Positions for Using the Knuckles During the Application of the Skin Pushing Technique

- **Common areas of use:** This is a relatively gentle technique, and it uses a variety of contact points. Therefore, it can be applied virtually anywhere on the body. In the deeper, more muscular areas, use the knuckles and elbows. Fingers can be used in the shallower and/or more sensitive areas.
- **Special considerations:** The skin pushing technique is very similar to the skin dragging technique described below. The technique chosen depends on the how the tissues accept the pressure. Skin pushing tends to be a bit deeper and can be harder to perform on less muscular areas or other softer tissue areas like the inside of the upper arms.

   The client will often report a scratching feeling or an uncomfortable pinching feeling as the technique is applied. This is due to the fascial fibers separating. While this is relatively normal, it is advised to be careful on sensitive areas, such as the insides of the arms and the inner thighs.

SKIN DRAGGING

- **Direction of stroke:** Multiple directions
- **Contact point:** The fingertips, elbows, and knuckles
- **Physical description:** Choose a contact point, and apply a slight downward and backward pressure to engage the fascia while pulling back a fold of tissue. Drag the fold of tissue toward you like a "wave" across the treatment area (see Figures 12.22 ■ through 12.24 ■ to see the

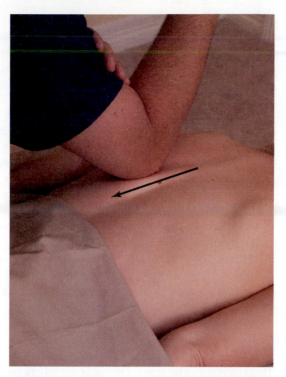

FIGURE 12.23

The Direction of Pressure and the Arm Position for Using the Elbow During the Application of the Skin Dragging Technique

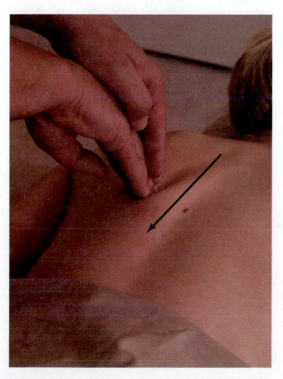

FIGURE 12.22

The Direction of Pressure and the Hand Positions for Using the Fingers During the Application of the Skin Dragging Technique

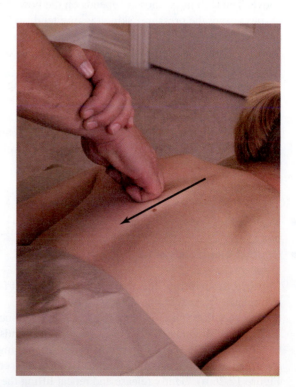

FIGURE 12.24

The Direction of Pressure and the Hand Positions for Using the Knuckles During the Application of the Skin Dragging Technique

direction of the stroke). The key is to move along the skin's surface, dragging the fold as you go. Repeat in several directions.

- ○ When using the fingertips, contact is made using the four fingers of one hand, while the four fingers of the other hand are placed on top of the first. This adds stability to the treating hand and decreases fatigue. It is important that the bones of the fingers are in a relatively straight line and the wrist is in line with the fingers. The elbows should be straight but not locked. It is important that the arms stay rigid enough to transfer the weight of your body into the client (Figure 12.22).
- ○ When using the elbows to contact the client, keep the shoulders low and firm (Figure 12.23).
- ○ When using the knuckles, keep them in a relatively straight line with the wrist. The elbows should be straight but not locked. It is important that the arms stay rigid enough to transfer the weight of your body into the client (Figure 12.24).

- **Common areas of use:** This is a relatively gentle technique, and it uses a variety of contact points. Therefore, it can be applied virtually anywhere on the body. In the deeper, more muscular areas, use the knuckles and elbows. Fingers can be used in the shallower and/or more sensitive areas.

- **Special considerations:** The skin dragging technique is very similar to the skin pushing technique described above. The technique chosen depends on the how the tissues accept the pressure. Skin dragging tends to be a bit lighter, so it may be better to use on less muscular areas or other softer tissue areas like the inside of the upper arms.

   The client will often report a scratching feeling or an uncomfortable pinching feeling as the technique is applied. This is due to the fascial fibers separating. While this is relatively normal, it is advised to be careful on sensitive areas, such as the insides of the arms and the inner thighs.

FASCIAL LIFT

- **Direction of stroke:** Lifting the tissues away from the body
- **Contact point:** Pads of fingers, the fingertips, and thumbs
- **Physical description:** It is important that the wrist is in a relatively straight line with the fingers. The elbows should be slightly bent. Grasp a fold of tissue between the fingers and thumbs of one or both hands (see Figure 12.25 ■). Gently lift the tissue up, pulling towards the ceiling, and hold for 5 to 10 seconds (see Figure 12.26 ■). Gently release and repeat lifting the fold of tissue in multiple different directions. Variation: Upon lifting the tissues, you may gently twist, move, or shake the fold.

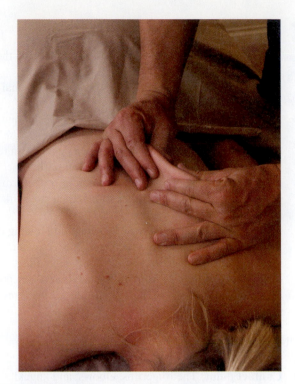

FIGURE 12.25

The Hand Positions for Grasping a Fold of Skin During the Fascial Lift Technique

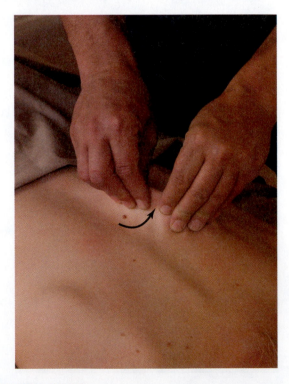

FIGURE 12.26

The Arrow Indicates the Lifting of the Skin During the Fascial Lift Technique

- **Common areas of use:** This technique may be applied anywhere a sufficient fold can be obtained. It is great for the fascia over joints, especially over the vertebral column. In those places the fascia can get tacked or glued down to the bone. Lifting the fascia up releases that bond.
- **Special considerations:** This is a relatively gentle technique and can be used throughout the body. It is especially useful over joints, including the spinal column (see Figure 12.27 ■). Sometimes the fascia is too tight or "glued down" to grasp a fold. This can be caused by adhesions or other factors such as excess adipose in the subcutaneous tissues. In this case other methods such as the standard release may be used to release the tissues first.

SKIN ROLLING

- **Direction of stroke:** Multiple directions
- **Contact point:** Pads of fingers, the fingertips, and thumbs
- **Physical description:** Skin rolling is a variation on the fascial lift that includes movement. It is important that the wrist is in a relatively straight line with the fingers. The elbows should be slightly bent. Grasp a fold of tissue between the thumbs and fingers, placing the hands close together (see Figure 12.28 ■). While maintaining a grip on the fold, "roll" the skin between your thumbs and fingers. The fingers "scoop up" new

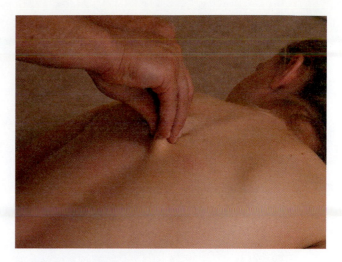

FIGURE 12.28

The Hand Position Used for Grasping a Fold of Skin to Perform Skin Rolling

skin and the thumbs "feed" it through in a continuous rolling motion. The rolling motion is used to move the hands across the area (see Figure 12.29 ■). Continue moving along in this fashion until you have covered the affected area. Repeat several times in multiple directions.

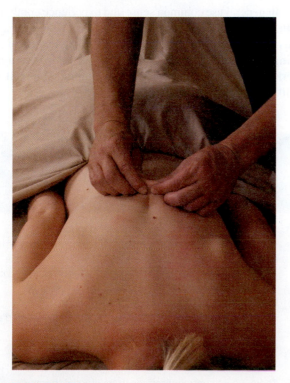

FIGURE 12.27

The Position Used to Perform the Fascial Lift Over the Vertebral Column

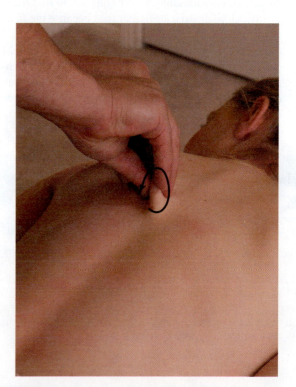

FIGURE 12.29

The Arrow Indicates the Finger Movement Used to Create the "Rolling" Motion During the Performance of Skin Rolling.

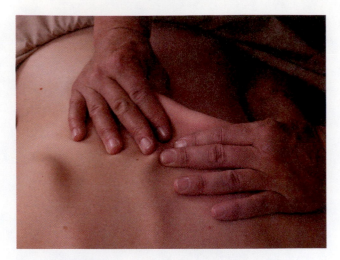

FIGURE 12.30

An Alternate Hand Position May Be Used to Grasp a Fold of Skin to Perform Skin Rolling.

- **Common areas of use:** Skin rolling can be performed anywhere a sufficient fold of skin can be lifted off of the surface of the body.
- **Special considerations:** Sometimes it is easier to grasp and roll the skin with the hands aligned so the fingers point toward each other and the fingertips of either hand are touching (see Figure 12.30 ■). Often it is difficult to grasp a sufficient fold because the fascia is too tight in a particular area. In this case, other methods can be used to release the fascia until a fold can be maintained. Like the drag and push, this technique can be uncomfortable for the client, therefore caution is recommended for sensitive skin and sensitive clients. Be sure the tissues are adequately warmed

up to minimize this possible reaction. If skin rolling is too uncomfortable for the client, the fascial lift may be indicated, as it is a gentler technique.

CONTRAINDICATIONS FOR MYOFASCIAL THERAPY

Myofascial therapy is a form of bodywork that uses a wide range of techniques. Some techniques are very gentle (such as the indirect methods), and some forms can be more intense (such as deep fiber friction). The contraindications will depend upon which technique is being used. Techniques such as deep fiber friction and skin rolling tend to apply a good deal of pressure to the small superficial blood vessels. Therefore, clients taking anticoagulant therapy (blood thinners or aspirin therapy) may be especially susceptible to severe bruising. Skin rolling is also contraindicated for those patients with thin, parchment-type skin (e.g., the elderly) because the therapy may tear the dry, brittle tissue.

Other techniques, such as the standard release, are very gentle, and the contraindications fall under the general common contraindications for all massage. These may include:

- Rashes
- Open wounds
- Recent injuries
- Infections

In general use common sense and experience combined with a sound knowledge of the basics of massage therapy. This should guide the therapy toward healing and not damaging the tissues. Generally speaking, as long as you are working below the client's pain threshold, you will be unlikely to do any harm.

QUICK QUIZ #24

1. The standard release is a very gentle technique and is very effective when used over areas of contracture.
   a. True
   b. False

2. Torquing is similar to the standard release technique in that they both use a twisting motion.
   a. True
   b. False

3. The drag and push technique is a relatively gentle technique, so it can be used without concern on areas of sensitive skin, such as the insides of the arms.
   a. True
   b. False

4. If you have trouble grasping a fold of skin for the skin rolling technique or for the fascial lift technique, you should: (Circle all that apply)
   a. use a different method to release the fascia to the point where a fold can be grasped.
   b. use more lubrication.
   c. ensure that the tissues have been adequately warmed up prior to using the method.
   d. All of the above
   e. None of the above

5. There are no contraindications to myofascial therapy techniques.
   a. True
   b. False

SUMMARY

Myofascial therapy requires focus and patience. The strokes are applied in a slow manner, allowing the tissues to move gently and completely. This also reduces discomfort to the client during therapy. Fascia is a continuous net, so it is important to work in multiple directions. No lubricant is used during treatment. It is very important to properly warm the tissues before therapy.

There are two categories of techniques: direct and indirect. The direct methods are applied directly over the pathology. The direct stretch technique is a gentle technique that can be used over local restrictions. Deep fiber friction is designed to break up adhesions and scars. It tends to cause some inflammation and should only be used directly over the site of adhesion.

The indirect methods generally contact a larger area. By working the larger surrounding areas, these techniques address compensations associated with the local areas of adhesion. The standard release is the most gentle technique and can be applied to any area where there is a restriction. It works very well across joints to release contracture. Torquing is a similar method which adds a twist to the pressure. It can be used almost anywhere and is slightly more intensive than the standard release.

This subset also includes the two moving techniques, skin dragging and skin pushing, which employ a deep glide. The fascial lift and its variant, skin rolling, round out this set.

The contraindications for MFR vary, depending on which techniques are used. Be sure to use the client history as a guide for appropriate therapy. Also, be sure to work below the client's pain threshold.

DISCUSSION QUESTIONS

1. Why is it important to apply myofascial techniques slowly with sustained pressure?
2. Why is it important to apply myofascial techniques in multiple directions?
3. What techniques may be used if it is difficult to grasp a fold of skin when applying the fascial lift or skin rolling techniques?

13 Sample Protocols for Myofascial Therapy

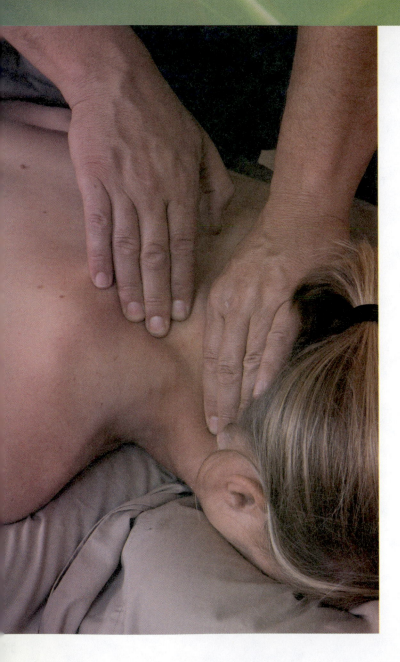

 CHAPTER HIGHLIGHTS

Chapter Objectives

Key Terms

Application of the Techniques

Sample Protocols

Summary

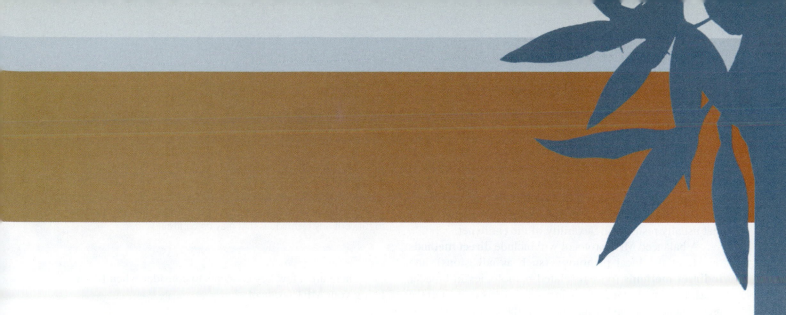

CHAPTER OBJECTIVES

- Understand how to combine the techniques of myofascial therapy
- Explore sample myofascial protocols for various body parts

- Rehearse assessment skills and practice myofascial techniques

KEY TERMS

Myofascial net 240

Direct methods 240

Indirect methods 240

Retinacula 240

Myofascial meridians 240

APPLICATION OF THE TECHNIQUES

The techniques of myofascial therapy (MFT) are designed to treat one of the largest and most complex systems in the entire body. The **myofascial net** is a web of specialized bands, sheaths, and netting that surrounds, supports, and separates all tissues of the body. Its structure is multidirectional and contains various levels of rigidity, tension, and thickness. When damaged, a variety of specific pathologies occur that usually restrict the flexibility of the entire net.

A balanced MFT protocol will include **direct methods** that treat the local pathology (such as adhesions), and **indirect methods** to treat related pathologies in broader areas. It is important to work in all directions as well as the recommended direction for applying the indirect methods. The recommended directions are based on the strokes of the connective tissue massage (CTM) tradition. These are particularly effective for treating the pathologies harbored by the **retinacula** (bands of fascia) described by Schultz and Feitis (1996). It is also helpful to use Thomas Myers' (2001) **myofascial meridians** ("lines of pull" among myofascial structures) as a frame of reference for your myofascial treatment strategy in each area of the body. If pathology is detected along a particular myofascial meridian, there is likely to be pathology elsewhere along that meridian which needs to be treated as well. Keep in mind that some techniques are inherently more invasive than others and should be used for more robust myofascia or in very tense *myogelotic* tissue. Other gentler techniques are best for sensitive or less tense tissues.

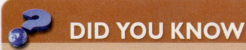

DID YOU KNOW

Before Every Massage

Remember to obtain a proper client history and perform a thorough assessment. This is important in order to develop a good plan and to rule out any techniques that may be contraindicated.

There are a few key concepts to consider when formulating your MFT protocol.

1. Know all the muscles in the area that will be treated.
2. Know the origins, insertions, and actions of each muscle.
   - Pay particular attention to the direction of the fibers of each muscle.
   - Note which muscles are layered over and under each other.
3. Know the layers of myofascia and how they relate to each other.
4. Know the major retinacula and the major myofascial meridians.

A suitable protocol will be easy to prepare if you match your understanding of the myofascia and types of pathology being treated to the relative benefits of the various techniques. Table 13.1 ■ provides a quick reference to the myofascial techniques and their common uses.

TABLE 13.1	Guide to Common Uses of Myofascial Techniques	
	Description	Common Uses
Direct Methods		
Direct stretch	Pressure is applied to a local area followed by stretching the fascia in multiple directions.	This is best for less robust myofascia or when there is more pain involved in the pathology.
Deep fiber friction	Pressure is applied to an adhesion followed by a linear, circular, or transverse grinding action to the area.	This is best for robust myofascia and more tense myogelotic adhesions.
Indirect Methods		
Standard release	Using two contact points, gentle pressure is applied in opposite directions for 2 to 10 minutes.	This is a gentle technique. It can be used most anywhere, even on sensitive or painful areas. It is good for working across joints.
Tourquing	Using two contact points, gentle pressure is applied in opposite directions with the addition of a twist to the area for 2 to 10 minutes.	This is a relatively gentle technique that is slightly deeper than standard release. It is to be used in slightly more robust areas.
Drag and push	A small contact point is used to press into the fascia, creating a fold of skin. The fold is then pushed or pulled along the area being treated.	This is a deep technique and should be used only on robust areas and clients.
Myofascial lift and skin rolling	A fold of myofascia is either simply lifted up or rolled along the surface of the treatment area.	Depending on the fascia, this technique may or may not be uncomfortable. Tissue with more tension will be more tender. The lift is better for sensitive tissue and clients.

SAMPLE PROTOCOLS

The Posterior Neck

☑ Review the muscles of the posterior neck (see Figure 13.1 ▪).

   • These muscles are responsible for moving the head and scapula.

☑ Review the layers of muscle of the posterior neck (see Table 13.2 ▪).

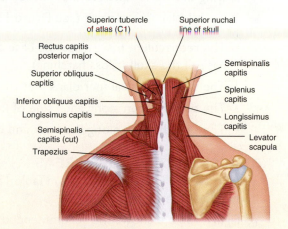

FIGURE 13.1

The Major Muscles of the Posterior Neck

TABLE 13.2	Layers of the Muscles of the Posterior Neck	
Myofascial Layer	Muscle Group	Name of Muscle
Superficial layer	Attaching to vertebra, scapula, and clavicle	*Trapezius*
Middle layer	Cervical vertebral	*Splenius capitus*
		Splenius cervicis
	Erector spinae	*Iliocostalis cervicis*
		Longissimus capitis
		Longissimus cervicis
		Spinalis capitis
		Spinalis cervicis
	Transversospinalis	*Semispinalis capitis*
		Semispinalis capitis
Deep layer	Suboccipital neck muscles	*Rectus capitis posterior major*
		Rectus capitis posterior minor
		Obliquus capitis inferior
		Obliquus capitis superior
	Vertebral muscles	*Multifidi*
		Rotatores
		Interspinalis
	Intertransversarii	*Intertransversarii posteriores*

WARM-UP AND ASSESS THE TISSUES

Using a selection of appropriate warm-up techniques, begin to warm the tissues and encourage circulation to the posterior neck. Make sure to work the entire area, including the upper back and shoulder. This is because the myofascia of the neck extends well into these areas.

IDENTIFY MYOFASCIAL PATHOLOGY

☑ During the warm-up, note the location of any restrictions and/or adhesions.

☑ Pay particular attention to (see Figure 13.2a ■):

- The retinaculum that wraps the base of the neck at the level of C7 and T12 and the one at the base of the skull (cross hatching)
- The two myofascial meridians that run along both sides of the spine (green)
- The two that run along each side of the neck and shoulder (blue)
- The two that run along the back and converge at the base of the neck (yellow)

ADDRESS THE BROADER AREAS

☑ Choose the indirect method(s) (Table 13.1) best suited to address the area, the pathology, and the needs of the client.

☑ Figure 13.2b ■ shows the recommended directions for applying the indirect methods to the posterior neck. The recommended directions are the minimum needed to release the major myofascial structures.

☑ Overall, it is important to apply the indirect methods in as many directions as possible to achieve the greatest therapeutic effect.

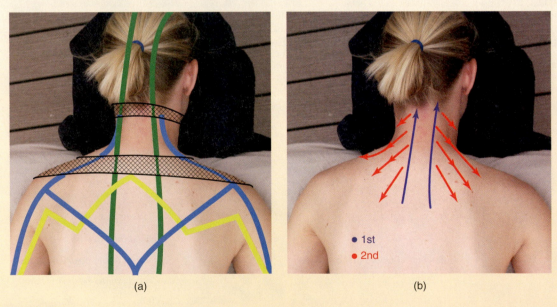

(a)   (b)

FIGURE 13.2a

The Retinacula and Myofascial Meridians of the Posterior Neck. Retinacula Are Represented by Cross Hatching. Myofascial Meridians Are Represented by Colored Lines.

FIGURE 13.2b

The Recommended Directions for Applying the Indirect Methods to the Posterior Neck

ADDRESS THE LOCAL ADHESIONS

☑ Select the direct method(s) best suited to treat the type of adhesions discovered during assessment (Table 13.1).

☑ Make sure to apply the technique(s) in as many directions as possible to achieve the greatest therapeutic effect.

☑ Treat as many adhesions as is practical during your session.

CLOSE

Use a selection of appropriate closing techniques to encourage circulation to the posterior neck. Also include some strokes to the shoulders and upper back to integrate these areas with the neck. Finish with effleurage strokes towards the core to encourage movement of blood and lymph through the area.

The Upper Back, Posterior Shoulder, and Upper Arm

☑ Review the muscles of the upper back, posterior shoulder, and upper arm (see Figure 13.3 ■).

  • These muscles are responsible for moving the scapula and upper arm.

☑ Review the layers of muscle of the upper back, posterior shoulder, and upper arm (see Table 13.3 ■).

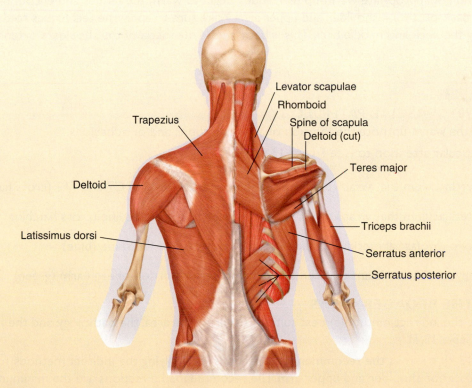

Levator scapulae
Rhomboid
Trapezius
Spine of scapula
Deltoid (cut)
Teres major
Deltoid
Triceps brachii
Latissimus dorsi
Serratus anterior
Serratus posterior

FIGURE 13.3
The Major Muscles of the Upper Back, Posterior Shoulder, and Upper Arm

TABLE 13.3   **Layers of the Muscles of the Upper Back, Posterior Shoulder, and Upper Arm**

Myofascial Layer	Muscle Group	Name of Muscle
Superficial layer	Attaching to trunk and arm	*Trapezius*
		Latissimus dorsi
	Attaching to scapula and arm	*Deltoid*
Middle layer	Attaching to scapula and trunk	*Levator scapulae*
	Attaching to scapula and arm	*Teres minor*
		Teres major
	Upper arm	*Triceps brachii*
Deep layer	Attaching to scapula and trunk	*Rhomboid major*
		Rhomboid minor
		Serratus anterior
	Rotators of the shoulder	*Supraspinatus*
		Infraspinatus
		Subscapularis
	Upper arm	*Anconeus*

WARM-UP AND ASSESS THE TISSUES

Using a selection of appropriate warm-up techniques, begin to warm the tissues and encourage circulation to the upper back, posterior shoulder, and upper arm. Make sure to apply the techniques to the entire area, including the neck and middle back. This is because the myofascia of the shoulders extend well into these areas.

IDENTIFY MYOFASCIAL PATHOLOGY

- ☑ During the warm-up, note the location of any restrictions and/or adhesions.
- ☑ Pay particular attention to (see Figure 13.4a ■):

  - The retinaculum that wraps the base of the neck at the level of C7 and T12 (cross hatching)

  - The retinaculum that wraps the chest just inferior to the nipple line (cross hatching)

  - The two myofascial meridians that run along both sides of the spine (blue)

  - The myofascial meridians that run along the posterior portion of each arm (green)

ADDRESS THE BROADER AREAS

- ☑ Choose the indirect method(s) best suited to address the area, the pathology, and the needs of the client (Table 13.1).
- ☑ Figure 13.4b ■ shows the recommended directions for applying the indirect methods to the upper back, posterior shoulder, and upper arm. The recommended directions are the minimum needed to release the major myofascial structures.
- ☑ Overall, it is important to apply the indirect methods in as many directions as possible to achieve the greatest therapeutic effect.

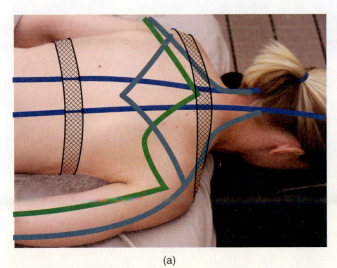

(a)

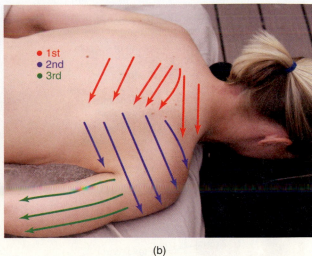

- 1st
- 2nd
- 3rd

(b)

FIGURE 13.4a

The Retinacula and Myofascial Meridians of the Upper Back, Posterior Shoulder, and Upper Arm. Retinacula Are Represented by Cross Hatching. Myofascial Meridians Are Represented by Colored Lines.

FIGURE 13.4b

The Recommended Directions for Applying the Indirect Methods to the Upper Back, Posterior Shoulder, and Upper Arm

ADDRESS THE LOCAL ADHESIONS

☑ Select the direct method(s) best suited to treat the type of adhesions discovered during assessment (Table 13.1).

☑ Make sure to apply the technique(s) in as many directions as possible to achieve the greatest therapeutic effect.

☑ Treat as many adhesions as is practical during your session.

CLOSE

Use a selection of appropriate closing techniques to encourage circulation to the upper back, posterior shoulder, and upper arm. Also include some strokes to the upper back to integrate this area with the shoulder. Finish with effleurage strokes towards the core to encourage movement of blood and lymph through the area.

The Posterior Forearm and Hand

☑ Review the muscles of the posterior forearm and hand (see Figure 13.5 ■).

- These muscles are responsible for moving the wrist, hand, and fingers.

☑ Review the layers of muscle of the posterior forearm and hand (Table 13.4 ■).

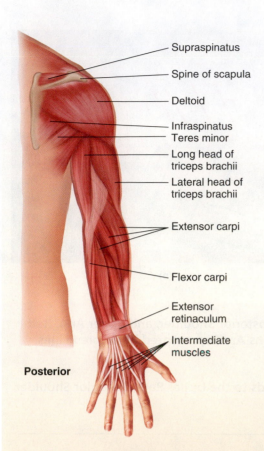

Supraspinatus

Spine of scapula

Deltoid

Infraspinatus
Teres minor

Long head of
triceps brachii

Lateral head of
triceps brachii

Extensor carpi

Flexor carpi

Extensor
retinaculum

Intermediate
muscles

Posterior

FIGURE 13.5

The Major Muscles of the Posterior Forearm and Hand

TABLE 13.4   Layers of the Muscles of the Posterior and Lateral Forearm and Hand

Myofascial Layer	Muscle Group	Name of Muscle
Superficial layer	Forearm/hand	*Brachioradialis*
		Extensor carpi radialis longus
Middle layer	Forearm/hand	*Extensor digitorum communis*
		Extensor digiti minimi
		Extensor carpi ulnaris
		Anconeus
Deep layer	Forearm/hand	*Supinator*
		Abductor pollicis longus
		Extensor pollicis brevis
		Extensor pollicis longus
		Extensor indicis
	Hand	*Dorsal interossei*

WARM-UP AND ASSESS THE TISSUES

Using a selection of appropriate warm-up techniques, begin to warm the tissues and encourage circulation to the posterior forearm and hand. Make sure to work the entire area, including the upper arm. This is because the myofascia of the forearm extend well into these areas.

IDENTIFY MYOFASCIAL PATHOLOGY

☑ During the warm-up, note the location of any restrictions and/or adhesions.

☑ Pay particular attention to (see Figure 13.6a ■):

- The retinaculum that wraps the elbow (cross hatching)
- The retinaculum that wraps around the wrist (cross hatching)
- The myofascial meridian that runs along the midline of the extensors of the forearm and hand (blue)
- The myofascial meridian along the medial portion (green)

ADDRESS THE BROADER AREA

☑ Choose the indirect method(s) (Table 13.1) best suited to address the area, the pathology, and the needs of the client.

☑ Figure 13.6b ■ shows the recommended directions for applying the indirect methods to the posterior forearm and hand. The recommended directions are the minimum needed to release the major myofascial structures.

☑ Overall, it is important to apply the indirect methods in as many directions as possible to achieve the greatest therapeutic effect.

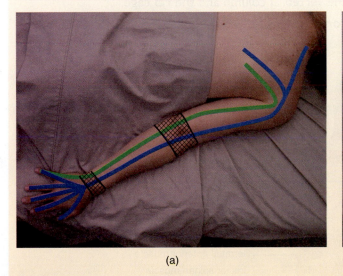

(a)

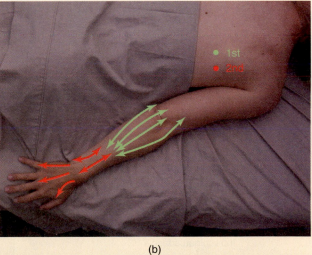

(b)

FIGURE 13.6a

The Retinacula and Myofascial Meridians of the Posterior Forearm and Hand. Retinacula Are Represented by Cross Hatching. Myofascial Meridians are Represented by Colored Lines.

FIGURE 13.6b

The Recommended Directions for Applying the Indirect Methods to the Posterior Forearm and Hand

ADDRESS THE LOCAL ADHESIONS

☑ Select the direct method(s) best suited to treat the type of adhesions discovered during assessment (Table 13.1).

☑ Make sure to apply the technique(s) in as many directions as possible to achieve the greatest therapeutic effect.

☑ Treat as many adhesions as is practical during your session.

CLOSE

Use a selection of appropriate closing techniques to encourage circulation to the posterior forearm and hand. Also include some strokes to the upper arm to integrate this area with the forearm. Finish with effleurage strokes towards the core to encourage movement of blood and lymph through the area.

The Posterior Torso (Back and Sacrum)

☑ Review the muscles of the posterior torso (see Figure 13.7 ■).

• These muscles are responsible for moving the vertebral column and the rib cage.

☑ Review the layers of muscle of the posterior torso (see Table 13.5 ■).

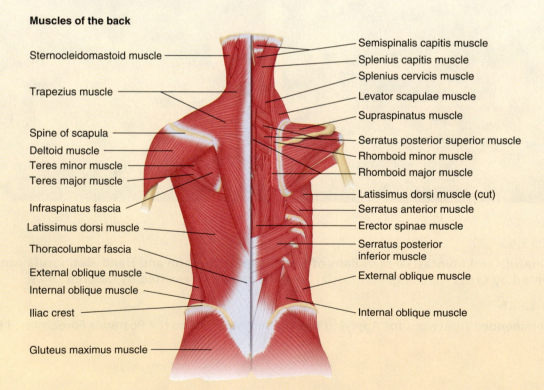

Muscles of the back

Sternocleidomastoid muscle
Trapezius muscle
Spine of scapula
Deltoid muscle
Teres minor muscle
Teres major muscle
Infraspinatus fascia
Latissimus dorsi muscle
Thoracolumbar fascia
External oblique muscle
Internal oblique muscle
Iliac crest
Gluteus maximus muscle

Semispinalis capitis muscle
Splenius capitis muscle
Splenius cervicis muscle
Levator scapulae muscle
Supraspinatus muscle
Serratus posterior superior muscle
Rhomboid minor muscle
Rhomboid major muscle
Latissimus dorsi muscle (cut)
Serratus anterior muscle
Erector spinae muscle
Serratus posterior inferior muscle
External oblique muscle
Internal oblique muscle

FIGURE 13.7
The Major Muscles of the Posterior Torso (Back and Sacrum)

TABLE 13.5	Layers of the Muscles of the Posterior Torso (Back and Sacrum)	
Myofascial Layer	Muscle Group	Name of Muscle
Superficial layer	Attaching to trunk and arm	*Trapezius*
		Latissimus dorsi
Middle layer	Erector spinae	*Iliocostalis thoracis*
		Iliocostalis lumborum
		Longissimus thoracis
		Spinalis thoracis
	Transversospinalis	*Semispinalis thoracis*
	Muscles of inspiration	*Serratus posterior inferior*
		Serratus posterior superior
Deep layer	Vertebral muscles	*Multifidi*
		Rotatores
		Interspinalis
	Intertransversarii	*Intertransversarii posteriores*
		Intertransversarii lateralis
		Intertransversarii medialis
	Prime mover	*Quadratus lumborum*

WARM-UP AND ASSESS THE TISSUES

Using a selection of appropriate warm-up techniques, begin to warm the tissues and encourage circulation to the back. Make sure to work the entire area, including the neck and hips. This is because the myofascia of the back extend well into these areas.

IDENTIFY MYOFASCIAL PATHOLOGY

☑ During the warm-up, note the location of any restrictions and/or adhesions.

☑ Pay particular attention to (see Figure 13.8a ■):

- The retinaculum that wraps the chest just inferior to the nipple line (cross hatching)

- The retinaculum that wraps the belly at a level with the navel (cross hatching)

- The retinaculum that wraps the pelvis (cross hatching)

- The two myofascial meridians that run along both sides of the spine (blue)

- The myofascial meridians that run along the side of the torso (green)

ADDRESS THE BROADER AREAS

☑ Choose the indirect method(s) (Table 13.1) best suited to address the area, the pathology, and the needs of the client.

☑ Figure 13.8b ■ shows the recommended directions for applying the indirect method(s) to the posterior torso. The recommended directions are the minimum needed to release the major myofascial structures.

☑ Overall, it is important to apply the indirect methods in as many directions as possible to achieve the greatest therapeutic effect.

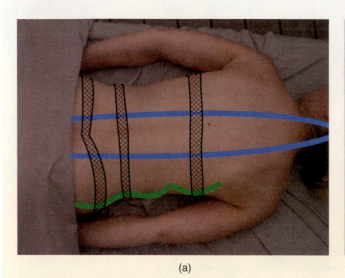

(a)

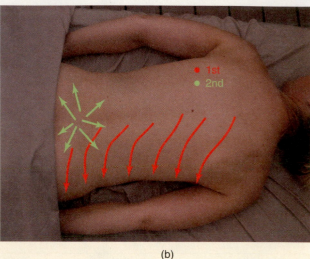

(b)

FIGURE 13.8a

The Retinacula and Myofascial Meridians of the Posterior Torso (Back and Sacrum). Retinacula Are Represented by Cross Hatching. Myofascial Meridians Are Represented by Colored Lines.

FIGURE 13.8b

The Recommended Directions for Applying the Indirect Methods to the Posterior Torso (Back and Sacrum)

ADDRESS THE LOCAL ADHESIONS

☑ Select the direct method(s) best suited to treat the type of adhesions discovered during assessment (Table 13.1).

☑ Make sure to apply the technique(s) in as many directions as possible to achieve the greatest therapeutic effect.

☑ Treat as many adhesions as is practical during your session.

CLOSE

Use a selection of appropriate closing techniques to encourage circulation to the posterior torso. Also include some strokes to the shoulders and neck to integrate these areas with the back. Finish with effleurage strokes to encourage movement of blood and lymph through the area.

The Posterior Hip and Thigh

☑ Review the muscles of the posterior hip and thigh (see Figure 13.9 ■).

- These muscles are responsible for moving the hip, knee and upper leg.

☑ Review the layers of muscle of the posterior hip and thigh (see Table 13.6 ■).

Muscles of the posterior left hip and thigh

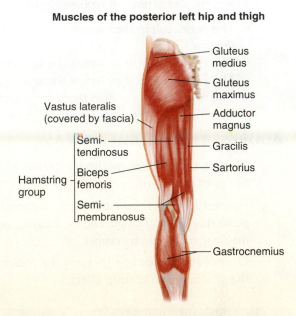

FIGURE 13.9

The Major Muscles of the Posterior Hip and Thigh

TABLE 13.6	Layers of the Muscles of the Posterior Hip and Thigh	
Myofascial Layer	Muscle Group	Name of Muscle
Superficial layer	Gluteal	*Gluteus maximus*
Middle layer	Posterior thigh	*Biceps femoris*
		Semitendinosis
		Semimembranosis
	Gluteal	*Gluteus medius*
Deep layer	Lateral rotators	*Piriformis*
		Obturator internus
		Gemellus superior
		Gemellus inferior
		Obturator externus
		Quadratus femoris
	Gluteal	*Gluteus minimus*

WARM-UP AND ASSESS THE TISSUES

Using a selection of appropriate warm-up techniques, begin to warm the tissues and encourage circulation to the posterior hip and thigh. Make sure to work the entire area, including the lower back and knee. This is because the myofascia of the hip and thigh extend well into these areas.

IDENTIFY MYOFASCIAL PATHOLOGY

☑ During the warm-up, note the location of any restrictions and/or adhesions.

☑ Pay particular attention to (see Figure 13.10a ■):

- The retinaculum that wraps the hip at the level of the sacrum and iliac crest (Figure 13.6a).
- The retinaculum that wraps the upper thigh at the base of the gluteal fold (cross hatching)
- The retinaculum that wraps the knee (cross hatching)
- The myofascial meridian that runs posteriorly along the hamstrings (blue)
- The meridian that runs from the gluteals along the iliotibial band (green)

ADDRESS THE BROADER AREAS

☑ Choose the indirect method(s) (Table 13.1) best suited to address the area, the pathology, and the needs of the client.

☑ Figure 13.10b ■ shows the recommended directions for applying the indirect method(s) to the posterior hip and thigh. The recommended directions are the minimum needed to release the major myofascial structures.

☑ Overall, it is important to apply the indirect methods in as many directions as possible to achieve the greatest therapeutic effect.

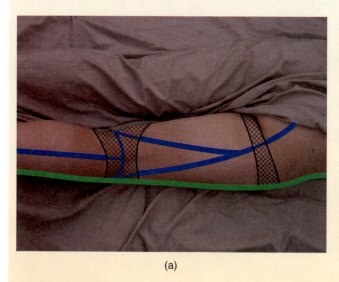
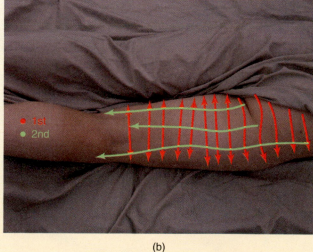

(a)   (b)

FIGURE 13.10a

The Retinacula and Myofascial Meridians of the Posterior Hip and Thigh. Retinacula Are Represented by Cross Hatching. Myofascial Meridians Are Represented by Colored Lines.

FIGURE 13.10b

The Recommended Directions for Applying the Indirect Methods to the Posterior Hip and Thigh

ADDRESS THE LOCAL ADHESIONS

☑ Select the direct method(s) best suited to treat the type of adhesions discovered during assessment (Table 13.1).

☑ Make sure to apply the technique(s) in as many directions as possible to achieve the greatest therapeutic effect.

☑ Treat as many adhesions as is practical during your session.

CLOSE

Use a selection of appropriate closing techniques to encourage circulation to the posterior hip and thigh. Also include some strokes to the lower back and knee to integrate these areas with the hip and thigh. Finish with effleurage strokes towards the core to encourage movement of blood and lymph through the area.

The Posterior Lower Leg and Foot

☑ Review the muscles of the posterior lower leg and foot (see Figure 13.11 ■).

- These muscles are responsible for moving the ankle, foot, and toes.

☑ Review the layers of muscle of the lower leg and foot (see Table 13.7 ■).

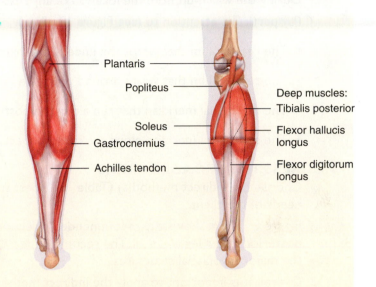

Plantaris

Popliteus

Soleus

Gastrocnemius

Achilles tendon

Deep muscles:
Tibialis posterior

Flexor hallucis longus

Flexor digitorum longus

FIGURE 13.11

The Major Muscles of the Posterior Lower Leg and Foot

TABLE 13.7	Layers of the Muscles of the Posterior Leg and Foot	
Myofascial Layer	Muscle Group	Name of Muscle
Superficial layer	Lower leg	*Gastrocnemius*
	Plantar surface of foot	*Abductor hallucis*
		Flexor digitorum brevis
		Abductor digiti minimi
Middle layer	Lower leg	*Soleus*
		Plantaris
	Plantar surface of foot	*Quadratus plantae*
		Lumbricales
		Flexor hallucis brevis
		Adductor hallucis
		Flexor digiti minimi brevis
Deep layer	Lower leg and foot	*Popliteus*
		Flexor hallucis longus
		Flexor digitorum longus
		Tibialis posterior
	Plantar surface of foot	*Dorsal interossei*
		Plantar interossei

WARM-UP AND ASSESS THE TISSUES

Using a selection of appropriate warm-up techniques, begin to warm the tissues and encourage circulation to the posterior lower leg and foot. Make sure to work the entire area, including the upper leg. This is because the myofascia of the lower leg extend well into these areas.

IDENTIFY MYOFASCIAL PATHOLOGY

☑ During the warm-up, note the location of any restrictions and/or adhesions.

☑ Pay particular attention to (see Figure 13.12a ■):

- The retinaculum that wraps the knee (cross hatching)

- The retinaculum that wraps around the ankle (cross hatching)

- The myofascial meridian that run along the posterior aspect of leg and foot (blue)

- The myofascial meridian along the lateral aspect of the leg and foot (green)

ADDRESS THE BROADER AREAS

☑ Choose the indirect method(s) (Table 13.1) best suited to address the area, the pathology, and the needs of the client.

☑ Figure 13.12b ■ shows the recommended directions for applying the indirect method(s) to the posterior lower leg and foot. The recommended directions are the minimum needed to release the major myofascial structures.

☑ Overall, it is important to apply the indirect methods in as many directions as possible to achieve the greatest therapeutic effect.

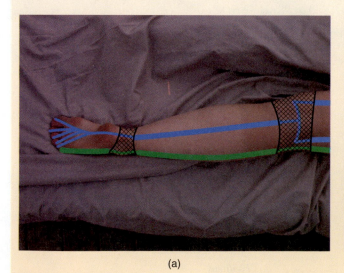

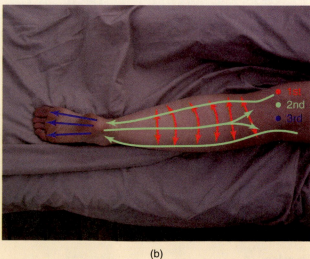

(a)   (b)

FIGURE 13.12a

The Retinacula and Myofascial Meridians of the Posterior Lower Leg and Foot. Retinacula Are Represented by Cross Hatching. Myofascial Meridians Are Represented by Colored Lines.

FIGURE 13.12b

The Recommended Directions for Applying the Indirect Methods to the Posterior Lower Leg and Foot

QUICK QUIZ #25

1. Deep fiber friction is best suited for: (Circle all that apply)
   a. sensitive and painful areas.
   b. very mild adhesions.
   c. less robust myofascia.
   d. more tense myogelotic adhesions.

2. The warm-up it is important because it allows you to: (Circle all that apply)
   a. encourage circulation to the local area.
   b. encourage circulation to nearby myofascia.
   c. note the location of restrictions, adhesions, or other pathology.
   d. note the location of the local retinacula and myofascial meridians.
   e. All of the above
   f. None of the above

3. The middle layer of myofascia in the area of the posterior neck includes the: (Circle all that apply)
   a. suboccipital neck muscles.
   b. cervical vertebral muscles.
   c. intertransversarii.
   d. transversospinalis.
   e. All of the above
   f. None of the above

4. In general, it is a good idea to apply both the indirect and the direct myofascial methods in as many different directions as possible.
   a. True
   b. False

ADDRESS THE LOCAL ADHESIONS

☑ Select the direct method(s) best suited to treat the type of adhesions discovered during assessment (Table 13.1).

☑ Make sure to apply the technique(s) in as many directions as possible to achieve the greatest therapeutic effect.

☑ Treat as many adhesions as is practical during your session.

CLOSE

Use a selection of appropriate closing techniques to encourage circulation to the posterior lower leg and foot. Also include some strokes to the upper leg to integrate this area with the lower leg. Finish with effleurage strokes towards the core to encourage movement of blood and lymph through the area.

The Head and Face

☑ Review the muscles of the head and face (see Figure 13.13 ■).

• These muscles are responsible for movement of the face and jaw.

☑ Review the layers of muscle of the head and face (see Table 13.8 ■).

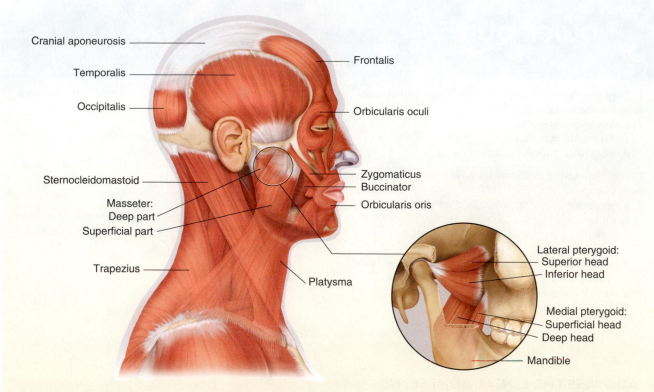

FIGURE 13.13

The Major Muscles of the Head and Face

TABLE 13.8	Layers of the Muscles of the Head and Face		
Myofascial Layer	Muscle Group	Name of Muscle	
Superficial layer	Muscles of eyelids	*Orbicularis oculi*	
		Levator palpebrae superioris	
		Corrugator supercilii	
	Muscles of nose	*Procerus*	
		Depressor septi	
		Nasalis	
	Muscles of scalp	*Epicranius*	*occipitalis*
			frontalis
		Temporoparietalis	
	Muscles of ear	*Auricularis anterior*	
		Auricularis posterior	
		Auricularis superior	
Middle layer	Muscles of the jaw	*Masseter temporalis*	
Deep layer	Muscles of the jaw	*Lateral pterygoid*	
		Medial pterygoid	

WARM-UP AND ASSESS THE TISSUES

Using a selection of appropriate warm-up techniques, begin to warm the tissues and encourage circulation to the head and face. Make sure to work the entire area, including the neck. This is because the fascia is continuous between the two areas.

IDENTIFY MYOFASCIAL PATHOLOGY

☑ During the warm-up, note the location of any restrictions and/or adhesions.

☑ Pay particular attention to (see Figure 13.14a ■):

- The retinaculum that wraps the head at the level of the eyes (cross hatching)

- The retinaculum located along the base of the chin (cross hatching)

- The two myofascial meridians that run along the top of the head from forehead to occiput along the epicranius (blue)

- The myofascial meridians that run along the side of the neck to the lateral cheek (green)

ADDRESS THE BROADER AREAS

☑ Choose the indirect method(s) (Table 13.1) best suited to address the area, the pathology, and the needs of the client.

☑ Figure 13.14b ■ shows the recommended directions for applying the indirect methods to the head and face. The recommended directions are the minimum needed to release the major myofascial structures.

☑ Overall, it is important to apply the indirect methods in as many directions as possible to achieve the greatest therapeutic effect.

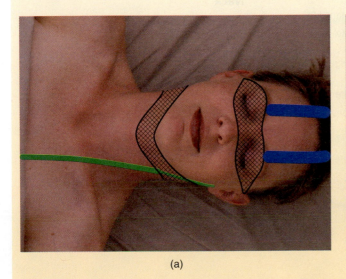
(a)

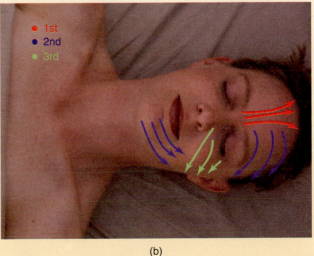
(b)

FIGURE 13.14a

The Retinacula and Myofascial Meridians of the Head and Face. Retinacula Are Represented by Cross Hatching. Myofascial Meridians Are Represented by Colored Lines.

FIGURE 13.14b

The Recommended Directions for Applying the Indirect Methods to the Head and Face

ADDRESS THE LOCAL ADHESIONS

☑ Select the direct method(s) best suited to treat the type of adhesions discovered during assessment (Table 13.1).

☑ Make sure to apply the technique(s) in as many directions as possible to achieve the greatest therapeutic effect.

☑ Treat as many adhesions as is practical during your session.

CLOSE

Use a selection of appropriate closing techniques to encourage circulation to the head and face. Also include some strokes to the neck to integrate this area with the head and face. Finish with effleurage strokes towards the core to encourage movement of blood and lymph through the area.

The Anterior Neck

☑ Review the muscles of the anterior neck (see Figure 13.15 ■).

• These muscles are responsible for swallowing and moving the head.

☑ Review the layers of muscle of the anterior neck (see Table 13.9 ■).

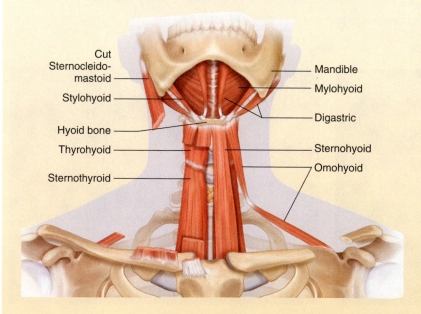

FIGURE 13.15

The Major Muscles of the Anterior Neck

TABLE 13.9	Layers of the Muscles of the Anterior Neck	
Myofascial Layer	**Muscle Group**	**Name of Muscle**
Superficial layer	**Superficial muscle**	*Platysma*
Middle layer	Suprahyoid muscles	*Digastricus*
		Stylohyoid
		Mylohyoid
		Geniohyoid
	Infrahyoid muscles	*Sternohyoid*
		Sternothyroid
		Thyrohyoid
		Omohyoid
	Prime mover	*Sternocleidomastoid*
Deep layer	Vertebral muscles	*Longus colli*
		Longus capitis
		Rectus capitus anterior
		Rectus capitus lateralis
		Intertransversarii anteriores
	Lateral vertebral muscles	*Scalenus anterior*
		Scalenus medius
		Scalenus posterior

WARM-UP AND ASSESS THE TISSUES

Using a selection of appropriate warm-up techniques, begin to warm the tissues and encourage circulation to the anterior neck. Make sure to work the entire area, including the chest and shoulders. This is because the myofascia of the neck extends well into these areas.

IDENTIFY MYOFASCIAL PATHOLOGY

☑ During the warm-up, note the location of any restrictions and/or adhesions.

☑ Pay particular attention to (see Figure 13.16a ■):

- The retinaculum that wraps the neck at the chin (cross hatching)

- The retinaculum that wraps the base of the neck at the level of C7 and T12 (cross hatching)

- The two myofascial meridians that run along both sides of the esophagus (blue)

- The myofascial meridians along each side of the neck (green)

ADDRESS THE BROADER AREAS

☑ Choose the indirect method(s) (Table 13.1) best suited to address the area, the pathology, and the needs of the client.

☑ Figure 13.16b ■ shows the recommended directions for applying the indirect methods to the anterior neck. The recommended directions are the minimum needed to release the major myofascial structures.

☑ Overall, it is important to apply the indirect methods in as many directions as possible to achieve the greatest therapeutic effect.

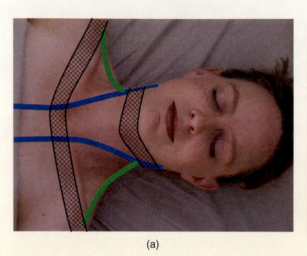
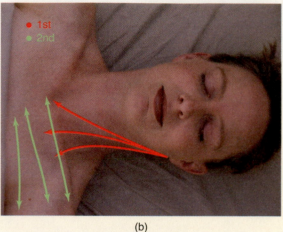

(a)   (b)

FIGURE 13.16a

The Retinacula and Myofascial Meridians of the Anterior Neck. Retinacula Are Represented by Cross Hatching. Myofascial Meridians Are Represented by Colored Lines.

FIGURE 13.16b

The Recommended Directions for Applying the Indirect Methods to the Anterior Neck

ADDRESS THE LOCAL ADHESIONS

☑ Select the direct method(s) best suited to treat the type of adhesions discovered during assessment (Table 13.1).

☑ Make sure to apply the technique(s) in as many directions as possible to achieve the greatest therapeutic effect.

☑ Treat as many adhesions as is practical during your session.

CLOSE

Use a selection of appropriate closing techniques to encourage circulation to the anterior neck. Also include some strokes to the chest and shoulders to integrate these areas with the neck. Finish with effleurage strokes towards the core to encourage movement of blood and lymph through the area.

The Chest, Anterior Shoulder, and Upper Arm

☑ Review the muscles of the chest, anterior shoulder, and upper arm (see Figures 13.17 ■ and Figure 13.19).

• These muscles are responsible for moving the clavicle and upper arm.

☑ Review the layers of muscle of the chest, anterior shoulder, and upper arm (see Table 13.10 ■).

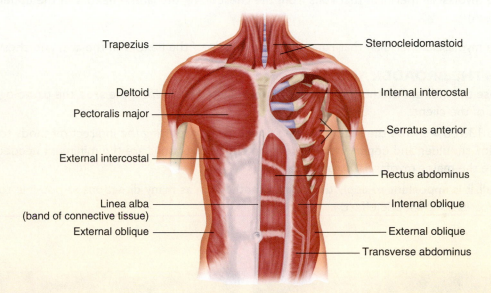

FIGURE 13.17

The Major Muscles of the Chest, Anterior Shoulder, and Upper Arm

TABLE 13.10	Layers of the Muscles of the Chest, Anterior Shoulder, and Upper Arm	
Myofascial Layer	Muscle Group	Name of Muscle
Superficial layer	Attaching to trunk and arm	*Pectoralis major*
	Attaching clavicle to arm	*Deltoid*
Middle layer	Attaching to arm and scapula	*Biceps brachii*
Deep layer	Attaching to scapula and trunk	*Pectoralis minor*
	Attaching to arm and scapula	*Coracobrachialis*
	Upper arm	*Brachialis*

WARM-UP AND ASSESS THE TISSUES

Using a selection of appropriate warm-up techniques, begin to warm the tissues and encourage circulation to the chest, anterior shoulder, and upper arm. Make sure to work the entire area, including the neck. This is because the fascia is continuous between the two areas.

IDENTIFY MYOFASCIAL PATHOLOGY

☑ During the warm-up of the anterior shoulder and upper arm, note the location of any restrictions and/or adhesions.

☑ Pay particular attention to (see Figure 13.18a ■):

- The retinaculum that wraps the base of the neck at the level of C7 and T12 (cross hatching)

- The retinaculum that wraps the elbow (cross hatching)

- The myofascial meridian that runs along the anterior neck and chest (red)

- The myofascial meridian that runs from the chest along the lateral flexors of the upper arm (green)

- The myofascial meridian that runs along the middle of the flexors of the arm and chest (blue)

ADDRESS THE BROADER AREAS

☑ Choose the indirect method(s) (Table 13.1) best suited to address the area, the pathology, and the needs of the client.

☑ Figure 13.18b ■ shows the recommended directions for applying the indirect methods to the chest, anterior shoulder, and upper arm. The recommended directions are the minimum needed to release the major myofascial structures.

☑ Overall, it is important to apply the indirect methods in as many directions as possible to achieve the greatest therapeutic effect.

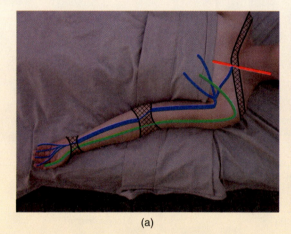
(a)

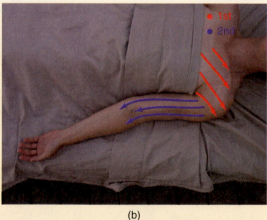
(b)

FIGURE 13.18a

The Retinacula and Myofascial Meridians of the Chest, Anterior Shoulder, and Upper Arm. Retinacula Are Represented by Cross Hatching. Myofascial Meridians Are Represented by Colored Lines.

FIGURE 13.18b

The Recommended Directions for Applying the Indirect Methods to the Chest, Anterior Shoulder, and Upper Arm

ADDRESS THE LOCAL ADHESIONS

☑ Select the direct method(s) best suited to treat the type of adhesions discovered during assessment (Table 13.1).

☑ Make sure to apply the technique(s) in as many directions as possible to achieve the greatest therapeutic effect.

☑ Treat as many adhesions as is practical during your session.

CLOSE

Use a selection of appropriate closing techniques to encourage circulation to the chest, anterior shoulder, and upper arm. Also include some strokes to the neck to integrate this area with the anterior shoulder. Finish with effleurage strokes towards the core to encourage movement of blood and lymph through the area.

The Anterior Forearm and Hand

☑ Review the muscles of the anterior forearm and hand (see Figure 13.19 ■).

• These muscles are responsible for moving the wrist, hand, and fingers.

☑ Review the layers of muscle of the anterior forearm and hand (see Table 13.11 ■).

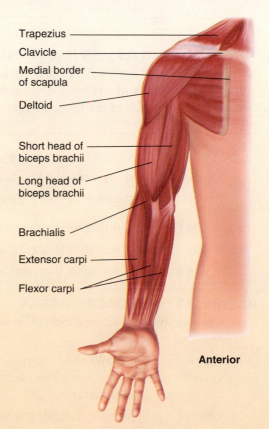

Trapezius

Clavicle

Medial border of scapula

Deltoid

Short head of biceps brachii

Long head of biceps brachii

Brachialis

Extensor carpi

Flexor carpi

Anterior

FIGURE 13.19

The Major Muscles of the Anterior Forearm and Hand

TABLE 13.11	Layers of the Muscles of the Anterior and Medial Forearm and Hand	
Myofascial Layer	Muscle Group	Name of Muscle
Superficial layer	Forearm and hand	*Pronator teres*
		Flexor carpi radialis
		Palmaris longus
		Flexor carpi ulnaris
	Hand	*Palmaris brevis*
		Abductor pollicis brevis
		Flexor pollicis brevis
		Opponens pollicis
Middle layer	Forearm and hand	*Flexor digitorum superficialis*
	Hand	*Adductor pollicis*
		Abductor digiti minimi
		Flexor digiti minimi brevis
		Opponens digiti minimi
Deep layer	Forearm and hand	*Flexor digitorum profundus*
		Flexor pollicis longus
		Pronator quadratus
	Hand	*Palmar interossei*
		Lumbricales

WARM-UP AND ASSESS THE TISSUES

Using a selection of appropriate warm-up techniques, begin to warm the tissues and encourage circulation to the anterior forearm and hand. Make sure to work the entire area, including the upper arm. This is because the myofascia of the forearm extends well into this area.

IDENTIFY MYOFASCIAL PATHOLOGY

☑ During the warm-up, note the location of any restrictions and/or adhesions.

☑ Pay particular attention to (see Figure 13.20a ■):

- The retinaculum that wraps the elbow and wrist (cross hatching)
- The myofascial meridian that runs along the midline of the forearm and hand (blue)
- The myofascial meridian that runs along the lateral aspect the arm and hand (green)

ADDRESS THE BROADER AREAS

☑ Choose the indirect method(s) (Table 13.1) best suited to address the area, the pathology, and the needs of the client.

☑ Figure 13.20b ■ shows the recommended directions for applying the indirect methods to the anterior forearm and hand. The recommended directions are the minimum needed to release the major myofascial structures.

☑ Overall, it is important to apply the indirect methods in as many directions as possible to achieve the greatest therapeutic effect.

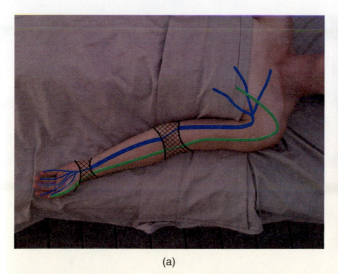

(a)

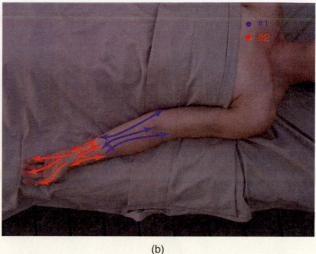

(b)

FIGURE 13.20a

The Retinacula and Myofascial Meridians of the Anterior Forearm and Hand. Retinacula Are Represented by Cross Hatching. Myofascial Meridians Are Represented by Colored Lines.

FIGURE 13.20b

The Recommended Directions for Applying the Indirect Methods to the Anterior Forearm and Hand

ADDRESS THE LOCAL ADHESIONS

☑ Select the direct method(s) best suited to treat the type of adhesions discovered during assessment (Table 13.1).

☑ Make sure to apply the technique(s) in as many directions as possible to achieve the greatest therapeutic effect.

☑ Treat as many adhesions as is practical during your session.

CLOSE

Use a selection of appropriate closing techniques to encourage circulation to the anterior forearm and hand. Also include some strokes to the upper arm to integrate this area with the forearm. Finish with effleurage strokes towards the core to encourage movement of blood and lymph through the area.

The Anterior Torso (Abdomen)

☑ Review the muscles of the anterior torso (see Figure 13.21 ■).

• These muscles are responsible for breathing and movement of the abdomen.

☑ Review the layers of muscle of the anterior torso (see Table 13.12 ■).

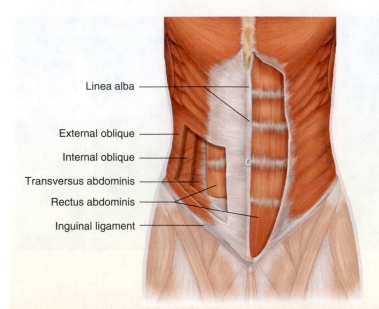

FIGURE 13.21

The Major Muscles of the Anterior Torso (Abdomen)

Labels:
- Linea alba
- External oblique
- Internal oblique
- Transversus abdominis
- Rectus abdominis
- Inguinal ligament

TABLE 13.12	Layers of the Muscles of the Anterior Torso (Abdomen)	
Myofascial Layer	**Muscle Group**	**Name of Muscle**
Superficial layer	Abdominal muscles	*Obliquus externus abdominis*
		Rectus abdominis
Middle layer	Thoracic muscles	*Intercostales externi*
	Abdominal muscles	*Obliquus internus abdominis*
Deep layer	Thoracic muscles	*Intercostales interni*
		Subcostales
		Transverses thoracis
		Levatores costarum
		Diaphragm
		Transverses abdominis
		Cremaster

WARM-UP AND ASSESS THE TISSUES

Using a selection of appropriate warm-up techniques, begin to warm the tissues and encourage circulation to the anterior torso. Make sure to work the entire area, including the chest and hips. This is because the myofascia of the anterior torso extend well into these areas.

IDENTIFY MYOFASCIAL PATHOLOGY

☑ During the warm-up, note the location of any restrictions and/or adhesions.

☑ Pay particular attention to (see Figure 13.22a ■):

- The retinaculum that wraps the chest just inferior to the nipple line (cross hatching)
- The retinaculum that wraps the belly at the level of the navel (cross hatching)

- The retinaculum that wraps the superior pelvis (cross hatching)
- The two myofascial meridians that run along both sides of the midline of the torso (blue)
- The myofascial meridian along the lateral side of the torso (green)

ADDRESS THE BROADER AREAS

☑ Choose the indirect method(s) (Table 13.1) best suited to address the area, the pathology, and the needs of the client.

☑ Figure 13.22b ■ shows the recommended directions for applying the indirect methods to the anterior torso. The recommended directions are the minimum needed to release the major myofascial structures.

☑ It is important to apply the indirect methods in as many directions as possible to achieve the greatest therapeutic effect.

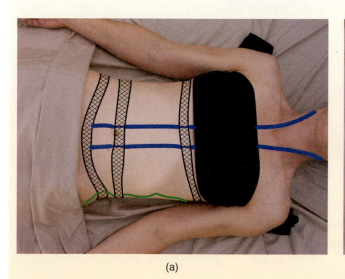 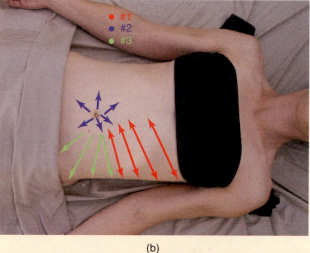

●	#1
●	#2
●	#3

(a)   (b)

FIGURE 13.22a

The Retinacula and Myofascial Meridians of the Anterior Torso (Abdomen). Retinacula Are Represented by Cross Hatching. Myofascial Meridians Are Represented by Colored Lines.

FIGURE 13.22b

The Recommended Directions for Applying the Indirect Methods to the Anterior Torso (Abdomen)

ADDRESS THE LOCAL ADHESIONS

☑ Select the direct method(s) best suited to treat the type of adhesions discovered during assessment (Table 13.1).

☑ Make sure to apply the technique(s) in as many directions as possible to achieve the greatest therapeutic effect.

☑ Treat as many adhesions as is practical during your session.

CLOSE

Use a selection of appropriate closing techniques to encourage circulation to the anterior torso. Also include some strokes to the chest and hips to integrate these areas with the torso. Finish with effleurage strokes towards the core to encourage movement of blood and lymph through the area.

The Anterior Hip and Thigh

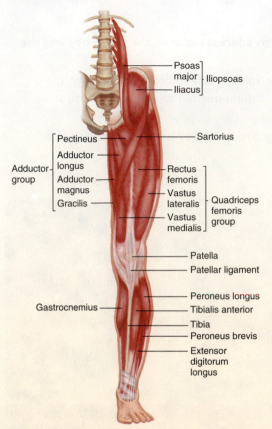

Psoas major — Iliopsoas
Iliacus

Pectineus — Sartorius

Adductor longus
Adductor group
Adductor magnus
Gracilis

Rectus femoris
Vastus lateralis — Quadriceps femoris group
Vastus medialis

Patella
Patellar ligament

Peroneus longus
Gastrocnemius — Tibialis anterior
Tibia
Peroneus brevis
Extensor digitorum longus

☑ Review the muscles of the anterior hip and thigh (see Figure 13.23 ∎).

• These muscles are responsible for moving the hip, knee, and upper leg.

☑ Review the layers of muscle of the anterior hip and thigh (see Table 13.13 ∎).

FIGURE 13.23

The Major Muscles of the Anterior Hip and Thigh

TABLE 13.13	Layers of the Muscles of the Anterior and Medial Hip and Thigh		
Myofascial Layer	Muscle Group	Name of Muscle	
Superficial layer	Anterior thigh	*Tensor fascia latae*	
		Sartorius	
	Medial thigh	*Gracilis*	
Middle layer	Anterior thigh	*Quadriceps femoris*	*rectus femorus*
			vastus lateralis
			vastus medialis
			vastus intermedius
	Medial thigh	*Adductor longus*	
		Adductor magnus	
Deep layer	Hip	*Psoas major*	
		Iliacus	
	Medial thigh	*Pectineus*	
		Adductor brevis	

WARM-UP AND ASSESS THE TISSUES

Using a selection of appropriate warm-up techniques, begin to warm the tissues and encourage circulation to the anterior hip and thigh. Make sure to work the entire area, including the abdomen and knee. This is because the myofascia of the anterior hip and thigh extend well into these areas.

IDENTIFY MYOFASCIAL PATHOLOGY

☑ During the warm-up, note the location of any restrictions and/or adhesions.

☑ Pay particular attention to (see Figure 13.24a ■):

- The major retinaculum that wraps the hip at the level of the pubis and along the iliac crest (previous Figure 13.22a)

- The retinaculum that wraps the upper thigh just inferior to the pubis (cross hatching)

- The retinaculum that wraps the knee (cross hatching)

- The myofascial meridian that runs anteriorly along the quadriceps to the center of the patella (blue)

- The myofascial meridian that runs along the lateral aspect of the thigh (green)

ADDRESS THE BROADER AREAS

☑ Choose the indirect method(s) (Table 13.1) best suited to address the area, the pathology, and the needs of the client.

☑ Figure 13.24b ■ shows the recommended directions for applying the indirect methods to the anterior hip and thigh. The recommended directions are the minimum needed to release the major myofascial structures.

☑ Overall, it is important to apply the indirect methods in as many directions as possible to achieve the greatest therapeutic effect.

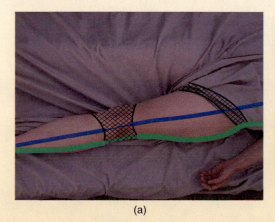
(a)

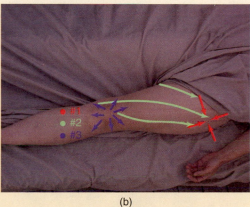
(b)

FIGURE 13.24a

The Retinacula and Myofascial Meridians of the Anterior Hip and Thigh. Retinacula Are Represented by Cross Hatching. Myofascial Meridians Are Represented by Colored Lines.

FIGURE 13.24b

The Recommended Directions for Applying the Indirect Methods to the Anterior Hip and Thigh

ADDRESS THE LOCAL ADHESIONS

☑ Select the direct method(s) best suited to treat the type of adhesions discovered during assessment (Table 13.1).

☑ Make sure to apply the technique(s) in as many directions as possible to achieve the greatest therapeutic effect.

☑ Treat as many adhesions as is practical during your session.

CLOSE

Use a selection of appropriate closing techniques to encourage circulation to the anterior hip and thigh. Also include some strokes to the abdomen and knee. Finish with effleurage strokes towards the core to encourage movement of blood and lymph through the area.

The Anterior Lower Leg and Foot

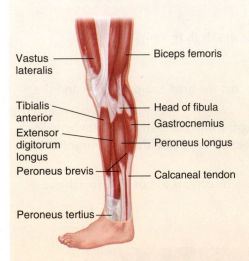

Vastus lateralis — Biceps femoris

Tibialis anterior — Head of fibula

Extensor digitorum longus — Gastrocnemius

Peroneus brevis — Peroneus longus

Peroneus tertius — Calcaneal tendon

☑ Review the muscles of the anterior lower leg and foot (see Figure 13.25 ■).

• These muscles are responsible for moving the ankle, foot, and toes.

☑ Review the the layers of muscle of the anterior lower leg (see Table 13.14 ■).

FIGURE 13.25

The Major Muscles of the Anterior Lower Leg and Foot

TABLE 13.14	Layers of the Muscles of the Anterior Lower Leg and Foot	
Myofascial Layer	Muscle Group	Name of Muscle
Superficial layer	Lower leg	*Tibialis anterior*
	Lateral lower leg and foot	*Peroneus longus*
	Dorsal foot	*Extensor digitorum brevis*
Middle layer	Lower leg and foot	*Extensor hallicus longus*
	Lateral lower leg and foot	*Peroneus brevis*
		Peroneus tertius
Deep layer	Lower leg and foot	*Extensor digitorum longus*

WARM-UP AND ASSESS THE TISSUES

Using a selection of appropriate warm-up techniques, begin to warm the tissues and encourage circulation to the anterior lower leg and foot. Make sure to work the entire area, including the upper leg. This is because the myofascia of the lower leg extend well into this area.

IDENTIFY MYOFASCIAL PATHOLOGY

☑ During the warm-up, note the location of any restrictions and/or adhesions.

☑ Pay particular attention to (see Figure 13.26a ■):

- The retinaculum that wraps the knee (cross hatching)
- The retinaculum that wraps around the ankle (cross hatching)
- The myofascial meridian that runs along the anterior lower leg and foot (blue)
- The myofascial meridian that runs along the lateral aspect of the lower leg and foot (green)

ADDRESS THE BROADER AREAS

☑ Choose the indirect method(s) (Table 13.1) best suited to address the area, the pathology, and the needs of the client.

☑ Figure 13.26b ■ shows the recommended directions for applying the indirect methods to the anterior lower leg and foot. The recommended directions are the minimum needed to release the major myofascial structures.

☑ Overall, it is important to apply the indirect methods in as many directions as possible to achieve the greatest therapeutic effect.

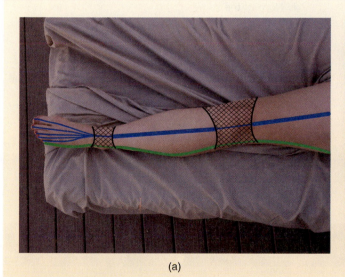
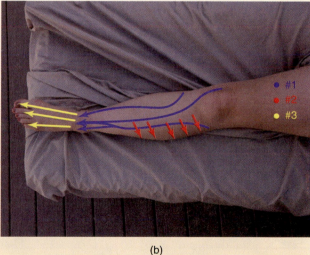

(a)   (b)

FIGURE 13.26a

The Retinacula and Myofascial Meridians of the Anterior Lower Leg and Foot. Retinacula Are Represented by Cross Hatching. Myofascial Meridians Are Represented by Colored Lines.

FIGURE 13.26b

The Recommended Directions for Applying the Indirect Methods to the Anterior Lower Leg and Foot

ADDRESS THE LOCAL ADHESIONS

☑ Select the direct method(s) best suited to treat the type of adhesions discovered during assessment (Table 13.1).

☑ Make sure to apply the technique(s) in as many directions as possible to achieve the greatest therapeutic effect.

☑ Treat as many adhesions as is practical during your session.

CLOSE

Use a selection of appropriate closing techniques to encourage circulation to the anterior lower leg and foot. Also include some strokes to the upper leg to integrate this area with the lower leg. Finish with effleurage strokes towards the core to encourage movement of blood and lymph through the area.

QUICK QUIZ #26

1. The standard release technique would be most suitable for more painful adhesions on the anterior lower leg, including the ankle and knee.
   a. True
   b. False

2. Which of the following techniques might be well suited for robust anterior thigh muscles with very tense mygelotic tissues? (Circle all that apply)
   a. Direct stretch technique
   b. Deep fiber friction
   c. Drag and push techniques
   d. Myofascial lift technique
   e. All of the above
   f. None of the above

3. The myofascia of the face exist primarily in a single layer.
   a. True
   b. False

4. The diaphragm is in a more superficial myofascial layer than the obliquus externus abodominis and the intercostals externi.
   a. True
   b. False

HOLISTIC CONNECTION

Hydrotherapy is a very general term for any type of therapy which involves the use of water. Some forms of hydrotherapy are commonly used in conjunction with massage, especially because water has the helpful property of maintaining a warm or cold temperature for long periods of time.

The following hydrotherapy tools can enhance the benefits of your massage. Use hot water packs to help warm tense areas before massaging them. Use ice cups to gently massage areas with mild inflammation and suggest ice packs at home for clients with minor injury or inflammation. Recommend the use of a hot tub with massaging jets before, after, or between massages. Don't forget yourself: As a therapist, hot tub therapy may be beneficial for you as well!

SUMMARY

When applying your myofascial therapy protocol, keep in mind the basic principles of this approach. Remember that you are treating all of the tissues that are integrated with the fascia and all of the structures that are connected by the fascial net. Think about the continuity of the net as you work through each body part. The various myofascial techniques use different strategies for treating pathology. If necessary, review the details of the techniques and structures you will be treating.

Before starting your protocol, determine if you will need any additional tools or supplies, such as an extra blanket, bolsters, a heat source, etc. Consider the order in which you will treat certain body parts. If the client has more severe adhesions in certain areas, you may want to begin by applying heat to the area while you work other tissues. Take care to use proper body mechanics for the most efficient use of your energy and to provide the best massage. Pay attention to subtle cues and changes in the client's body. Communicate with the client regularly during the protocol.

As you become more practiced, you will develop more variable protocols. MFT protocols for a specific body part or set of body parts can be combined with other methods such as deep tissue massage, neuromuscular therapy, acupressure, and more.

DISCUSSION QUESTIONS

1. Why is it important to review the major retinacula and myofascial meridians before applying MFT?

2. What factors should you consider when selecting the best indirect method(s) to use on the posterior neck?

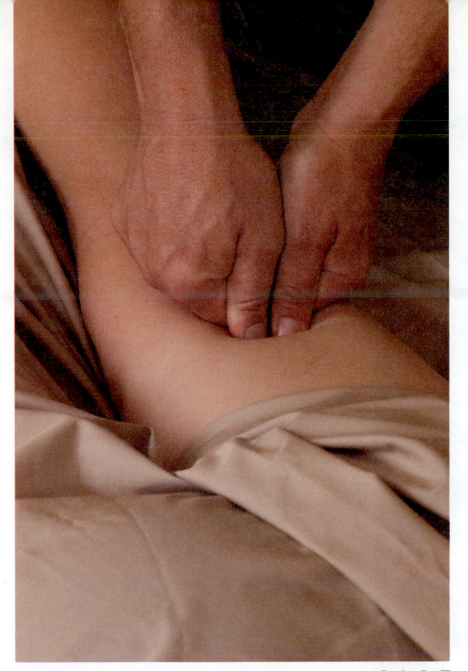

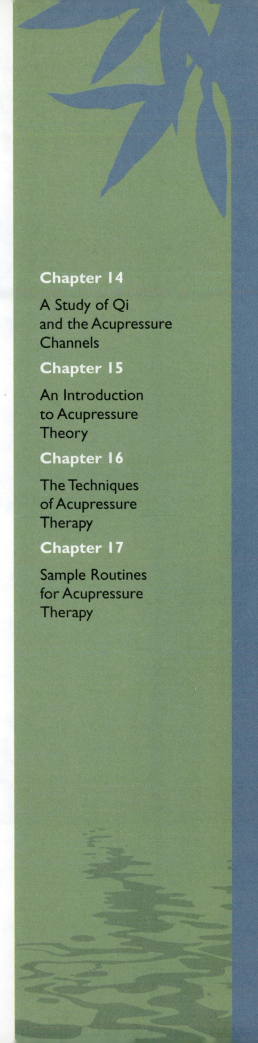

PART

5

The Acupressure Approach

14 A Study of Qi and the Acupressure Channels

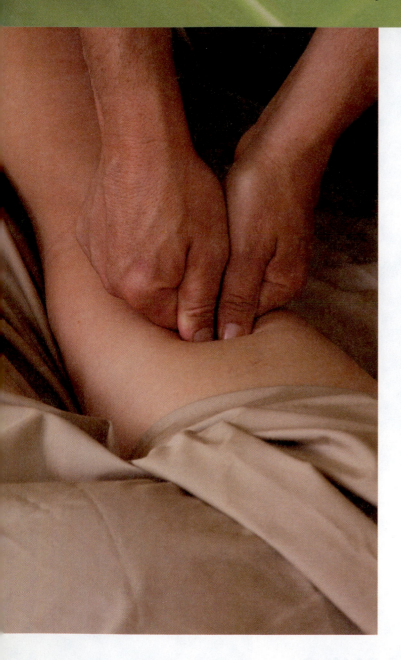

CHAPTER HIGHLIGHTS

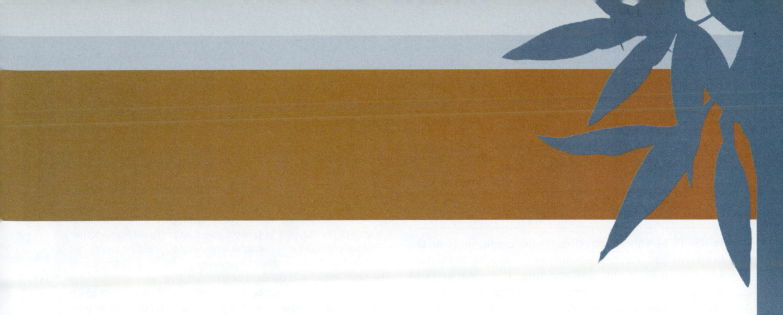

 CHAPTER OBJECTIVES

- Understand the Chinese holistic view of the body
- Explore the three treasures: Qi, Jing, and Shen
- Discover the Chinese concept of blood and body fluids
- Investigate the channel system and how it functions within the body

- Locate the pathways of the 12 major channels
- Learn the classifications and functions of acupoints
- Examine the individual channels and their functions

 KEY TERMS

Traditional Chinese Medicine (TCM) is complex and varied. Its roots lie in ideas thousands of years old, yet it still flourishes today. The concepts, theories, and principles in TCM can seem daunting in their complexity. However, many of the techniques, such as acupressure, can be applied effectively with a solid understanding of a few key concepts.

FUNCTION VS. STRUCTURE

In the TCM view of physiology, the emphasis is on the functions and interrelationships of the organs and tissues and not on their physical structure. It's not that TCM doesn't recognize the physical structure of the body's organs, tissues, and fluids; it's just that it places more significance on how each functions within the context of the whole body. This contrasts with Western medicine, which has an emphasis on specialization and dissection.

Western theory tends to focus on the physical and chemical details of each tissue, organ, or system. Its emphasis is on distinguishing between different types of cells tissues and their structure. Western science typically tries to understand the whole by analyzing each and every part. Although this approach is profound in its ability to understand how the body is physically ordered, it sometimes falls short in its ability to evaluate the interrelationships between the structures.

Chinese theory takes into account the structure of the body's parts, but mainly in relation to how the parts are working together. Thus, we might say the Chinese emphasis is on functional interrelationships, while Western medicine's emphasis is on structural relationships.

For example, TCM understands that blood is the physical substance that circulates through the vessels. However, according to TCM, its function of nourishing the body is more important than the physical microscopic components of it. Furthermore, in order for the blood to perform its function of nourishing the body, it needs help from a variety of other organs and systems. The blood obtains the nutrients to nourish the

DID YOU KNOW

Theories of quantum physics discuss the nature of the universe in energetic terms. Everything, even material structures, are understood to be energy vibrating at different frequencies. It is the specific frequency of the vibration that makes one object different from another. For example, rocks and plants have two very different structures, but both are made up of differing amounts of electrons, protons, and neutrons vibrating at different frequencies. Thus, all matter is energy in motion. Qi can be described as this infinite vibration from which all energy and matter arises. Energy condensed becomes material (Fritz, 2000).

body from the digestive system and the lungs. It then relies upon the heart to pump it through the vessels to the rest of the body. Blood also needs the function of the liver and spleen to help keep it clean.

From this perspective, blood cannot properly perform its functions without other organs doing their part. The functions of each tissue, organ, and fluid are intricately tied to the functions of all the others. They are all part of a coordinated system of interconnecting activities that all contribute to the whole. Blood is just a component of the system and thus can only function in context of the system. If the rest of the system is working well, then blood can perform its role. Conversely if blood is not performing its functions well, the rest of the system will be adversely affected.

Since it is the interrelationships of the organs, tissues, and fluids that make up the function of the whole body, any analysis of organs, tissues, and fluids is seen through this cooperative lens. TCM views the whole body in terms of active principles that embody harmonized groups of functions working together. This is a holistic framework that uses a generalized perspective of anatomy.

In other words, Chinese theory attempts to describe the whole by understanding how its parts work together to make it whole. Each tissue, organ, and system works to the benefit of the whole. In fact, no body part is greater than any other. The body is an intricate biomachine, and each element must be doing its job or a system breakdown will occur.

This generalized perspective led the Chinese to use a very simplified system of categorizing the body's various organs, tissues, and substances. In the TCM system there are five elemental substances important to sustaining all aspects of life. Three of the substances are collectively known as the three treasures: Qi, Jing, and Shen. The other two elemental substances have a very close relationship to each other, as they are the two major fluids in our bodies: blood and body fluid. These five substances embody the primary components that make up a living being according to TCM theory.

DID YOU KNOW

Another example of organ cooperation is in the digestion of fats. When an ingested fat makes its way to the small intestine, it stimulates the liver and gallbladder to secrete bile. The bile breaks down the fat in the small intestine. The broken-down fats are then absorbed from the small intestine into a series of vessels called *lacteals*. The lacteals carry the predigested fat over to the liver for more processing, before it is sent to the rest of the body. The digestion of fats involves the collaboration of the small intestine, the liver, and the gallbladder, none of which can perform the entire function alone.

THE THREE TREASURES: QI, JING, AND SHEN

Qi

Qi, sometimes written as *Chi* and pronounced "Chee," is the perfect example of how the Chinese synthesize multiple concepts into a holistic view that emphasizes function over structure. Understanding the concept of Qi is crucial to any basic understanding of traditional Chinese medicine.

Qi is often described as "life force," or bioelectric energy. However, Qi is much more than just electric energy. It is best understood, simply, as energy—all forms of energy. This includes the substances from which the body's energy is derived as well as the driving force behind all of the body's activities.

In other words, Qi is at once a substance circulating through all living things and the energy from which the living thing feeds. It is energy that exists simultaneously on the material or physical level as well as on the ethereal or subtle level. Qi is constantly changing forms. It manifests physically and at the same time as the power behind that manifestation.

In Western physical science, energy is categorized according to its location and function. For example, kinetic energy is associated with the movement of things, and thermal energy is energy that creates heat. Physical science also recognizes chemical, electrical, and stored forms of energy. Each one of these categories still refers to the same substance, energy. It is simply categorized based upon its observed manifestation. The Chinese categorize Qi in much the same way. They classify different forms of Qi based on its location and function. It's important to remember no matter how it is categorized, all forms of Qi are still made up of the same basic energy matrix.

CATEGORIES OF QI

Figure 14.1 ■ compares the many different categories of Qi. Qi, in the living being, originates as *Prenatal* Qi, or as the Chinese call it, *Yuan Qi*. Yuan Qi is the starting energy derived from our parents. It is responsible for fetal growth and sets the stage for early development as a child. The mother provides the fetus with most of this energy, as it is derived from her food, drink, and exercise habits.

Once born, our Yuan Qi is augmented from the environment and our health habits. This is classified as the *Postnatal Qi* or *Zong* Qi. Zong Qi is derived from the food we eat called *Gu Qi* and the air we breathe called *Kong Qi*.

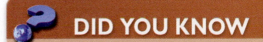

DID YOU KNOW

Yuan Qi is also translated as "Original Qi." Zong Qi can be translated as "Gathering Qi."

Yuan Qi and Zong Qi combine to form *Zheng Qi*. Zheng Qi is circulated in the channels of the body and flows to the organs where it becomes the basis for all physiological activity. To the Western mind, Zheng Qi can best be understood as nutrients and oxygen that circulate in the blood and lymph, as well as the electric current that flows through the nerves and fascia. Therefore, Zheng Qi supports the functions of all the tissues, organs, and systems.

Since Zheng Qi is the basis for all of the body's functions, the Chinese felt it useful to further categorize it based upon the organ where it is functioning. The Qi of each organ manifests according to the functions attributed to that specific organ. Heart Qi functions to perform the act of circulating the blood, Liver Qi performs those duties required by the liver, and so on. In addition, some whole systems are categorized as forms of Qi. One such system is the system of immune function, which is categorized as *Wei Qi*. Wei Qi represents all aspects of immunity, such as preventing pathological influences such as colds or flu from attacking.

Even though there are all these different classifications of Qi, it's all still just basic energy being created, consumed, and circulated to and from the different structures of the body. In a nutshell, Qi is the energy that supports all activity and movement in the body. All motor functions rely on Qi to create their

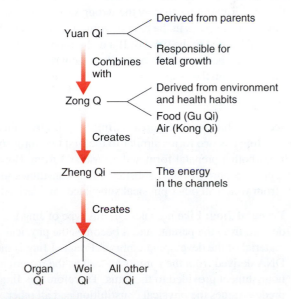

FIGURE 14.1

The Origin and Organization of Qi

movement. All of the body's internal activities—electrical, hormonal, and glandular—rely on Qi. Even thinking uses Qi.

In his book, *The Complete Illustrated Guide to Chinese Medicine* (1996), Tom Williams states, "Qi is constantly ascending, descending, entering, and leaving the body, and health and well-being are dependent on this continuous dynamic activity" (p. 33). Qi ascends and descends as it circulates through our vessels feeding our organs and tissues. Qi enters the body via the food we eat and the air we breathe. It leaves the body via the energy we expend in our daily activities. Qi is in a constant flow, and as long as it stays that way the body is healthy. When the flow of Qi is disrupted it can manifest in four basic ways.

THE DISHARMONY OF QI

- **Deficient Qi:** When Qi is depleted due to overwork or illness, there isn't enough Qi to carry out the body's functions. This can manifest as tiredness or weakness. It may even affect a large system such as the Wei Qi, which may result in a chronic infection. If a specific organ's Qi is depleted, then it will affect that organ's ability to perform its various functions. Deficient Qi anywhere can result in disharmony that can eventually affect the entire body.
- **Sinking Qi:** If the Qi is not strong enough to carry itself to the head, the Qi is said to be *sinking*. This may result in memory issues and or foggy brain functioning. The Qi also holds the body together. If the Qi sinks, disorders such as a prolapsed organ may result. This most commonly affects the uterus and colon.
- **Stagnant Qi:** Qi may become blocked or stagnant due to injury, illness, or deficiency. Tissue damaged from an injury or poor nutrition blocks the Qi flow. When the Qi is blocked in the channels, pain or internal disharmony is the result.
- **Rebellious Qi:** Rebellious Qi occurs when Qi is forced, through disharmony, to flow the wrong way. The most obvious example is in the case of vomiting. Stomach Qi should descend to the bowels. If a disharmony sets in, the Qi may become rebellious and go the wrong way going back up the esophagus carrying food up with it.

Jing

The second of the three treasures is **Jing.** Jing is also called *essence.* Jing has two forms similar to the first two forms of Qi: It has both a prenatal form and a postnatal form. However, Jing is a pure physical substance that constitutes the basis from which all other physical substances are derived.

- **Prenatal Jing:** Like prenatal Qi, this type of Jing is derived from the parents and it becomes the physical material of the developing embryo. Prenatal Jing is the DNA derived from the parents as well as the maternal nourishment provided to the fetus. Therefore this Jing predetermines the physical constitution and all other foundations of our bodies. It determines generally how an individual responds to the rigors of life both physically and mentally.

- **Postnatal Jing:** Postnatal Jing, according to the Chinese, is the special essence derived from food and liquids. This is the physical substance the body uses to nourish growth and development. Western correlations may be proteins, vitamins, and nutrients.

Both prenatal and postnatal Jing combine to assist and/or direct the Qi to help the child grow and develop into an adult. In adulthood, Jing is also responsible for the body's ability to produce offspring. The Chinese believe that Jing is the substance from which semen, sperm, ova, and vaginal secretions are derived. Therefore the stronger one's Jing, the more fertile they will be. Furthermore, strong Jing is passed on (as prenatal Jing) to the offspring.

As well as providing the original constitution from our parents and continually supporting growth, Jing is also said to have a special relationship with our brain and spinal cord. It is said that Jing provides the substance and growth of these two structures.

DISORDERS OF JING

The main disorder of Jing is deficiency. If the parents don't have enough Jing to pass on to the fetus, then childhood development will be affected, often resulting in learning disabilities such as delayed speech and coordination problems. As we age, weak or deficient Jing shows up as infertility and other sexual malfunctions. Conversely, strong Jing will have a positive influence on brain development and sexual function.

Shen

The third treasure is known as **Shen.** Shen is the aspect of a person that involves thinking and self-expression. In the West, we would call this the "spirit," or the demeanor, of a person. Shen is reflected in the general feeling or impression we project to others. The average person can often tell how somebody is feeling both physically and mentally at first glance of that individual. They immediately see if they are feeling ill or mentally "under the weather."

The Shen is expressed through the general skin color, physical presentation, and overall temperament of the person. A person with strong Shen will come across as vibrant, alive, and happy. Conversely, a person with weak Shen will be withdrawn, sullen, and depressed. Since Shen is partly the thinking mind, disorders of the Shen often manifest as muddled and confused thinking or in mental disorders such as mania or schizophrenia.

The three treasures work together as three essential components of living things. To summarize:

- Qi is energy and is responsible for giving the body life and maintaining the functions of the body.
- Jing is the essence, the deepest component, of the physical body and is responsible for growth and reproduction.
- Shen is our consciousness, our thinking mind, and our personality and spirit.

Although Jing, Qi, and Shen are considered the three treasures, there are two additional elemental substances that carry as much importance. They are blood and body fluids.

Blood

Blood is an extremely important concept in Chinese medicine. **Blood,** like all the substances according to Traditional Chinese Medicine, is not only that red stuff which flows through the vessels. It is also a concept of function. According to TCM theory, the spleen and stomach, transform food and liquids into a clear usable form. This clear substance combines with Jing and Qi to produce blood. Blood's primary function is to nourish the entire body by bringing Qi and nutrients to the various tissues. The blood is also responsible for hydrating the tissues and viscera. Blood and Qi have a special relationship. Blood is a substance that uses the energy of Qi for its movement around the body. Yet blood also carries the Qi throughout the body. This is the classic example of a functional interrelationship; both Qi and blood must be healthy for both to function properly. There are three common disorders of the blood.

DISORDERS OF BLOOD

- **Deficient blood:** This disorder manifests as pale skin, weakness, confusion, and often times dizziness. Mental and/or emotional problems are common with blood deficiency because of blood's responsibility of nourishing the brain.
- **Stagnant blood:** This is the result of blunt trauma, weak Qi, or insufficient blood volume. Symptoms of stagnant blood often include pain (usually of a sharp stabbing variety), stiffness, and bruising. Tumors are considered to be the most severe type of blood stagnation.
- **Heat in the blood:** If heat enters into the blood this causes "reckless" moving of the blood. This causes excessive bleeding issues, such as chronic bloody noses and heavy menses for women.

Body Fluids

Body fluids in TCM include all other fluids and secretions aside from blood. Sweat, tears, and gastric juices are some examples. Together the spleen and stomach digest food, and the body fluids also separate the pure fluids from the impure fluids. These are called *clear/thin fluids* and *thick/turbid fluids*, respectively. The clear/thin fluids are turned into interstitial fluid, tears, and sweat. The thick/turbid fluids flow into the joint spaces and help fill the bone marrow. They also become organ fluids such as bile in the liver. Therefore, the function of each body fluid depends upon where it is found. One of the main responsibilities of body fluid is to moisten the tissues and organs as well as to assist in their function.

These five basic elements (the three treasures, the blood, and body fluids) are part of the simplified system of Chinese anatomy and physiology. Having a firm grasp of these five concepts puts you well on your way to understanding the TCM point of view.

THE CHANNELS

Another concept that is critical for understanding TCM is the nature of the channels. The system of channels is one of the hallmarks of traditional Chinese medicine. According to TCM theory, the **channels** (sometimes called *meridians*) form a pervasive network that is responsible for carrying the blood, Qi, and body fluids to all parts of the body. This network also connects the various organs, neurological structures, tissues, and senses of the body together.

From a Western medical perspective, this network of channels involves a variety of systems, including the circulatory system, the nervous system, the lymph system, and the myofascial system.

The Chinese recognize and understand these Western systems as well. However, they also have a different way of organizing and categorizing the body. They consider all of those Western systems to be components of the channel system.

The Chinese view the channels as collections of functional groupings rather than simple physical structures. The channel represents all of the tissues and structures that run along its path. In other words, they include the nerves, blood vessels, muscles, connective tissue, and organs that follow their pathways.

The traditional meridian charts that are most commonly seen only display a thin, superficial line to show the trajectory of the channels. However, in textbooks as early as the *NeiJing Internal Classic* of 221 BCE, there are references to the channels being more than a superficial structure. This ancient text describes superficial aspects of the channels as well as aspects that lie deep within the body. It goes on to describe how the entire channel can only be seen in dissection (O'Connor & Bensky, 1981).

The channels are described as having both width and depth. They extend from the superficial tissues down to the bone and also spread out to meet each other. The traditional channel maps show only the center of the channel (see Figure 14.2 ■). This is done to keep the picture clean and

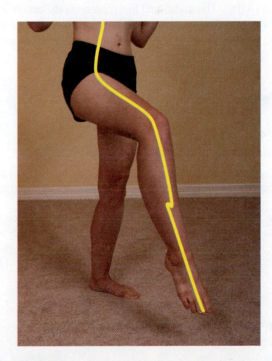

FIGURE 14.2

Representation of the Stomach Channel Focused on Illustrating Only the Centerline of the Channel

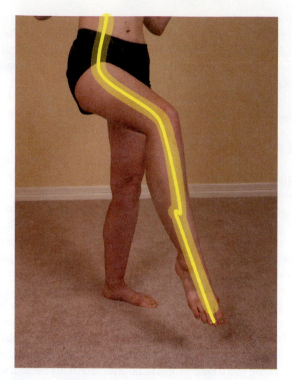

FIGURE 14.3

Representation of the Stomach Channel Showing that the Channel Includes the Broader Area That Spreads to the Adjacent Channels on Either Side

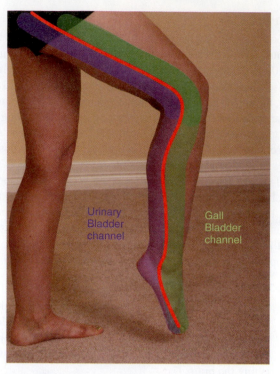

FIGURE 14.4

The Border Between the Urinary Bladder Channel and Gall Bladder Channel

simple. Additionally, the centerline is where the major acupoints are found.

In reality, each channel is really more like a band (see Figure 14.3 ■). The traditional line represents the center of the band—its thickest, most conductive part. However, as mentioned, each channel spreads to meet the adjacent channels.

They can be drawn as wide swaths that extend out from the narrow center of the traditional line to border on the adjacent channels. Figure 14.4 ■ shows how the Gall Bladder channel and the Urinary Bladder channel share a common border along the lateral leg. When the extended bands are added to a chart of the traditional paths, the channels cover the entire body.

QUICK QUIZ #27

1. Traditional Chinese medicine places great emphasis on analyzing how well the various parts of the body are functioning together because: (Circle all that apply)
   a. the health of the body is viewed from a holistic perspective.
   b. the Chinese do not understand much about the physical structure of the organs.
   c. no organ or system can perform its function without the proper functioning of the others.
   d. All of the above
   e. None of the above

2. Qi, blood, and body fluid are three elemental substances important to sustaining life.
   a. True
   b. False

3. Qi: (Circle all that apply)
   a. has the function of warming the body.
   b. represents all forms of energy inside and outside of the body.
   c. transforms food into nutrients.
   d. protects the body from infection.
   e. All of the above
   f. None of the above

4. The TCM channels, or meridians, include nerves, muscle, blood vessels, and organs.
   a. True
   b. False

THE CLASSIFICATION OF CHANNELS

Jing Luo

The Chinese call the channel system the **Jing Luo** (see Figure 14.5 ■). The Jing are the major channels most people are familiar with as they are often seen in the charts, pictures, and diagrams about acupressure. The Jing are the primary focus of acupressure therapy and will be discussed fully in this text.

The Luo are a series of small connecting channels that link the flow of Qi between the major channels. Luo literally translates as "net" because these small channels are distributed like a net throughout the body and help carry the Qi into all tissues. The Luo are not categorized, as it would be impractical because they are so plentiful and so dispersed.

THE JING CHANNELS

Jing refers to a group of 20 major channels that run along the torso and out to the limbs. These channels are labeled, categorized, and evenly distributed in the body. These are the channels that practitioners use for diagnosis and treatment. The 20 Jing channels are broken into two subgroups, the 12 primary channels and the 8 extra channels.

The 12 Primary Channels   The **12 primary channels** are bilateral—there is an exact "mirror-image" copy of each channel on the right and left sides of the body. This means that there are 12 primary channels on the right side and

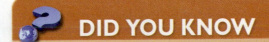

DID YOU KNOW

Chinese is a tonal language. The word written in PinYin for English readers as "Jing" has many different pronunciations and many different meanings in Chinese. The word *jing* which means "essence" and the word *Jing* which refers to the "Jing Luo" may look the same to an English reader. However the two words have completely different pronunciations and meanings.

12 mirror copies on the left side. Figure 14.6 ■ shows the Lung channels as they are located on both sides of the body.

The 12 primary channels, along with the organs and many other elements of the body, are categorized according to Yin/Yang principles. The principles of Yin/Yang are discussed more completely in Chapter 15. For the purposes of understanding the organization of channels, it is important to know that Yin and Yang represent the concept of opposites, which balance each other. The channels are arranged to reflect this balance.

Channels are grouped into 6 Yin and Yang pairings. The pairs coincide with the Yin/Yang pairing of the major organs. Six of the channel pairs (3 Yin and 3 Yang) run through the

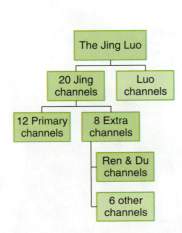

FIGURE 14.5

The 12 Primary Jing Channels Are Most Relevant to Bodywork. Of the 8 Extra Channels, the Ren Channel and the Du Channels Are Most Important to Bodywork.

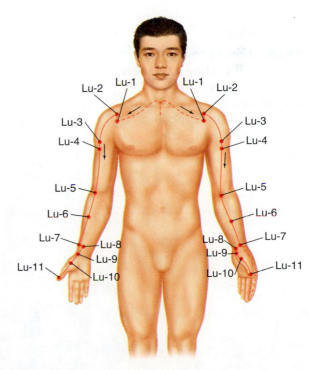

FIGURE 14.6

The Mirror Copies of the Lung Channel on the Left and Right Sides of the Body

hands, arms, torso, and head. The other 6 channel pairs (3 Yin and 3 Yang) run through the feet, legs, torso and head. (It is common to find these groups referred to as the "hand Yin channels," "arm Yang channels," "foot Yang channels," "leg Yin channels" etc.). Each channel of a Yin/Yang pair is positioned on the opposing side of a particular body part or body area from its complement. Each complement supports and controls the body area where it is found.

Take for example, the Heart and Small Intestine channels. The Heart channel (Yin) is paired with the Small Intestine channel (Yang) to form a Yin/Yang pair. The Heart channel is located on the anterior medial wrist, arm, and torso, so it carries the Qi, blood, and body fluids through that area. The Small Intestine channel is directly opposite, on the posterior medial side of the wrist, arm, and torso, so it is responsible for carrying Qi, blood, and body fluids through its area. The location of the Heart and Small Intestine channels so close together on the same body part yet on opposing sides means that they both oppose each other and rely on each other for support (see Figure 14.7 ■). The rest of the channels are organized in the same fashion.

This balanced relationship is also represented by the relative location of the channels on the body. The Yin channels are located on the anterior and medial aspects of the body (see Figure 14.8 ■), and the Yang channels are located on the posterior and lateral aspects (see Figure 14.9 ■). These are the respective Yin and Yang areas of the body.

A portion of each channel is located close to the surface of the body. This is where it is possible tap into the Qi through **acupoints,** which are access points located along

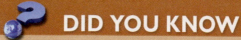

DID YOU KNOW

In the upper torso, there is a correlation between Western anatomy and the flow of Qi. The nerves that connect to the anterior horn of the spinal cord are motor nerves that send signals out to the periphery of the body. This can be understood as Qi flowing out along the anterior Yin channels. Conversely, the nerves that connect to the posterior horn of the spinal cord are sensory and receive signals from the periphery. This can be seen as the Qi flowing in along the Yang channels (Marieb, 2004).

the surface portion of the channels. The channels also have a portion that flows deep inside and connects to the internal organs. The deep internal connection is what allows the channel to be used to treat its namesake organ in addition to treating the local myoskeletal area along its pathway.

The Chinese say that the Qi flows out from the torso to the ends of the hands along the Yin channels (the anterior side of the body) and flows back from the hands to the torso along the Yang channels (the posterior side of the body). The Qi flows out from the head and torso to the feet along the Yang channels. It flows inward from the feet to the torso and head along the Yin channel (see Figure 14.10 ■).

FIGURE 14.7

The Location of the Heart and Small Intestine Channels. These Channels Form a Yin/Yang Pair and Are Therefore Located on Opposing Sides of the Hand, Arm, and Torso.

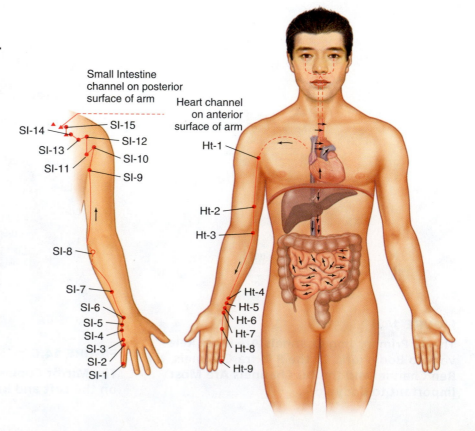

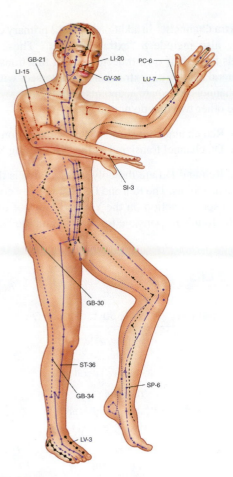

FIGURE 14.8

The Location of the Yin Channels on the Body

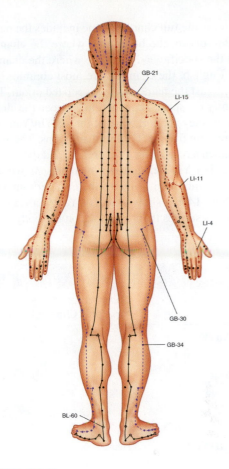

FIGURE 14.9

The Location of the Yang Channels on the Body

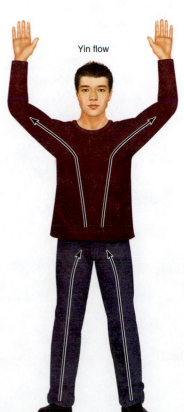

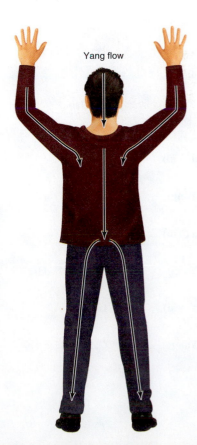

FIGURE 14.10

Qi Flows from the Head and Hands towards the Feet on the Yang Surfaces of the Body, and from the Feet towards the Torso and Hands on the Yin Surfaces of the Body.

In Chinese, the full channel name includes the name of its associated organ, the body area where the channel is found, and the specific body surface where the channel is located. In English, the channels are most commonly represented with just the name of the associated organ. This is done to signify the special connection between the channels and the organs they support. Five of the six Yin/Yang channel pairs represent five pairs of familiar organs. These organ pairs are known as the **Zang** (Yin organs) and the **Fu** (Yang organs). The sixth Yin and Yang pairing represent two important, but more ambiguous, organs, the Pericardium and the San Jao. Table 14.1 ■ shows the Yin/Yang pairing of the channels and describes their locations on the body.

The 8 Extra Channels In addition to the 12 primary channels, the Jing also include 8 "extra channels." These **8 extra channels** have their own trajectories and functions and are not bilateral. Six of the extra channels intersect with the 12 major channels and share acupoints with them.

The other two that do not intersect are:

- The Ren channel translated as the "Conception Vessel"
- The Du channel translated as the "Governing Vessel"

The Ren and Du are the only extra channels that have their own acupoints. The Ren and Du channels are considered to have a special action on the Yin and Yang of the entire body. The Ren is responsible for the Yin and the Du for the

TABLE 14.1	The Zang/Fu–Yin/Yang Pairing of Organs and Channels		
Zang/Fu Designation	Complementary Yin/Yang Channel Pair	Body Areas of Channel	Body Surface Area Description
Zang Organ (Yin)	Lung	Hand Arm and chest	Taiyin "Greater Yin" Anterior lateral arm
Fu Organ (Yang)	Large Intestine	Hand Shoulder, neck, and face	Yangming "Yang brightness" Posterior lateral arm
Zang Organ (Yin)	Heart	Hand Arm and chest	Shaoyin "Lesser Yin" Anterior medial arm
Fu Organ (Yang)	Small Intestine	Hand Shoulder, neck, and face	Taiyang "Greater Yang" Posterior medial arm
Zang Organ (Yin)	Pericardium	Hand Arm and chest	Jueyin "Absolute Yin" Anterior middle arm
Fu Organ (Yang)	San Jao	Hand Shoulder, neck, and face	Shaoyang "Lesser Yang" Posterior middle arm
Zang Organ (Yin)	Spleen	Foot Leg, torso, and chest	Taiyin Anterior medial leg
Fu Organ (Yang)	Stomach	Foot Leg, torso, and face	Yangming Anterior lateral leg
Zang Organ (Yin)	Kidney	Foot Leg, torso, and chest	Shaoyin Posterior medial leg
Fu Organ (Yang)	Urinary Bladder	Foot Leg, back, neck, and head	Taiyang Posterior middle leg
Zang Organ (Yin)	Liver	Foot Leg, torso, and chest	Jueyin Medial middle leg
Fu Organ (Yang)	Gall Bladder	Foot Leg, torso, neck, and head	Shaoyang Lateral middle leg

Yang. The Ren and Du channels are often used for meditation because they run along what is the traditional path of the *Chakras*. The Ren channel, being Yin, is positioned on the anterior surface along the midline. The Du channel, being Yang, is positioned along the spine.

All of the extra channels have additional working theories that are beyond the scope of this text. Our discussion of the channels will focus on the 12 primary Jing channels, as they are more accessible and likely to be involved with myoskeletal problems. They are also the primary channels used in acupressure treatment.

HOW DO THE CHANNELS WORK?

It is possible to affect all levels of physiological function by tapping into the correct channel using acupuncture and acupressure. This is because the channels are made up of the circulatory, nervous, lymphatic, and myofascial systems. The 12 main channels represent the main thoroughfares of the nerves, lymph, and blood vessels, while the smaller channels (Luo) represent the smaller nerves, vessels, and capillaries.

The channels are kind of like a freeway system in a city. The freeways are the large main roads that run through all of the important areas of the city. The side roads either feed into or exit from the freeways and connect to the lesser areas of the city. To get around the city quickly, one uses the freeways. This is because the freeway is the fastest and connects the far reaches of the city in the most efficient way. The Jing channels are like the freeways because they follow the major nerve, blood, and lymph pathways while the Luo are more like the side roads. The major channels connect the far reaches of the body together in the fastest and most efficient way. This is why applying acupuncture to the Stomach channel on the leg affects the functioning of the stomach. The channel passes through the stomach and the leg and therefore connects both areas. Stimulation on one section of a channel will have an effect on the distant sections that are connected to it.

This is also how channels can reflect disorders in their namesake organ. If the stomach is ill, any structure along the Stomach channel such as the anterior leg may also become affected. The reverse can also occur. A blockage in the channel (the Lower Leg, for example) can cause a problem with the associated organ (the stomach) because the Qi needs to flow freely through the whole channel in order to promote proper health.

THE MUSCLE-CHANNEL CONNECTION

Just as the channels follow the main nerves, blood, and lymph vessels, they also follow functional muscle groupings and their related fascia. In this way, channels also represent major "lines of pull" of muscular contraction. Like Thomas Myers' anatomy trains (described in Chapter 9), the channels represent groups of muscles that are aligned and perform movement patterns. Each channel reveals an individual line of movement along its pathway.

For example, the three Yin channels located on the anterior arm pass through the lateral, middle, and medial portions of all of the muscles of flexion (see Figure 14.11 ■). Each channel represents a direction of pull performed by this muscle group.

- The Lung channel is active when the arm is flexed at the elbow and shoulder (as when lifting a glass to the mouth, for example).
- The Pericardium channel is active when the arm is horizontally adducted and flexed at the elbow (as when pulling something towards the chest like playing tug of war).
- The Heart channel is active when pulling the arm toward the waist (like pulling on a rope to ring a bell).

If there is an injury along any of these channels, simply follow the pathway of the channels, looking for compensation in the muscles along the way. If one portion of the flexors is damaged, it is likely that the other muscles along that same contraction line (channel) are also affected.

Whenever there is injury to the myoskeletal system, the Chinese describe it as pathology located in the channel. Injury or trauma, according to the Chinese, causes Qi and blood to stagnate in the channel. This makes sense, as swelling and tissue damage disrupt the nerves, blood, and lymph vessels (the structures that carry Qi). The Chinese say that when there is restriction, there is Qi stagnation. When there is Qi stagnation, there is pain.

The Qi should not only flow through each channel smoothly, but it should also flow freely from one channel to the next. When it does not flow freely there can be widespread dysfunction because of the connectivity of the channels. The Chinese maintain that the Qi does not just flow randomly through the channels. There is a specific sequence in which the Qi moves through the channels. According to

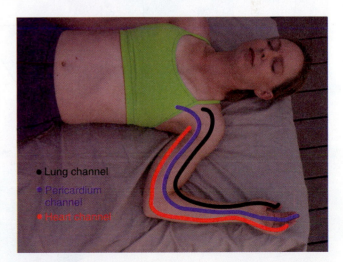

- Lung channel
- Pericardium channel
- Heart channel

FIGURE 14.11

The Location of the Three Yin Channels of the Arm and Hand. The Lung Channel (Black), the Pericardium Channel (Blue), and the Heart Channel (Red).

TCM, the Qi becomes full in a separate channel every two hours and therefore circulates through the entire body in 24 hours (see Figure 14.12 ■). The **24-hour flow of Qi** occurs in the following sequence:

- 🕐 3–5 a.m. Lung
- 🕐 5–7 a.m. Large Intestine
- 🕐 7–9 a.m. Stomach
- 🕐 9–11 a.m. Spleen
- 🕐 11 a.m.–1 p.m. Heart
- 🕐 1–3 p.m. Small Intestine
- 🕐 3–5 p.m. Urinary Bladder
- 🕐 5–7 p.m. Kidney
- 🕐 7–9 p.m. Pericardium
- 🕐 9–11 p.m. San Jao

- 🕐 11 p.m.–1 a.m. Gall Bladder
- 🕐 1–3 a.m. Liver

The 24-hour cycle explains why the full effects of an acupressure treatment may not be felt until a day later. It takes 24 hours for the Qi to fully circulate and to affect the entire body. The 24-hour cycle helps when diagnosing disease that tends to appear only at a certain time of day. It can also be used in myoskeletal assessment. (See Chapters 15 and 16 for more about TCM assessment.)

A complete understanding of the influences of the major channels and those of the many connecting, minor channels is a huge undertaking. Though it is worthwhile to understand all the correlations, a full understanding is not necessary for the application of acupressure when treating myoskeletal issues. When using channel theory to treat myoskeletal pathology, there are just a few fundamental concepts to keep in mind.

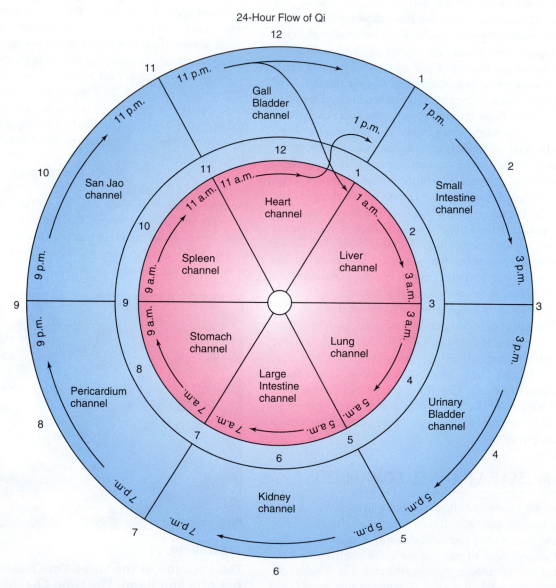

FIGURE 14.12

The 24-Hour Cycle of Qi Flow Through the Channels

The most important questions to answer are:

- What is the path of the exterior portion of the channel? Note the muscles, vessels, nerves, and connective tissue structures which lay along that path.
- Is the channel Yin or Yang? This helps you to keep track of the location and relationship that each channel has with its Yin/Yang counterpart.
- What is the corresponding organ of the channel? Noting the channel's organ is not only important because it is part of the channel's name, but also because it reminds you of the channel's far reaching influences on the body.
- Where does the affected channel lie in the 24-hour flow of Qi? This will help with assessing related pathology.

ACUPOINTS

Acupoints are points in the skin, muscles, and joints that commonly reflect pathology and are used to access the Qi for treatment. Most acupoints are primarily found along the traditional centerline of the channel. Many of these points have been mapped for years and have specific names, classifications, and clearly defined influences on the rest of the body. Generally speaking, stimulating the acupoints is said to have a powerful influence on the flow of Qi, blood, and body fluids.

In fact, modern research has shown that most traditional acupoints are located close to a major *nerve plexus* (a network of converging and diverging nerve fibers), major blood and lymph vessels, and specific myofascial structures.

In 1960, a study conducted by the Anatomical Teaching and Research Group of Shanghai found that 324 acupoints have direct nerve supplies. Out of the main 324 points, 304 are supplied directly by superficial *cutaneous* nerves. While 155 have deep neural connections, interestingly, 137 points have both superficial and deep neural connections. These studies and microscopic observations show the strong connection between acupoints and anatomical locations of neural structures (O'Connor & Bensky, 1981).

Other studies by the same group have explored the relationship between acupoints and blood vessels. In a study of 309 points, 24 were shown to be directly over arterial branches, while 262 points were shown to be within 0.5 cm of either arterial or large venous branches (O'Connor & Bensky, 1981).

The acupoints also have been shown to have a structural relationship with the myofascia. Stanley Rosenberg, a certified Rolfer and author, described the relationship between myofascia and acupoints. He noted that acupoints were "located where two muscles overlapped each other" (Rosenberg, 2003, p. 16). He went on to say,

> When I explored [the acupoint] with my fingers, I found that I could easily dive through a tunnel. The margin of one muscle was on one side of my finger and the margin of the other muscle was on the other side of my finger. (Rosenberg, 2003, p. 16)

Here, Rosenberg is describing the fascial septum between muscles, which is one of the most effective places to treat the myofascia.

Additionally, the piezoelectric current that flows through all fascia may be the basis for the Chinese description of the subtle flow of Qi that flows in the superficial portion of the channels. If an electric probe is run along the channel on the surface of the skin, we discover that acupoints are areas where there is a high level of electrical conductivity. The electrical conductivity extends into the subcutaneous fascia and eventually into the deeper layers of fascia within the muscles and joints via the piezoelectric current (O'Conner & Bensky, 1981).

As noted, some acupoints have a specific impact on the body's processes or functions when stimulated. An example of this is the acupoint Pericardium #6, which is found on the wrist (see Figure 14.13 ■). When this acupoint is stimulated, it will prevent and/or alleviate motion sickness, nausea, and even morning sickness from pregnancy.

DID YOU KNOW

Research using an fMRI to observe changes in brain activity provides interesting insight into how acupoints work. Bladder 60, an acupoint located on the ankle and which is associated with the eyes, was stimulated with acupuncture. The stimulation registered in the occipital lobe of the brain just as visual information from the eyes would. Interestingly, although the ankle is much farther away, the signal traveled from the ankle to the brain many times faster than the neural signal from the eyes (O'Connor & Bensky, 1981).

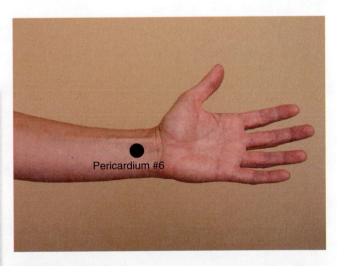

Pericardium #6

FIGURE 14.13

The Location of the Acupoint Pericardium #6 on the Anterior Wrist

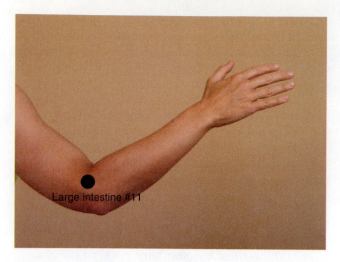

FIGURE 14.14

The Location of the Acupoint Large Intestine #11 on the Lateral Elbow

Some acupoints have a wide range of special actions. They can treat specific symptoms, affect tissues and organs, and have a general effect on the whole body. The acupoint Large Intestine #11, for example, is a powerful point for treating elbow pain (see Figure 14.14 ■), but is also effective for releasing heat, such as fever, as well as treating constipation.

There are a variety of ways a traditional Chinese medicine practitioner can stimulate acupoints. Though there is some evidence that massaging the points may be the oldest form of stimulation (O'Conner & Bensky, 1981), acupuncture (which uses needles) and moxibustion (which uses a burning herb over the point) are also popular methods. Some suggest that massage is the best way to stimulate the points because the practitioner uses his or her own Qi in the therapy. The focus of this text is on stimulating acupoints and channels using bodywork methods such as compression, kneading, and static pressure.

Locating Acupoints

Acupoints are located based on their position relative to other body structures and landmarks. Since every person's physical dimensions are so different, it would be impossible to find acupoints using standard measurements such as inches or millimeters. A person who is six feet tall has much longer leg bones than a person who is four feet tall. Therefore it would be impossible to say that the patella is 22 inches proximal to the ankle on every person. The same is true for acupoints.

For this reason there is a special system for locating acupoints along the channels. This system uses "body inches" called **cun** (pronounced "chun"). Each cun is equivalent to the width of the knuckle of the client's thumb. In addition to using the thumb as a ruler, other body parts have consistent measurements of cun. (Figure 14.15 ■ shows the common cun

FIGURE 14.15

A Chart of the Cun (or "Body Inch") Measurements According to Acupressure Theory

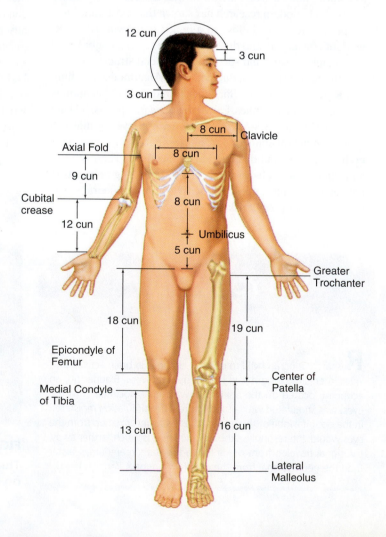

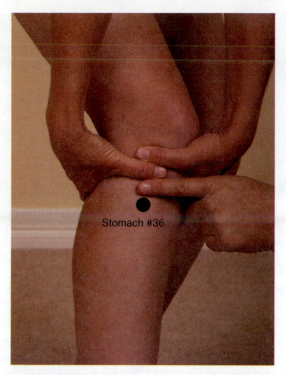

FIGURE 14.16

Stomach #36 Is About 3 Cun Below the Knee on the Anterior Lateral Surface of the Lower Leg.

measurements.) The specific location of an acupoint can be found counting distances, in cun, along a channel. For example, the point Stomach #36 can be located 3 cun inferior to the lower lateral border of the kneecap (see Figure 14.16 ■).

Often acupoints are not found by measuring cun, but by locating bony landmarks and the tissues between them. Many acupoints are found in areas where bones come together or in natural grooves along the body's surface. An example is Gall Bladder #34. This point is located by finding the head of the fibula and moving just inferior and anterior to that head (see Figure 14.17 ■).

Classifying and Naming Acupoints

Traditional Chinese medicine practitioners have many ways of classifying acupoints. They may be classified based on a variety of reasons, such as having similar functions or similar locations. One group of acupoints, called *Xicleft* acupoints,

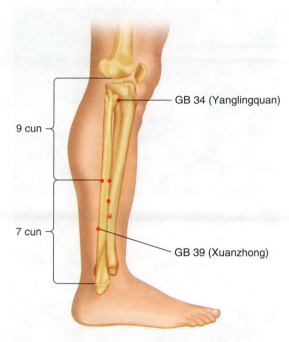

FIGURE 14.17

Gall Bladder #34 Is Located Just Inferior to the Head of the Fibula on the Lower Leg.

is organized according to similar functions. These points are especially effective for acute problems such as pain. These points are found on all 12 major channels. Another group of acupoints, called *Back Shu,* demonstrates both types of classification. They are grouped together because of their location (along both sides of the spine) and their ability to treat specific organs.

Oftentimes, using specific combinations of acupoints will produce results surpassing the use of a single acupoint or a large number of acupoints. One of the most popular combinations is called the *four gates.* It combines Liver #3, located between the big toe and second toes of each foot (see Figure 14.18 ■), with Large Intestine #4, located between the thumbs and index fingers (see Figure 14.19 ■). The four gates combination has the special function of relaxing the entire body and clearing the mind.

The classification of acupoints often dictates how they are used, and the combining of different acupoints is an art form unto itself.

HOLISTIC CONNECTION

Mu points and Shu points are important groups of acupoints. Interestingly, these points coincide with certain "Head's zones" (areas described by Sir Henry Head which reflect internal pathology as local skin tenderness). In fact, Head also described "maximum points" within these zones, which coincide closely with these

diagnostic and therapeutic acupoints of traditional Chinese medicine (Beissner, Henke, & Unschuld, 2009). The independent discovery of these areas shows how different perspectives build a more complete view of the whole body.

See Chapters 6–9 for more about Head's zones.

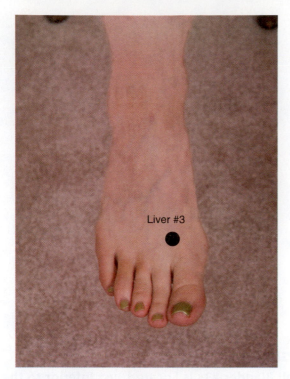

FIGURE 14.18
The Location of the Acupoint Liver #3

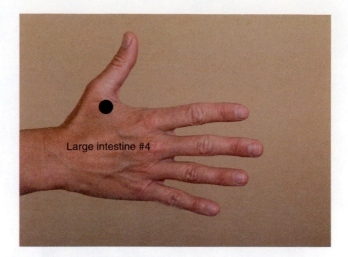

FIGURE 14.19
The Location of the Acupoint Large Intestine #4

As bodyworkers, there are only two major categories that we need to be concerned with: traditional channel acupoints and Ashi acupoints. **Traditional channel acupoints** are acupoints found along a channel. They are listed by the name of the channel in which they are located and by the number in which they are found along that channel. For example, Lung #1 is the first acupoint on the Lung channel; Lung #2 is the second, etc. This name is often abbreviated to just the first letter or two of the corresponding channel and the number. For example, Heart #1 becomes H1, Spleen #6 becomes Sp6 and so on (see Table 14.2 ■).

In the Chinese language, almost all acupoints have poetic names that either describe the acupoint's location or tell something significant about it. For example, Sp6 is called *three Yin crossing* because the three Yin channels of the leg meet at this acupoint.

Most traditional acupoints are found along the course of a channel, but not all of them. Some acupoints, called *extra acupoints*, are found in very specific locations throughout the torso and limbs that do not correspond to a specific channel. *Taiyang* are two extra acupoints found in the temple region between the lateral end of the eyebrow and the outer corner of the eye (see Figure 14.20 ■).

TABLE 14.2	Channel Abbreviations
Channel Abbreviations	
Lungs	Lu
Large Intestine	LI
Spleen	Sp
Stomach	St
Liver	Lv
Gall Bladder	GB
Heart	H
Small Intestine	SI
San Jao	SJ
Pericardium	P
Urinary Bladder	UB

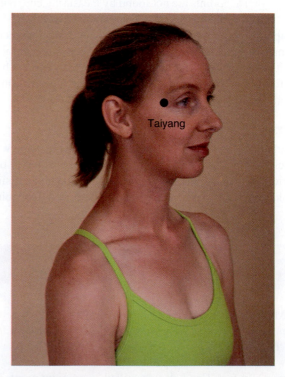

FIGURE 14.20
The Location of Taiyang

QUICK QUIZ #28

1. The 12 primary channels: (Circle all that apply)
   a. intersect with the ren and du channels.
   b. are bilateral.
   c. are grouped into Yin and Yang pairings based upon their functions.
   d. share acupoints with some of the extra channels.
   e. All of the above
   f. None of the above

2. The Yang channels are found on the posterior and medial surfaces of the body.
   a. True
   b. False

3. The Qi moves through the body in a set sequence in a 24-hour period.
   a. True
   b. False

4. Acupoints: (Circle all that apply)
   a. have a specific impact on the function of the body when stimulated.
   b. tend to be areas with a high level of electrical conductivity.
   c. tend to be located in areas supplied by important neurological structures.
   d. tend to be in areas with little or no blood vessels nearby.
   e. All of the above
   f. None of the above

5. Ashi acupoints are found along the path of the traditional channels, and they have specific names and numbers according to their location on a particular channel.
   a. True
   b. False

Finally, some acupoints, called *Ashi* **(pronounced aahh-shee) acupoints,** have no specific location. Ashi acupoints are found wherever there is a painful spot on the body.

There are about 350 commonly used acupoints. This number includes all channel acupoints and extra acupoints but not Ashi acupoints. There can be an infinite number of Ashi acupoints.

MAP OF THE MAJOR CHANNELS AND ACUPOINTS

The following figures illustrate the paths of the 12 major channels. Keep in mind that the diagrams, and the descriptions, only present the channel on one side of the body. There is an exact duplicate (*mirror channel*) on the other side of the body. The internal (or deep) portions of the channel are indicated by a dotted line in the diagrams. The external (or superficial) portions are a solid line with the acupoints in dots indicated along their course.

Lung Channel
- Location name: Hand/Arm Taiyin (meaning "greater Yin"). The greater Yin area of the body in this case is along the anterior, lateral aspect.
- Time of day the Qi in the channel is full: 3–5 a.m.
- This channel begins with an internal section deep inside the torso that flows through the lungs. The exterior portion emerges at the anterior crease of the shoulder and travels down the anterior/lateral portion of the arm, past the wrist ending on the thumb (at the corner of the nail).
- It has roughly 11 acupoints along its course and treats disorders of the Lungs, Large Intestine, nose, skin, wrist, forearm, and anterior shoulder (see Figure 14.21 ■).

Large Intestine Channel
- Location name: Hand/Arm Yangming (meaning "Yang brightness"). The bright Yang area of the body in this case is along the posterior, lateral aspect.
- Time of day the Qi in the channel is full: 5–7 a.m.

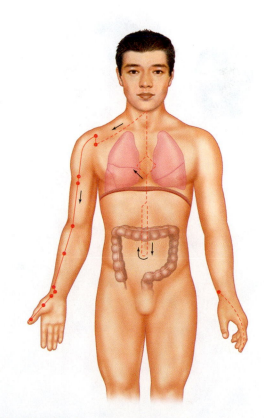

FIGURE 14.21
The Path of the Lung Channel

- The exterior section begins at the radial side of the tip of the index finger and travels up the lateral/posterior side of the arm past the superior portion of the shoulder. From there it travels up the lateral neck and onto the face going around the lips, teeth, and gums to end just below the nostril on the opposite side of the face. It also has an internal section running to the Large Intestine.
- It has 20 acupoints and treats disorders of the nose, teeth, Lungs, Large Intestine, elbow, and forearm (see Figure 14.22 ■).

Stomach Channel

- Location name: Foot/Leg Yangming (meaning "Yang brightness"). The bright Yang area of the body in this case is along the anterior, lateral aspect.
- Time of day the Qi in the channel is full: 7–9 a.m.
- The external section begins just below the pupil of the eye and travels down the cheekbone and along the jaw. Then it travels superior along the face (in front of the ear) to the lateral forehead. An internal section takes it down to the neck, where it emerges externally at the neck and travels down the chest and abdomen to the leg. In the leg, it travels down the lateral quadriceps to the lateral edge of the tibia and ends at the lateral tip of the second toe.
- It has 45 acupoints and treats the Stomach, Spleen, muscles, some systemic issues, the knees, hip, and ankle (see Figure 14.23 ■).

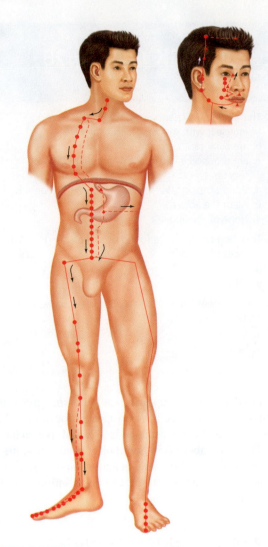

FIGURE 14.23
The Path of the Stomach Channel

The Spleen Channel

- Location name: Foot/Leg Taiyin (meaning "greater Yin"). The greater Yin area of the body in this case is along the anterior, medial aspect.
- Time of day the Qi in the channel is full: 9–11 a.m.
- The external section begins at the medial end of the big toe and runs along the medial edge of the foot to travel the medial portion of the entire leg. From there, it travels to the abdomen and up into the chest, where an internal section terminates at the base of the tongue.
- It has 21 acupoints along its path and treats disorders of the digestive process, the muscles, the knee, and ankle (see Figure 14.24 ■).

The Heart Channel

- Location name: Hand/Arm Shaoyin (meaning "lesser Yin"). The lesser Yin area of the body in this case is along the anterior, medial aspect.
- Time of day the Qi in the channel is full: 11 a.m.–1 p.m.
- It begins with an internal branch in the Heart organ and runs upward to the eye and downward to the

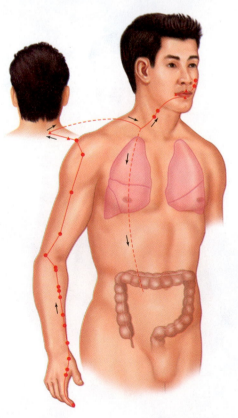

FIGURE 14.22
The Path of the Large Intestine Channel

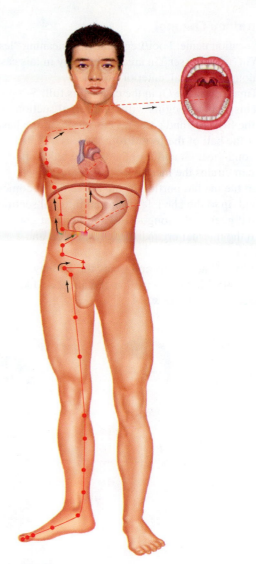

FIGURE 14.24

The Path of the Spleen Channel

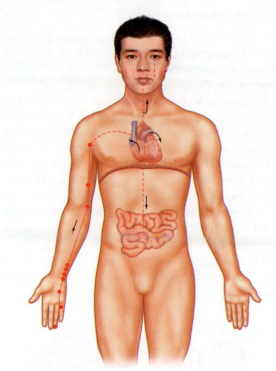

FIGURE 14.25

The Path of the Heart Channel

It also has an internal section that flows deep through the Heart and to the Small Intestine organ.

● It has 19 acupoints and treats disorders of the face, shoulders, elbows, wrist, and neck (see Figure 14.26 ■).

Small Intestine. It runs laterally to the axilla, where it emerges to the exterior and then travels the anterior medial surface of the arm through the medial wrist terminating at the tip of the pinky finger.

● It has 9 acupoints and treats disorders of Heart, Small Intestine, mind, Shen, elbow, forearm, and wrist (see Figure 14.25 ■).

The Small Intestine Channel

● Location name: Hand/Arm Taiyang (meaning "greater Yang"). The greater Yang area of the body in this case is along the posterior, medial aspect.
● Time of day the Qi in the channel is full: 1–3 p.m.
● It begins with an external section at the tip of the pinky finger and travels along the posterior/medial arm to the posterior deltoid. From there, it zigzags across the scapula, and moves up to the lateral portion of the neck and into the face. On the face, it travels below the eye and along the cheekbone to end just anterior to the ear.

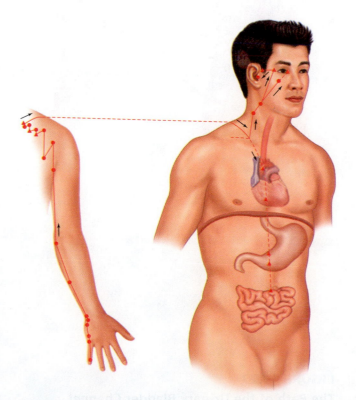

FIGURE 14.26

The Path of the Small Intestine Channel

The Urinary Bladder Channel

- Location name: Foot/Leg Taiyang (meaning "greater Yang"). The greater Yang area of the body in this case is along the posterior, aspect.
- Time of day the Qi in the channel is full: 3–5 p.m.
- It begins with an external section at the medial corner of the eye and travels over the head to the posterior portion of the neck. Then the channel divides into a portion that travels next to the spine and another parallel portion that travels lateral to the first. Both sections travel down to the buttocks and upper leg. The two parts converge at the back of the knee and continue as one, down the calf to the lateral foot to end at the lateral tip of the little toe. It has an internal section that travels to the urinary bladder organ.
- It has 67 acupoints and can treat disorders of the head, neck, back, knees, ankles, eye, and every organ system (see Figure 14.27 ■).

The Kidney Channel

- Location name: Foot/Leg Shaoyin (meaning "lesser Yin"). The lesser Yin area of the body in this case is along the medial, anterior aspect.
- Time of day the Qi in the channel is full: 5–7 p.m.
- This channel begins with an internal section at the little toe and emerges externally at the base of the ball of the foot. From there it travels along the arch and into the medial ankle. It then circles the medial maleolus and travels up the medial portion of the leg to the abdomen and up to the clavicle. It has an internal section that goes to the tongue and another that goes to the internal organs: Kidneys, Liver, and Lungs.
- It has 27 acupoints and treats the Kidneys, Urinary Bladder as well as the ankle and knee. (see Figure 14.28 ■).

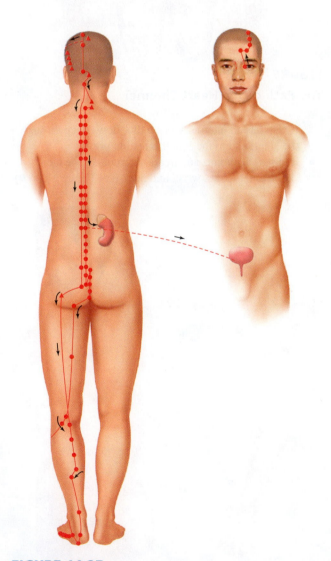

FIGURE 14.27

The Path of the Urinary Bladder Channel

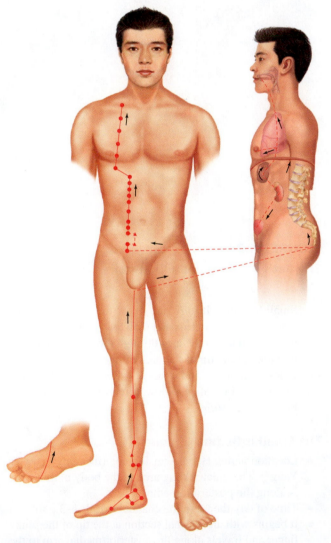

FIGURE 14.28

The Path of the Kidney Channel

The Pericardium Channel

- Location name: Hand/Arm Jueyin (meaning "absolute Yin"). The absolute Yin area of the body in this case is along the anterior aspect.
- Time of day the Qi in the channel is full: 7–9 p.m.
- It begins with an internal section in the center of the chest and has a section that descends down through the diaphragm. The exterior section emerges at the chest just lateral to the nipple. From there it travels down the middle of the anterior arm between the Heart channel and the Lung channel. It continues through the wrist to terminate at the end of the middle finger with an internal section extending to the ring finger.
- It has 9 acupoints and treats disorders of the Heart, Stomach, wrist, and elbow (see Figure 14.29 ■).

The San Jao Channel

- Location name: Hand/Arm Shaoyang (meaning "lesser Yang"). The lesser Yang area of the body in this case is along the posterior, lateral aspect.
- Time of day the Qi in the channel is full: 9–11 p.m.

- It begins with an external section at the tip of the ring finger and travels up the posterior arm to the posterior deltoid. From there it travels up over the superior shoulder to the lateral neck, over the ear, and into the temple. It has an internal section that travels down through the Heart and diaphragm.
- It has 23 acupoints and treats disorders of the wrist, elbow, shoulder, neck and ear (see Figure 14.30 ■).

The Gall Bladder Channel

- Location name: Foot/Leg Shaoyang (meaning "lesser Yang"). The lesser Yang area of the body in this case is along the lateral aspect.
- Time of day the Qi in the channel is full: 11 p.m.–1 a.m.
- It begins with an external section at the outer corner of the eye. Then it zigzags along the side of the head (around the ear) to eventually travel down the neck to the side of the torso. It zigzags along the side of the body down to the thigh. It travels the lateral thigh to the lower leg where it again zigzags a little until it meets with the lateral foot and finally ends at the tip of the fourth toe. It has a deep internal section

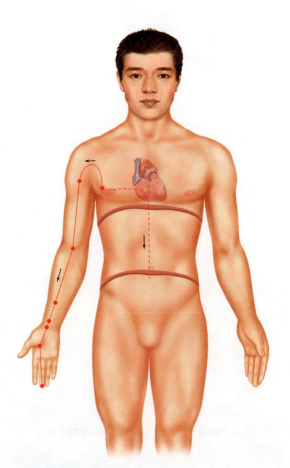

FIGURE 14.29

The Path of the Percardium Channel

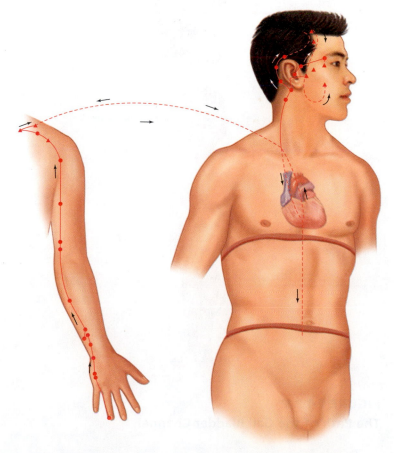

FIGURE 14.30

The Path of the San Jao Channel

that travels from the face down to the liver and gall bladder organs.

- It has 44 acupoints and treats disorders of the eyes, sinews, gall bladder, liver, sides of knees, and ankles (see Figure 14.31 ■).

The Liver Channel

- Location name: Foot/Leg Jueyin (meaning "absolute Yin"). The absolute Yin area of the body in this case is along the medial, anterior, aspect.
- Time of day the Qi in the channel is full: 1–3 a.m.
- This channel begins with an external section at the lateral big toe and travels along the medial

top of the foot towards the medial portion of the leg. From there it continues up along the inside of the leg to enter the groin. It has an internal section that travels to the lateral abdomen and emerges with an external branch and the end of the 11th rib to terminate in the chest just below the nipple. It also has an internal section that travels the chest to the head and face. The Liver channel connects to the Lung channel to complete the 24-hour cycle of Qi.

- It has 14 acupoints and treats disharmony of the liver and blood. It also treats the eyes, sinews, ankles, and knees (see Figure 14.32 ■).

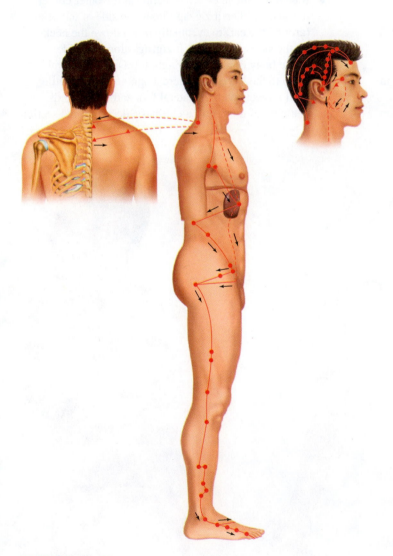

FIGURE 14.31

The Path of the Gall Bladder Channel

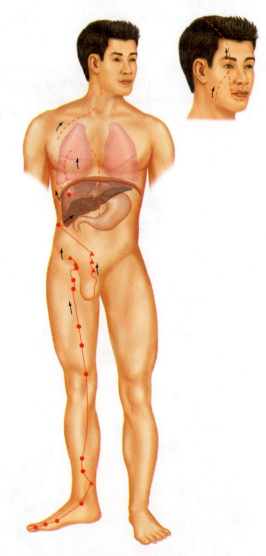

FIGURE 14.32

The Path of the Liver Channel

SUMMARY

Traditional Chinese medicine views the body from a holistic perspective. TCM focuses on the function and interrelationships of organs and systems rather than on their physical structure. The system understands the body in terms of how each part generates, supports, and shares function with all other parts.

There are five elemental substances important to sustaining all life. These include the three treasures—Qi, Jing, and Shen—as well as blood and body fluid.

The word Qi represents all forms of energy, including those formed in the body and those used by it. The Chinese discuss Qi in terms of where it is functioning or which structure is generating it.

Jing is "essence." It is the fundamental physical substance. Jing can be understood as the physical constitution passed on from our parents and derived from the food and liquids that nourish our bodies. Shen is "spirit." Shen represents a person's mind and demeanor. Shen can be seen in a person's outward presentation.

Blood is responsible for hydrating and nourishing the organs and tissues. Blood carries Qi and at the same time Qi moves the blood throughout the body. Body fluid includes the clear/thin fluids such as tears and sweat, as well as the thick/turbid fluids found in the bone marrow, joint spaces, and bile. Body fluids moisten the tissues and help in their function.

These five substances each have their own important functions. If they are deficient, excessive, or out of balance, specific symptoms will be expressed in the overall health of the body system.

The channels make up an elaborate network that carries Qi and blood through the whole body. The channels have a superficial route and a deep route that provide communication to all tissues and structures.

The network of channels is divided into the Jing and the Luo. The Jing include the 12 major channels (named for the organs) and the 8 extra channels. The Luo are a smaller network, a sort of net that connects the major channels. The Qi circulates in the channels over a 24-hour time span. The channels can reflect internal pathology and can also be used to treat it. They also reflect the outer structure of the body.

Each channel includes the skin, muscles, nerves, and blood vessels that follow its pathway. The channels are bands that represent muscular lines of pull, the flow of blood, and the flow of neural information along their pathways.

Acupoints are areas of high electrical conductivity. They are located along the channels and can also be found in the space between. Traditional channel acupoints are located by landmarks and by measuring the cun or "body inches." Acupoints can be used to treat local areas and other specific structures, such as the corresponding organs.

DISCUSSION QUESTIONS

1. How are the Lung channel and Stomach channel related to each other?
2. Name four types of Qi and their specific functions.
3. How do the channels in the body differ from the channel lines seen in traditional diagrams?
4. List four major functions of the channels.
5. Explain two methods for locating acupoints.

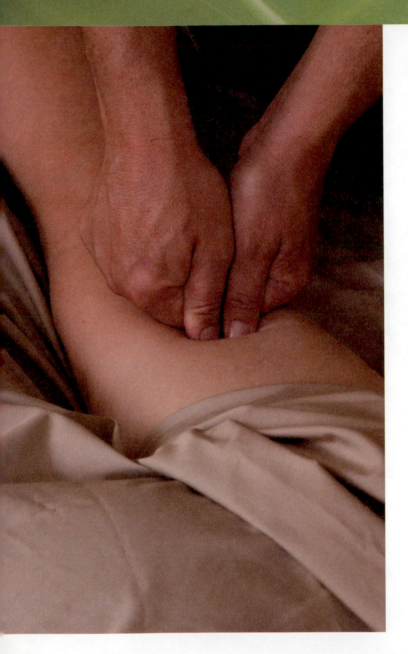

15 An Introduction to Acupressure Theory

 CHAPTER HIGHLIGHTS

Chapter Objectives

Key Terms

The Origins of Chinese Massage (Tui-na)

Acupressure

Chinese Theories of Nature and the Body

The Generating and Controlling Cycles in Acupressure

Channel Theory

Using Acupoints

Using Qi in Therapy

Summary

Discussion Questions

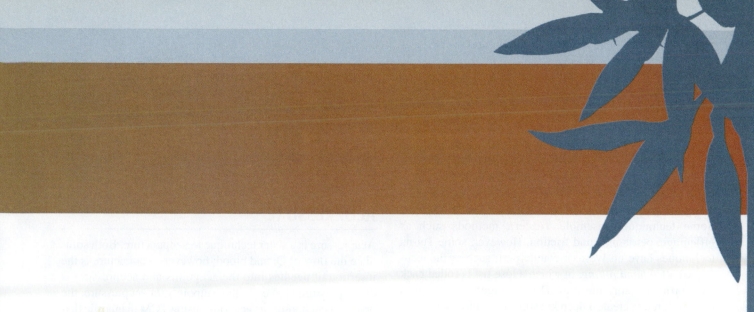

 CHAPTER OBJECTIVES

- Survey the history and modern uses of acupressure
- Consider the traditional Chinese understanding of nature, the body, and medicine
- Explore channel theory and the flow of Qi
- Understand the use of acupoints

 KEY TERMS

THE ORIGINS OF CHINESE MASSAGE (TUI-NA)

The Chinese system of massage and joint manipulation is called **Tui-na.** Pronounced "Twee-naa," the words translate as "push-grasp" or "poke-pinch" in English.

Tui-na employs a series of techniques including pressing, tapping, and kneading. These techniques may be applied using the palms, fingertips, knuckles, or handheld tools. Some techniques resemble Western methods such as effleurage, petrissage, and friction. However, some Tui-na techniques have no Western counterpart, such as the technique called *hand rolling*, in which a lose fist is rolled back and forth over sore muscles. Done correctly, it provides enough force to create a deep kneading effect in the muscle.

Tui-na techniques range from light pressure to very deep work, some of which can be very vigorous, even quite uncomfortable. All are designed to stimulate the flow of Qi and blood and to remove blockages along the channels of the body.

As mentioned, joint manipulation techniques are also a part of Tui-na. Some of these techniques are very similar to Western chiropractic and osteopathic techniques and others employ a very dynamic form of joint mobilization. This dynamic form uses multiple movements performed by the doctor and the patient together. This active movement is very beneficial in freeing up restricted joints.

In addition to the hands-on therapies, clinical practitioners often use liniments, plasters, herbal packs, and compresses to aid in the healing process. Overall, Tui-na stresses integration of the whole body through balancing the muscles, bones, and channels.

Pediatric Tui-na

Pediatric Tui-na is a subdivision formulated for the treatment of small children, usually those younger than 8 years of age. It uses traditional Chinese medical diagnoses to understand the nature of the imbalance and then attempts to correct the imbalance using a variety of strokes and techniques to encourage Qi flow. According to the Chinese, young children's channels are easily stimulated. So instead of using specific acupoints, they use a series of strokes along small portions of the channels. The strokes are applied mainly to the hands and feet, although they are not limited to those areas. For example, to boost the overall health of a child, a common pinch and roll technique (similar to skin rolling) is applied to both sides of the spine from the sacrum to the cervical region. This technique may be applied daily 1 to 10 times per session. It stimulates all organ systems and encourages brain function (Ya-li, 1994).

ACUPRESSURE

Acupressure is a sister technique to acupuncture. Both stimulate the flow of Qi and blood; however, acupuncture is the insertion of needles into the acupoints and acupressure is direct pressure applied to the acupoints. In acupressure, the practitioner chooses the acupoints using TCM diagnostic theory. Once chosen, each point is pressed for a few seconds and then released. The pressure is often applied to the same point a number of times. Sometimes light vibration may be applied to the acupoints along with the pressure for especially stubborn blockages. The depth of pressure depends on the treatment area. Large muscles may require more depth while thinner, less muscular areas may require less depth. Pressure may be applied using the fingers, palms, thumbs, knees, and feet. In standard traditional treatments, the practitioner must concentrate his or her own Qi to help direct the Qi of the patient to the areas that are imbalanced or blocked.

The Origins of Acupressure

Acupressure is probably one of the oldest treatment modalities found within the Chinese system. It is widely believed that the use of acupressure to stimulate acupoints predated the use of needles and other implements to stimulate them. There are many theories as to the origins of the use of acupoints for healing. They range from the bizarre to the plausible. One theory paints a picture of ancient people sitting around a campfire. They may have noticed that placing heated stones from the campfire on sore or injured parts of their bodies had a soothing effect and sped up the healing process. They might also have discovered that the heated stones helped internal complaints as well. They may have begun to experiment and discover that various scratches on the surface of the skin often had similar effects as the heated stones. Thus, they began practicing with various types of heating or skin pricking to see how it affected the body (O'Connor & Bensky, 1981).

Other theories about the origins of this amazing method surmise that ancient people noticed that rubbing certain spots on the body's surface helped to alleviate pain and encouraged the resolution of internal disorders. This observation may have lead to experimentation with more aggressive methods, such as scratching and eventually poking the skin with sharp stones or bones (O'Connor & Bensky, 1981).

Still, there are other stories of how ancient warriors would return from battle with amazing cures for chronic problems. It appeared that after having received a battle wound in a specific spot on the body, the warrior received a remarkable cure for an old chronic problem. Perhaps a

DID YOU KNOW

Some Tui-na methods are very unfamiliar to Western practitioners. Nonetheless, they can be very effective. I once watched a TCM practitioner apply a therapy to a Chinese patient. The therapy involved using a short stick to aggressively rub the spinous processes of the vertebral column. It looked very painful, yet the patient reported great relief from the treatment.

discovery such as this prompted the ancient Chinese to experiment with piercing the skin, to try to correct similar chronic imbalances (O'Connor & Bensky, 1981).

Regardless of how acupuncture and acupressure were first discovered, we do know from archaeological evidence that ancient people used stones, bones, and later metals to prick, poke, and even puncture the skin in an effort to heal themselves. In fact, archaeologists recently discovered an ancient man buried in the ice. He had peculiar tattoos on his skin that remarkably correspond to modern acupoints. He also had a pouch that contained bone implements that appear as though they could have been used as acupuncture needles (Huihe, 1992).

Although the ancient origins are lost or are not yet discovered by archaeology, there are written texts and traditions that go back thousands of years. Remarkably, these thousand-year-old texts are still relevant today and are used by those who study and practice this healing art.

A Chronology of the Major Early Texts

In the earliest days, techniques and theories were handed down from generation to generation through apprenticeships. Each family had its own methods and classifications of acupoints and herbs. These methods were considered sacred, and the healing secrets were kept within each family's circle. It wasn't until the Warring States Period of 770 to 221 BCE that a general compilation of information called the *NeiJing Internal Classic* was completed. Also known as *The Yellow Emperor's Internal Classic of Medicine*, the *NeiJing* is the oldest known text. It provides the general foundation for the techniques of Chinese medicine and its herbal pharmacology. Following in the footsteps of the *NeiJing*, the *NanJing*—or *Classic on Difficult Medical Problems*—was also written during this time period. This incredible resource outlines the Chinese perspectives on physiology, pathology, diagnosis, and treatment. This text was intended to supplement the *NeiJing* as a theoretical foundation (O'Connor & Bensky, 1981).

During the Han Dynasty (206 BCE to 220 CE), the famous doctor Zhang Zhongjing expanded on the *NeiJing* and *NanJing* with his *Treatise on Febrile and Miscellaneous Diseases*. This text discussed the theory of "exterior invasions." Zhang Zhongjing believed that natural factors, such as heat, could invade the body and cause disease. This theory is similar to Western medicine's view about communicable diseases, such as colds and flu. Zhang Zhongjing also wrote *Prescriptions from the Golden Cabinet*. Here he classifies disease on the basis of the internal organs. He describes over 40 diseases and 262 prescriptions (Huihe, 1992).

During the Sui Dynasty (58–618 CE) and the Song Dynasty (960–1279 CE), many more texts were written which elaborated on the earlier treatises. It wasn't until the Jin and Yuan dynasties (1271–1368 CE) that distinctively different schools of thought developed. There were four schools that were collectively known as the "Four Major Schools." Each had its own unique approach; yet all four schools used the earlier written texts as their foundation. This was a time of great creativity, for it was the first time that physicians had more than one major approach from which to choose. It was during this time of diversity that the book, *Treatise on the Spleen and Stomach*, was written by Li Dong-Yuan. This famous text brought to the forefront the idea that much of disease comes from internal imbalances. Li Dong-Yuan discussed the value of harmony between the internal organs and the importance of the spleen and stomach in that balance. He felt that external invasions could only be present if the body was weak and its defenses were down (Huihe, 1992).

During the next few generations, many medical advances and famous books were written, including the *Treatise on Pestilence* completed during the Ming Dynasty (1368–1644 CE). This book further elaborated on the work of Zhang Zhongjing and discussed the sources of diseases that arise from outside the body. As time progressed and more information was collected, masters began to examine the various shortcomings of earlier texts and tried to correct the earlier misconceptions. One such book, called *Errors in Medicine Corrected*, was written during the Qing Dynasty (1644–1911 CE). This text, written by Wang Qingren, attempted to clear up the anatomical errors of the ancient texts. Wang Qingren also originated the idea that blood stagnation is a major cause of internal ailments (Huihe, 1992).

Throughout the following decades, and with the influx of Western scientific methodology, China continued expanding on the knowledge of the old texts and still carries on that work today. In fact, other countries have been contributing greatly to the advancement of acupuncture and acupressure for quite some time. Germany and France have been experimenting with and using these methods for a few hundred years, perhaps even as long as they have been trading with the East. America had its first widely publicized introduction to acupuncture during President Nixon's visit to China. During that visit, Americans got to see firsthand how acupuncture was being used during medical procedures. It has been many years since that first introduction, but finally there is a growing national interest in the methods of acupressure and acupuncture. The recent endorsement of acupuncture from the World Health Organization has been instrumental to this newfound interest (Williams, 1996).

 DID YOU KNOW

In 1972, *New York Times* correspondent James "Scotty" Reston received acupuncture as postoperative treatment while he was covering Nixon's visit to China. He wrote at length about his experience and was instrumental in introducing this healing system to the United States (Williams, 1996).

Modern Acupressure

Acupressure and acupuncture found their way into the United States through a variety of popular approaches. One such approach is a technique called "Touch for Health." This technique was created by John F. Thie, D.C. He published his first manual in 1973. It is a practical guide to natural health that uses acupressure, touch, and massage to improve postural balance and reduce physical tension and mental stress. Touch for Health relies heavily on the traditional Chinese channels in its therapy. It also refers to seven different types of points called *touch reflexes*. One of these is the series of points called the *neurolymphatic points*, which were discovered in the early 1930s by Frank D. Chapman, D.O. and his wife Ada Hinckley Chapman, D.O. (Thie, 1994).

In 1937, Dr. Ada Hinckley Chapman and a colleague named Charles Owens, D.O. wrote the book *An Endocrine Interpretation of Chapman's Reflex*. It described the system of reflex points first used by Dr. Frank Chapman.

According to the Chapmans, these reflex points are predictable fascial tissue abnormalities that reflect *visceral* dysfunction or pathology. Dr. Chapman felt that the special relationship of these points to both neural and lymphatic function was the key to the profound effects they had on all systems of the body. Neurolymphatic points can be used for diagnosis, for influencing the motion of fluids (mostly lymph), and for influencing visceral function (Thie, 1994).

In the early 1970s, Mary Burmeister popularized an ancient form of acupressure known as *Jin Shin Jyutsu*. This form descends from ancient techniques that were developed in the Taoist and Buddhist temples of China and then brought to Japan by Jiro Murai in the early 1900s. Jiro Murai discovered these ancient Chinese techniques and created the form of acupressure called *Jin Shin Jyutsu*. Mary Burmeister, a student of Jiro Murai, eventually brought these techniques back to California and taught them to Western students. One such student was Iona Marsaa Teeguarden (Burmeister & Monte (see p. 412) 1997).

Teeguarden took these teachings and developed her own special style she calls *Jin Shin Do*. Teeguarden's approach differs from Jin Shin Jyutsu by emphasizing classic Chinese acupuncture theory. In Teeguarden's writings she makes use of 12 major channels, which she calls the *organ meridians*, and the 8 extra channels, which she calls the *strange flows*. She also integrates Reichian's theories about emotions and attitudes with acupressure theories about how the emotions relate to the meridians. Finally, Teeguarden emphasizes the use of ancient movement and breathing exercises called *Qi gong* (Teeguarden, 1978).

Another technique that has helped to popularize acupressure in the West is a technique called *Tapas acupressure technique (TAT)*. Tapas Fleming, a licensed acupuncturist in California, developed the method in 1993. TAT incorporates elements of traditional Chinese acupressure techniques and emphasizes the clearing of negative emotions and beliefs. TAT is carried out by applying light pressure to four areas (the inner corner of each eye, one half an inch above the space between the eyebrows, and one on the back of the head).

Acupressure is a mainstay in most Asian health care systems and is growing in popularity in the United States. It is a popular form of self-therapy as it has very few contraindications. Some people believe that acupressure is superior to acupuncture because the touch carries with it a sharing of Qi between the therapist and client, which may have more profound effects on the movement of Qi.

CHINESE THEORIES OF NATURE AND THE BODY

As mentioned, the Chinese medical system is thousands of years old. At its inception, there were no microscopes to study cells or modern imaging technologies such as radiographs or MRIs (magnetic resonance imaging) to look inside the body. Instead, practitioners used observation and careful analysis of symptoms in order to understand disease and its processes. They observed how the health of the internal organs is reflected in the skin, muscles, and joints. They observed that the health of the skin, muscles, and joints could indicate the health of the internal organs. The Chinese paid close attention to how an individual's emotions and thoughts impacted their bodies and influenced the healing process. They also took into account the impact of the environment and how our bodies are constantly adjusting to it. They evaluated how all of these elements combine together to promote or discourage health. Through this type of careful observation, they developed basic theories about the internal workings of the body and its relationship to the outside environment.

Yin/Yang is the Way of heaven and earth,	The fundamental principle of the myriad things,	The father and mother of change and transformation,	The root of inception and destruction. ~ *Su Wen, Yellow Emperor's Classic*

Yin and Yang

Yin and Yang is the most basic classification system for looking into the interrelationships of all things. Early Chinese theorists noticed that all things have an opposite. Just like a coin has two sides, so does everything in the universe. Day does not exist without night, nor does heat without cold, soft without hard, etc. The Chinese organized these dualities into two distinct groups. One they called *Yin*, and the other they called *Yang*. This essentially created two categories for dividing everything in the world.

TABLE 15.1	Common Yin/Yang Counterparts	
	Yin	Yang
In Nature	Night	Day
	Winter	Summer
	Moon	Sun
	Water	Fire
	Dark	Light
	Earth	Sky
	Contraction	Expansion
	Descending	Rising
In the Body	Anterior/front	Posterior/back
	Female	Male
	Rest	Action
	Blood	Qi
	Organs	Skin
	Solid	Hollow
	Structure	Function
	Interior	Exterior
In Disease	Chronic	Acute
	Gradual onset	Rapid onset
	Chills	Fever
	Depression	Anxiety
	Hypo-function	Hyper-function

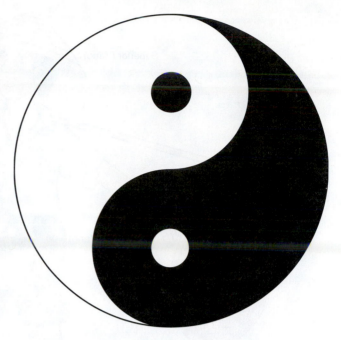

FIGURE 15.1

Symbolic Representation of Yin/Yang

Table 15.1 ■ provides a list of some common Yin/Yang counterparts. This list is by no means exhaustive. It is just a sample of which types of things are normally classified as Yin and which are classified as Yang.

When looking at lists of Yin and Yang categories, it is easy to get the impression that this is a static concept and all things are either one or the other. The reality is that Yin and Yang are opposite ends of a continuum, and really everything actually falls somewhere in between the ends. Nothing is either all hot or all cold; it is always somewhere in between these two extremes. Often it is in dynamic flux between the two. This constant change is a very important idea and will be elaborated upon later in this chapter.

The concept of Yin and Yang is often written as Yin/Yang. This is to emphasize that each component makes up part of a whole rather than being two distinct entities. To understand this dynamic relationship, it is helpful to look at the symbol for Yin/Yang (see Figure 15.1 ■). The Yin/Yang symbol is a whole circle that is split into halves. One half represents Yin, the other Yang. Together, they make up the whole. The dark half of the symbol represents the Yin nature of things, and the light half represents the Yang nature of things.

In addition to showing the Yin/Yang halves, the symbol illustrates that the opposing sides are dependent upon each other for their very existence. Like a coin, in order to have one side the other side must also exist. The symbol represents this relationship by having a small spot of dark (Yin) within the white (Yang) side, and a small spot of white (Yang) within the dark (Yin) side. The symbol shows that it is the interdependence of these opposites that creates the balanced whole. Balance of Yin and Yang is the key.

In regards to medical theory, health and illness are understood over the backdrop of Yin/Yang theory. Giovanni Maciocia (1989) states that, "Every physiological process and every symptom or sign can be analyzed in the light of the Yin-Yang theory" (p. 7). The regulation of body temperature is a good example. As soon as the body's temperature rises above normal, which would be a Yang state, the body counteracts that process by adding Yin to cool it down. It does this by turning on the cooling mechanisms, like sweating and dilating blood vessels. This cools the system, boosts the Yin, and brings the body into balance.

In addition to bodily processes, areas of the body are also categorized according to Yin/Yang principles. Figure 15.2 ■ illustrates some common Yin/Yang divisions of the body. Some examples include:

- The superior portions of the body are more Yang in relation to the inferior portions of the body, which are considered Yin.
- The lateral surfaces are more Yang and the medial surfaces are more Yin.
- The posterior half is more Yang compared to the anterior half of the body, which is Yin.
- The exterior of the body is more Yang, while the interior is more Yin.

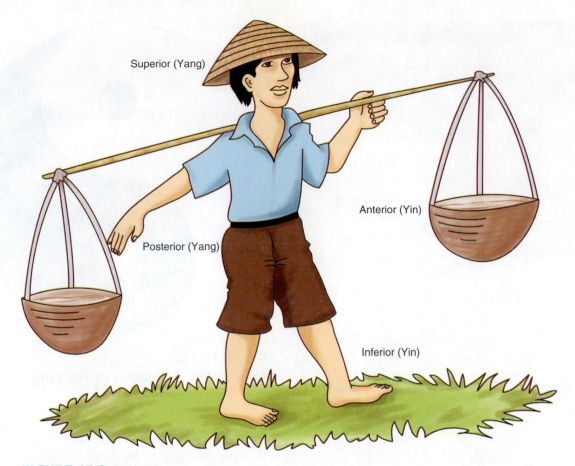

Superior (Yang)

Anterior (Yin)

Posterior (Yang)

Inferior (Yin)

FIGURE 15.2

Yin and Yang Areas of the Body

These comparisons can go on and on because Yin/Yang is infinitely divisible and all of the body's structures are relative to each other.

For example, some organs such as the gastrointestinal (GI) tract are more Yang than other organs (such as the heart). This is because the GI tract opens to the outside (through the mouth and anus), which is considered more Yang relative to the deeper position of the heart located deep inside the chest. However, all internal organs (GI tract included) are Yin in comparison to the skin. This is because the skin is entirely on the outside and exposed to light relative to the internal organs in the deep dark regions of the body. The skin itself has Yang areas (posterior and lateral) and Yin areas (anterior and medial).

DID YOU KNOW

Take a look at your forearm. You will notice that the skin on the lateral/posterior half is rougher, durable, and less sensitive, which is Yang in nature. The medial/anterior aspects are soft and sensitive, which is Yin in nature.

Yin/Yang analogies are also used when diagnosing and treating pathology. For example, an inflamed joint is described as an excessive Yang condition because of the heat that is often felt around the area of pain due to the increased vascular response. Too much Yang results in the Yin/Yang being out of balance. For proper health, the two must be brought back into balance. The analogy works because in order to bring down the excessive Yang (heat/inflammation), a therapist can add Yin (i.e., ice) to cool and balance the Yin/Yang. Conversely, when there is lack of circulation to an area due to tension or injury, the tissues become cold. This is described as excessive Yin. In this case, the therapist adds Yang (i.e., heat) to the area to encourage circulation.

Understanding the Yin/Yang divisions and the ways that they complement and counteract each other helps to simplify the complexity of the world with more manageable concepts. It also reminds us of the natural balancing act of all things and processes in the world.

TRANSFORMATION OF YIN/YANG

Everything in the universe is constantly moving between the two extremes of Yin and Yang, balancing and counterbalancing and ever changing.

Nature contains many examples of the constant flow of Yin into Yang. Winter, which is Yin, transforms into spring, which is more Yang. Then, spring transforms into summer which is even more Yang. Summer becomes fall, which is more Yin. Eventually, fall transforms back into winter again. There is never really a time when a particular season is totally and completely that one season. It is always transforming into the next phase. This dynamic interchange reveals the truth that all things are ever changing, constantly moving, and that change is the only constant. Even the mountains, which seem as though they are unchanging, are both growing from underneath and simultaneously being eroded by wind and rain. It is just happening so slowly that it is hard to see the change.

This idea of constant flow, flux, or change is essential to all Chinese theory. It is rooted in the Chinese concept called the **Tao.**

The Tao ("The Way")

Tao (pronounced "dao") means "the path" or "the way." It is a universal principle that underlies everything from the creation of the universe to the interactions of all things. All things in the world are considered to be manifestations of the Tao as well as contained within it. The Tao is often referred to as "the nameless" because neither it, nor its principles, can ever be adequately expressed in words. The Tao has neither shape nor form. Often it is simply understood as change, both the process of change and the thing being changed.

A river is often used as a metaphor for the Tao. Like the Tao, the movement of the river defines its existence. A river is constantly flowing, moving, and carrying life along with it. Its life is in its movement and its ability to keep flowing. The Tao is the movement that constantly propels our lives forward, and as we move, we are also in constant change.

The Tao is like a well: used but never used up. It is like the eternal void: filled with infinite possibilities.	The Tao doesn't take sides; it gives birth to both good and evil.	The Tao is like a bellows: it is empty yet infinitely capable. The more you use it, the more it produces; the more you talk of it, the less you understand. *Lao Tzu*

TAOISM

While the Tao cannot be expressed in simple terms, the school of thought called *Taoism* holds that it can be known, and its principles can be followed. Taoists use the Yin and

> Beyond the gate of experience flows the Way, Which is ever greater and more subtle than the world.
>
> *Lao Tzu*

DID YOU KNOW

One system of exercise and martial art that springs from Taoist principles is *Tai chi*. Tai chi uses a routine of combined movements to promote coordination, strength, and flexibility. In some styles, there are hidden martial arts defense moves within the routines.

Being true to Taoist principles, Tai chi emphasizes softness and yielding instead of forceful techniques. An attacking force is not met with force, but rather by yielding and allowing the force to pass through without causing harm. In Tai chi, it is better to be the "cork in water." No matter how hard it is pushed into the water, the cork yields. By not resisting, the cork is not broken.

Yang paradigm to understand the principles of the Tao. The Tao represents the unity of the Yin/Yang opposites and is also the force behind one's constant transformation into the other.

The founder of Taoism, Lao Tzu, wrote the definitive source on Taoism, called the *Tao Te Ching* (pronounced "Dao De Jing"). It is a practical philosophical manual that includes principles for achieving fulfillment in life. Much of the text focuses on the value of following the Tao and of the ultimate uselessness of trying to understand and/or control it outright.

According to Taoist thinking, resisting change (the Tao) is impossible. Change is inevitable—you cannot stop it. When you try, you have to stiffen up against it and use considerable effort. Even then you will be standing still while everything else is moving. Think about standing in a river and resisting the current. You can tighten up and hold still, yet the river keeps flowing, effortlessly bending around you and not slowing down. Even if you resist harder, the river bends and moves on. The Tao is the river of change. You cannot stop it. When you resist change, you cause tension inside yourself without having any effect on the constant change. It is better to go with the river, get into its flow, and ride the waves of change.

The ability to accept, adjust to, and promote change is the key to longevity in Taoist theory. Flexible muscles, tendons, ligaments, and joints ensure that the body can manage the rigors and constant demands that life can put on it. Flexible vessels ensure the constant flow of blood and lymph to the whole body, keeping all structures nourished and clean. A flexible mind allows constant learning and growth and prevents stagnation in old thoughts of the past. The Taoists would say "enjoy the process, nothing is permanent so enjoy the impermanence, embrace the change."

The basic ideas of "being in the moment," "embracing constant change," and "going with the flow" are essential to bodywork. Being in the moment during bodywork means that you will be aware of the subtle effects of your therapy. You will then be able to quickly adjust your methods to keep the therapeutic process on the right track.

"Embracing the change" and "going with the flow" means allowing and not resisting. This is important whenever you apply pressure to the body. If you push into the muscle like an adversary (fast and hard), it will push back. If you relax and allow your pressure to be accepted by the client, you encounter less resistance. Then you will be able to work deeper and more effectively.

Like the Tao, healing is a process, and is subject to a constant barrage of influences, both good and bad, in and out of the therapy session. You should embrace the process; don't push for results. If you try too hard to make a change in your client's body, you run the risk of overworking it. That often leads to a setback. It is much better to work *with* your client's body than *against* it. Sometimes this means less is more. Coach your client about the healing process. Help your client realize that it is a progression with both ups and downs. This encourages patience and will help the client to stick with the therapy.

The Five Elements

Five element theory is a classification system that goes hand in hand with Taoist thought and Yin/Yang principles. It attempts to classify the interactions within nature itself and between nature and the body. It also classifies interactions within the body, the mind, and the inner organs.

The five elements are Wood, Fire, Earth, Metal, and Water. They represent the major substances as well as the functions, characteristics, and dynamic processes that make up the universe.

- Wood represents all plant matter, the process of growing and spreading, and the characteristics of flexibility and being rooted.
- Metal represents all minerals, the process of cutting, and the characteristics of hardness and conductivity.
- Fire represents heat from all sources, the process of burning and drying, and the characteristics of rising and motion.

- Water represents its many forms (liquid, solid, and vapor), the process of wetting and cooling, and the characteristics of descending, flowing, and yielding.
- Earth represents food nourishment, the process of support for growth, and the characteristics of production and fertility.

The five element model is efficient because it uses only a few categories to classify all of the structures and processes and their interactions. This makes it very useful for memorizing and keeping track of the correlations between mind, body, and nature.

In traditional Chinese medicine, each of the five elements correspond with a **Zang** (Yin) organ and a **Fu** (Yang) organ (see Table 15.2 ■). Each element also corresponds with a particular season, emotion, taste, color, and more. Most of these correlations make sense intuitively and they are very important in TCM diagnosis and treatment.

It is important to remember that the organs of the body are viewed as systems of function, not simply as a single physical structure. The organs are seen to parallel the function of the five elements in nature. Therefore the organs are assigned to a particular element based on the Chinese understanding of how the organ system functions within the body (Table 15.2).

The heart and its function of circulating blood is associated with warming and therefore belongs to the Fire element. The Earth permits sowing, growing and reaping. Therefore the spleen, which in Chinese theory is the organ responsible for digestion and absorption of food, is the Earth's corresponding organ. The kidneys control water metabolism. Thus they belong to the Water element.

The liver is given the Wood element because it is said to spread the Qi throughout the body, which is like a tree spreading its leaves. The last element is Metal. Metal is responsible for conducting and is associated with the lungs. The lungs conduct Qi throughout the body through the process of breathing.

QUICK QUIZ #29

1. The Chinese system of massage called Tui-na includes:
   a. bone and joint manipulation.
   b. acupuncture.
   c. acupressure.
   d. herbal treatments.
   e. All of the above
   f. None of the above

2. The techniques and theories of acupressure and acupuncture were developed exclusively in China.
   a. True
   b. False

3. Which of the following are considered to be Yin? (Circle all that apply)

   a. Rising
   b. Light
   c. Back
   d. Expansion
   e. All of the above
   f. None of the above

4. The body's regulation of temperature demonstrates: (Circle all that apply)
   a. the constant fluctuation between Yin and Yang.
   b. the body's innate ability to balance Yin and Yang.
   c. the fact that the body is flexible and always changing.
   d. All of the above
   e. None of the above

Element	Wood	Fire	Earth	Metal	Water
Zang Organ	Liver	Heart	Spleen	Lung	Kidney
Fu Organ	Gall Bladder	Small Intestine	Stomach	Large Intestine	Bladder
Season	Spring	Summer	None	Autumn	Winter
Color	Green	Red	Yellow	White	Black
Climate	Wind	Heat	Damp	Dryness	Cold
Sense Organ	Eyes	Tongue	Mouth	Nose	Ears
Tissue	Sinew	Vessels	Muscle	Skin	Bone
Emotion	Anger	Joy	Worry	Sadness	Fear
Sound	Shouting	Laughing	Singing	Crying	Groaning
Taste	Sour	Bitter	Sweet	Pungent	Salty

TABLE 15.2   The Five Elements in Nature and in the Body

The focus of TCM is on quality of function and how well the organs are working together. Five element theory uses the metaphor of the elements to describe interactions between the organs. The theory describes how each organ either generates and supports another organ, or how it controls and keeps another organ in check. Organs and elements support one another through the **generating cycle (Sheng cycle).** They are understood to keep one another in check through the **controlling cycle (Ke cycle).**

THE GENERATING CYCLE (SHENG CYCLE)

The following diagram clarifies the supporting and generating relationships between the five elements in the world and between the organs within the body (see Figure 15.3 ■).

Fire creates Earth as ashes fall to the ground.

Earth creates Metal as it uses the minerals from the ground to melt into Metal.

Metal creates Water as Water condenses on cold Metal surfaces.

Water nourishes Wood as Wood draws upon Water to help it grow.

Wood creates Fire, as it is the fuel from which it burns.

The sequence of relationships between the five elements in the world is mirrored in the relationships between the organ functions of the body.

- The heart (Fire) generates the spleen (Earth). The spleen uses the blood and Qi circulated by the heart to perform its function of digestion.
- The spleen (Earth) generates the lungs (Metal). The spleen helps moisten the lungs and provides Qi to the lungs from the food and liquids it digests.
- The lungs (Metal) generate the kidneys (Water). The lungs are the source of the chest Qi that the kidneys draw upon to perform their functions.
- The kidneys (Water) generate the liver (Wood). The kidneys are the source of Yin fluids including the blood, which the liver is said to store.
- The liver (Wood) generates the heart (Fire). The liver stores the blood that the heart circulates around the body.

The generating sequence shows how the organs support and nourish each other. It shows how each organ's structure and function creates, and is dependent upon, the structures and functions of the others. Harmony is the natural state in the environment and in the body. Along with generating one another, each organ system must also prevent a different organ system from becoming too prevalent.

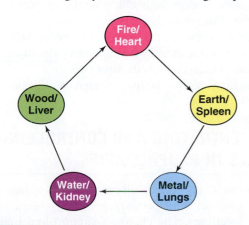

FIGURE 15.3

The Generating Cycle (Sheng Cycle)

DID YOU KNOW

The connection between health and emotions is also appreciated by Western science. Laughter is known to affect blood pressure. Worry will frequently cause stomach distress, and extreme fear has been known to affect the bladder.

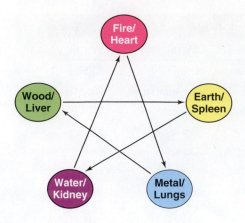

FIGURE 15.4

The Controlling Cycle (Ke Cycle)

THE CONTROLLING CYCLE (KE CYCLE)

The following diagram clarifies the limiting or controlling relationships between the five elements in the world and between the organs within the body (see Figure 15.4 ■).

Fire controls Metal as intense heat can melt Metal.

Metal controls Wood as Metal in the form of an axe chops Wood.

Wood controls Earth as the roots from trees hold Earth in place.

Earth controls Water as an Earthen dam blocks a river.

Water controls Fire as Water can douse and extinguish a Fire.

The controlling sequence as it relates to organ interactions

- Liver (Wood) controls the spleen (Earth).
  The liver/gallbladder controls the spleen by regulating fat digestion through bile secretion.
- Spleen (Earth) controls the kidney (Water).
  The spleen controls the kidney by regulating the absorption of water into the body through digestion.
- Kidney (Water) controls the heart (Fire).
  The Kidney controls the heart by regulating blood pressure through the juxtaglomerular apparatus.
- Heart (Fire) controls the lung (Metal).
  The heart controls the lungs by regulating the rate of blood moving through the pulmonary circuit.
- Lung (Metal) controls the liver (wood).
  The lungs control the liver through its influence on the flow of blood.

THE GENERATING AND CONTROLLING CYCLES IN ACUPRESSURE

Sometimes it may be difficult or too painful to treat a particular channel with primary pathology (e.g., broken bones, swelling). The channels support and limit one another just as the organs do, through the generating and controlling sequences. These principles can be used effectively in acupressure therapy to provide indirect treatment to related areas.

Generating Cycle

When choosing an acupressure strategy, the generating cycle can be used to address a lack of function or weakness in a channel. When a channel is deficient, applying therapy to its generating channel will boost the therapeutic effect.

As seen in Table 15.2, each element governs not just one channel, but a Yin/Yang pair of channels. These pairs can be used to guide treatment as well. For example, if there is weakness along the muscles of the Urinary Bladder channel (water element), you may stimulate the channels belonging to the metal element (the Lung and Large Intestine channels) as metal is the element that generates the water element.

Controlling Cycle

The controlling cycle can be used to plan a treatment strategy in much the same way. If there is an excessive condition in the tissues along a particular channel, then treatment of the channel which corresponds to the controlling element will enhance therapy. Excessive conditions are the result of the body's overreaction to an injury, irritation, or other condition. This can manifest as pain, swelling, inflammation, and/or a rash.

For example, if there is inflammation along the leg section of the Stomach channel (earth), you may apply therapy to either of the channels belonging to the wood element (Liver and Gall Bladder) to help control the overactive response in the Stomach channel.

As before, replacing the elements with corresponding organs shows how these concepts can be used to assess as well as formulate a treatment plan. For example, if the Liver/Wood is deficient, then treatment may focus on the Liver itself or on the Liver's generating organ, the Kidney/Water. By boosting the Kidney/Water, the Liver/Wood also benefits.

If the Liver/Wood has an excess, then treatment may focus on the controlling organ Lungs/Metal. The Lungs are said to keep the Liver in check. If both cycles are working together, then the body is in a state of balance or optimal health.

CHANNEL THEORY

As described in Chapter 14, the channels include all of the tissues and vessels located below the surface, including the muscles. The channels also represent a chain of interconnected muscular structures. Remember that each channel follows a line of pull in a functional muscle grouping. If there is pathology in a muscle anywhere along the chain, then the rest of the chain will most likely be affected.

Tension, trigger points, and other pathologies shorten the structure and the movement of the affected muscle. The rest of the muscles of the same chain (along the channel) will be the first to be affected through compensation. Their movement is now challenged because the movement of the damaged muscle is restricted. Therefore, it is important to investigate the entire channel for pathology. When treating,

HOLISTIC CONNECTION

Ayurveda is an ancient form of medicine that originated in India and has been developed over centuries. Although slightly different than that of traditional Chinese medicine, Ayurvedic medicine also has a five element system at its core. Ayurveda bases its system of health and well-being on the elements, Earth, Water, Fire, Air, and Ether.

Like the Chinese system, Ayurveda maintains a holistic view of the body and is mindful of the body's connection to nature. Healing takes place by bringing the body into its natural and perfect state of balance. Investigate Ayurveda as another way of helping your clients achieve health and wellness.

---

it is important to focus on the local area as well as the distant parts of the channel. This way all of the pathology as well as its immediate compensations are addressed. If parts of the channel are left untreated, they will slow the progress of healing the original pathology.

Because all of the body's muscles work together to produce even small movements, pathology in one muscle can be evident beyond the affected channel. It is therefore important to investigate the other channels that may be affected.

Mirror Channels

Keep in mind that the channels are bilateral—meaning that there is a duplicate of each channel on both sides of the body. For the purposes of this text, these channels will be called **mirror channels.** Each channel has the capacity to reflect pathology located within its mirror channel on the other side of the body. For example, pathology along the Lung channel of the right arm may over time show up as pathology along the Lung channel of the left arm.

Understanding Yin/Yang Complementary Channels

As previously discussed, the anterior and inferior aspects of the body are more Yin than the superior and posterior aspects. Therefore, the anterior is where the Yin channels are found, and the posterior is where the Yang channels are found. The head is the most superior aspect of the body, so all the Yang channels either begin or end there. The beginnings and ends of the Yin channels are distributed over the Yin aspects of the

chest, hands, feet, and face. (Refer to diagrams in Chapter 11 for locations of channels.)

Remember, the channels are distributed so that each one is paired with its **Yin or Yang complement.** According to Yin/Yang theory, all things are moving on a continuum between the two sides. Yin is flowing into Yang while Yang is flowing into Yin. The Yin/Yang channel pairing also represents this ebb and flow of Yin/Yang. The Yin channels are found in direct opposition to their Yang complement on the body. The muscles of each channel oppose each other in movement; so while one is working, the other is relaxed, and vice versa.

The Lung channel, for example, is a Yin channel. It is found along the anterior portion of the hand, wrist, arm, neck, and head (see Figure 15.5 ■). The muscles which are associated with the Lung channel are the flexors of the arm and chest. The Large Intestine channel is the Lung's Yang compliment, and it runs along the lateral, posterior aspect of the hand, wrist, arm, neck, and head. The muscles associated with the

DID YOU KNOW

Think of a person bent over working in the fields. Their front will be in the shade and be cooler, which is Yin. Their back will be warm and bright, which is more Yang.

HOLISTIC CONNECTION

The process by which pathology moves from one side of the body across to the other side is partly due to compensation. When it becomes painful for one arm to perform a movement, the other will often take over. The side that takes over can become overworked and develop its own pathology.

Pathology can also be transmitted across the body via the nerves. Pfluger's law of symmetry and the segmented

structure of spinal nerves help to explain the transmission of pathology across the spine.

For more about compensation, see Chapters 2–4. For additional information about the nervous system and massage, see Chapters 6–9.

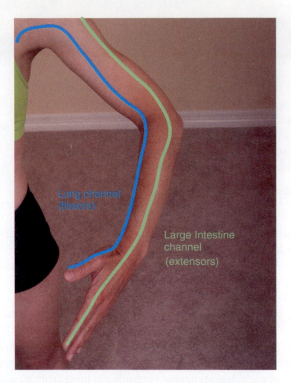

FIGURE 15.5

The Locations of the Lung Channel and the Large Intestine Channel on the Arm

Large Intestine channel are the antagonists of the flexors—the extensors of the arm and back. True to the dynamics of Yin/Yang, as the flexors along the (Yin) Lung channel contract, they will pull and cause the extensors along the (Yang) Large Intestine channel to relax, which allows movement of the arm. There is a true embodiment of the give and take of Yin and Yang as the limb moves back and forth.

As long as this give and take of movement is in balance, the body part will be healthy. In other words, the Yin and Yang channels must be in balance. The relative strength, tension, and flexibility should be equal on both sides. If the Yang muscles are too strong or tense, the muscles of the Yin channels are affected, and vice versa.

Use this concept when assessing injury or dysfunction in the myoskeletal system. Look for imbalance between the complementary channels of Yin/Yang pairs. Sometimes, when there is an excessive contraction or trigger point on one side of the pair, the opposite side will be stressed in one way or another and will develop its own pathology.

CASE STUDY #1

Sally, a local factory worker, complains of pain in her right posterior upper arm and shoulder. Assessment reveals tension in the muscles of the posterior arm and shoulder (i.e., the triceps and the teres major and infraspinatus). Furthermore, these muscles are beginning to knot up with trigger points and myofascial adhesions. The primary presentation of the pathology is along the San Jao channel, which runs along the posterior arm and upper back (see Figure 15.6 ◼).

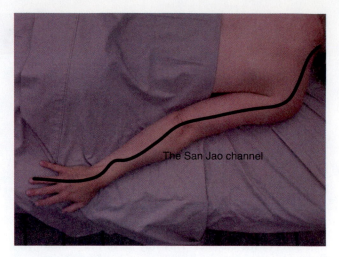

FIGURE 15.6

The Location of the San Jao Channel

With the primary channel identified, the next step is to assess the Yin complement: in this case, the Pericardium channel. The Pericardium channel runs along the anterior chest and arm (see Figure 15.7 ◼). Upon palpation it is discovered that the muscles along the Pericardium channel (biceps, forearm flexors, pectoralis) are in severe contracture. Sally's job at the factory requires that she hold a heavy drill in her right hand. She does this 8 hours a day, 5 days a week. It is no wonder her anterior arm muscles are in chronic flexion. The chronic flexion has caused the antagonist muscles in the posterior arm and shoulder to become overstretched and to develop painful pathology.

In this case, tension in the Pericardium channel caused the San Jao channel to be chronically affected due to the fact that the muscles of the San Jao channel were constantly resisting the tension caused by the flexion in muscles of the Pericardium channel.

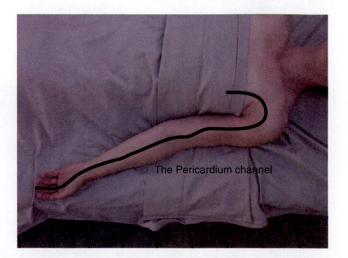

FIGURE 15.7

The Location of the Pericardium Channel

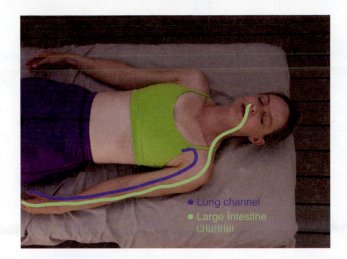

FIGURE 15.8

The Locations of the Lung Channel and the Large Intestine Channel

TABLE 15.3	The 24-Hour Flow of Qi Through the Channels
🕐 3–5 a.m. Lung	🕐 3–5 p.m. Urinary Bladder
🕐 5–7 a.m. Large Intestine	🕐 5–7 p.m. Kidney
🕐 7–9 a.m. Stomach	🕐 7–9 p.m. Pericardium
🕐 9–11 a.m. Spleen	🕐 9–11 p.m. San Jao
🕐 11 a.m.–1 p.m. Heart	🕐 11 p.m.–1 a.m. Gall Bladder
🕐 1–3 p.m. Small Intestine	🕐 1–3 a.m. Liver

In some cases, the channels of a Yin/Yang pair may not have any portions that cross the same body part. Nonetheless, they may still affect each other.

CASE STUDY #2

Bob, a data analyst, complains of pain and tension in his chest and shoulder. Assessment finds trigger points in his pectoralis and anterior deltoid along the Lung channel. It also reveals tension in the lateral neck along the Large Intestine channel which is the Lung channel's Yang complement. The Lung channel is located along the anterior chest and arm, but does not pass over the neck. The Large Intestine channel follows the posterior arm and has a section that passes along the lateral side of the neck (see Figure 15.8 ■). Although these portions of the two complementary channels are not very close together in this location, they will still influence one another. Bob was working extra hours, which was causing some extra stress. In addition to the long hours in front of his computer, the stress caused his shoulders to be pulled higher and higher to his ears. This caused the muscles along the Large Intestine channel to become chronically short and tense. The neck tension eventually affected his anterior chest and shoulder muscles. This is because tension in the lateral neck and shoulder affects the movement of the scapula. Over time, the restriction in the scapula affected the muscles of the shoulder and anterior chest, which attach to it.

Using the Flow of Qi Chart

Table 15.3 ■ and Figure 15.9 ■ show the flow of Qi as described in Chapter 14. It depicts the Chinese concept of how the Qi flows from channel to channel during a 24-hour day. The chart illustrates another important concept. It reveals how Qi is transmitted between the agonist/antagonist muscles of Yin/Yang complementary channels.

For example, the Lung channel is the Yin counterpart to the Large Intestine channel. The Lung channel runs along the anterior arm through the flexor muscles. The Large Intestine channel runs along the posterior arm through the extensor muscles (see Figure 15.10 ■). According to the chart, Qi flows from the Lung channel to the Large Intestine channel. The Qi flowing into the Large Intestine channel from the Lung channel is a metaphor explaining how when one muscle group (agonist) is using energy to contract, the other muscle group (antagonist) must relax to allow for the movement of the arm.

In addition to describing the flow of Qi through the Yin/Yang pairs, the chart also describes the flow of Qi as it moves from one area of the body to the next. For example, according to the chart the Qi flows from the Large Intestine channel to the Stomach channel, then from the Stomach channel to the Spleen channel. Upon observation of the location of these channels, we see that the Large Intestine channel ends in the face where the Stomach channel begins and the Stomach channel ends on the foot where the Spleen channel begins. The flow continues to cycle this way and begins over again each 24 hours.

This concept can also be understood from a myoskeletal perspective. Using the flow of Qi as a guide, this chart shows the muscular connections between body parts. Almost all movements involve multiple muscle groups and require at least some adjustment from the rest of the body. A simple act, such as bringing a fork to the mouth, involves muscles of the hand, arm, shoulder, back, and neck to act in unison.

For example, the Spleen channel is a Medial Leg channel that ends in the chest. According to the chart, the Heart channel is next. The Heart channel goes from the chest, down the medial arm to the hand. These channels collectively cover the muscles of the medial leg, the anterior torso, and the anterior medial arm. Many activities, such as throwing a ball, engage the chain of muscles embodied by this sequence of channels (see Figure 15.11 ■). The connection between the muscle groups is evident when tracing the flow of Qi through the channels.

Overall, the chart can be used to trace the trail of pathology as it spreads along the channels, through the Yin/Yang pairs, and then through the rest of the body. The key is to follow the flow of Qi through the channels, to identify the next channel for possible pain and dysfunction. For example, the Qi flows from the Large Intestine channel into the Stomach channel. Therefore, if the Large Intestine channel has pathology, look to the Stomach channel next for additional compensatory pathology.

FIGURE 15.9

The 24-Hour Cycle of Qi Flow Through the Channels

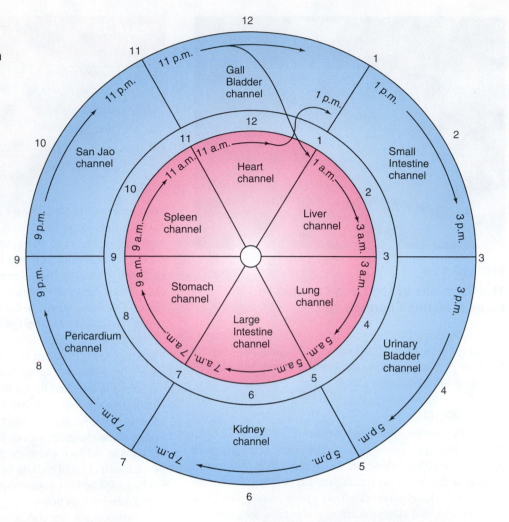

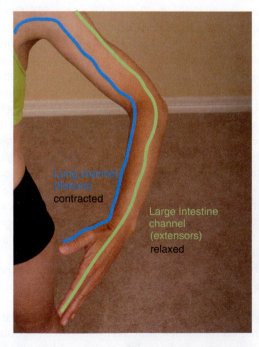

FIGURE 15.10

When the Muscles of the Lung Channel Contract, the Muscles of the Yang Counterpart (Large Intestine Channel) Will Be Relaxed.

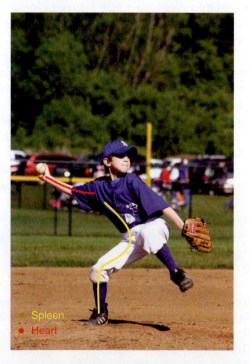

FIGURE 15.11

When Throwing a Ball, the Spleen and Heart Channels Are Activated Together.

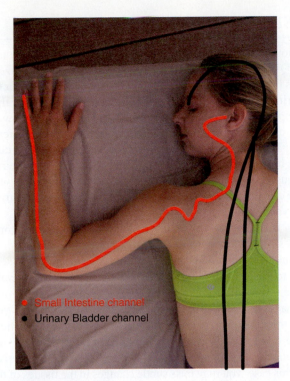

FIGURE 15.12

The Location of the Small Intestine Channel and Its Proximity to the Urinary Bladder Channel

CASE STUDY

Jack, a local carpenter, was experiencing pain on the posterior shoulder blade, probably stemming from repetitive use at work. Assessment revealed the Small Intestine channel (which runs along the back of the arm, the posterior shoulder, and the side of the neck; Figure 15.11) was affected. According to the flow of Qi chart, the next channel to assess is the Urinary Bladder channel. The Urinary Bladder channel runs over the back of the head, down the neck, and the entire spine (see Figure 15.12 ■). The assessment showed that there were a number of adhesions and a lot of tension along the Urinary Bladder channel from the neck to the low back. From a myoskeletal point of view, it makes sense that pain and restriction in the shoulder will affect the neck and spine. The scapula is anchored to the spine through muscles such as the trapizeus and rhomboids. The Urinary Bladder channel covers the muscles of the spine, so it makes sense to check there for signs of pain and tension.

Using the flow of Qi chart in this way provides insight into the progression of pathology through the myoskeletal system that may not otherwise be readily apparent.

USING ACUPOINTS

Acupoints can have a wide range of complex and powerful effects throughout the body. As massage therapists, our focus is on treating myoskeletal pathology. To this end, there are two simple categories of acupoints that should be understood—traditional acupoints and Ashi acupoints.

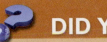

DID YOU KNOW

In addition to treating whole channels, sometimes certain traditional acupoints are chosen for specific purposes. For example, the acupoint Pericardium #6 (P6) is classified as a Luo connecting point, which means it has the special purpose of connecting the channels. It is also classified as a *confluent acupoint*, which means it is used in combination with the other confluent acupoints for specific conditions. In addition to these two classifications, this acupoint is also used to treat the simple symptom of nausea. This can make the selection of acupoints for treatment a very complex subject. However, as massage therapists, our primary concern is treating disease of the myoskeletal system. In this context, P6 is used as a local acupoint to treat pathology in the anterior forearm and wrist and to help clear its channel. In this way, the points are used as locations of interest along the channel. Using the acupoints as reference locations in order to search for and treat local pathologies is the simplest way to use them.

When treating pathology located in a particular channel, pay special attention to the traditional acupoints along that channel. These acupoints are located at strategic points along the channel where the Qi can be accessed most easily.

- **Traditional channel acupoints** These are the classic acupoints located along the channels. These acupoints have a long history of use and have very specific locations. Traditional acupoints are used to treat the channel itself and the surrounding areas and can also affect its related organ or systems. The acupoints are used to stimulate function along the channel by encouraging Qi flow. When treating myoskeletal pathology, traditional acupoints are divided into local or distant points (see Figure 15.13 ■).
  1. A **local acupoint** is any traditional acupoint, on any channel, that is close to or running through the area of pathology. It is very important to treat these acupoints, as this will draw the circulation of blood and Qi directly to the most affected area.
  2. **Distant acupoints** are traditional acupoints that are located along the affected channel, but found away from the location of pathology. These acupoints

DID YOU KNOW

The Yin/Yang symbol shows the constant movement of the moment. Often described as "being in the now," focusing your Qi means that you are present, participating in what is unfolding before you and not thinking about other things. This is where life happens.

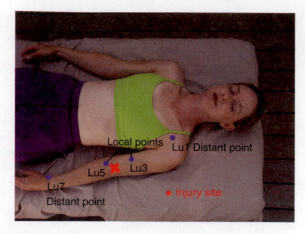

FIGURE 15.13

The Local and Distant Points to Be Used When Treating Pathology Located on the Lung Channel at the Elbow

represent compensation and will help stimulate the whole channel when treated. A common technique is to include the most distant acupoints (located at the ends of the channels) in a treatment plan. This will ensure that the entire channel has been addressed.

- **Ashi acupoints** Translated as, "Ah, that's it," these acupoints may correlate with trigger points or knots in the muscle. They may simply be points that hurt when palpated. Ashi points are important to the bodyworker as they represent acute myoskeletal pathology. Ashi points can be found anywhere along the channel center-lines and/or just adjacent to them. They are not mapped out on the traditional channel system because they are variable. All of the Ashi acupoints should be treated in addition to the traditional acupoints associated with the pathology. By addressing both Ashi and traditional acupoints, the therapist ensures better success in healing.

USING QI IN THERAPY

Another important concept in acupressure theory is the use of Qi in the therapy. For the greatest benefits to be realized, it is important that the therapist and client both focus their Qi during the treatment and healing. The Chinese believe that the properly focused practitioner actually exchanges Qi with the client and uses their Qi to influence the Qi of the client.

Remember, Qi is energy, and focusing your energy during bodywork prevents it from being wasted. If you are not focused, you may not use energy efficiently, and you will tire quickly. In order to focus your Qi, you must concentrate on your breathing.

Breathing is a rhythmic body movement that never stops. By simply concentrating on this sensation, the random thoughts of the mind can be ignored. A clear mind is essential to focusing Qi. Without the internal chatter, you are available to put all of your Qi and focus completely on the task at hand. It is easy to be distracted by outside thoughts. If you are thinking about plans for the weekend or some other stress like money, bills, etc., your hands may be performing the treatment, but your mind (and Qi) will be somewhere else. In this case, you may miss subtle changes in the tissues of the client. You may miss a tense area or an active acupoint. It is essential to let go of outside thoughts and truly be in the moment. By putting your thoughts and Qi into the moment of each session, you will be aware of all the variables involved in treating the client.

Furthermore, distraction during the session may take attention away from body mechanics and will adversely affect your leverage. If you are not using proper leverage, you will have to work harder to get the proper results. Working harder will leave you with less Qi to perform the therapy. Breathing deeply and slowly stabilizes the torso, which gives a better base to apply pressure. It also ensures that you are getting enough oxygen (called *Kong Qi*) to nourish your tissues and help maintain stamina throughout the therapy.

QUICK QUIZ #30

1. According to the generating and controlling cycles, Earth/Spleen: (Circle all that apply)
   a. are supported by Fire/Heart.
   b. support the Metal/Lung.
   c. are supported by the Liver/Wood.
   d. control the Water/Kidney.
   e. All of the above
   f. None of the above

2. The pattern of the flow of Qi through the channels can be used to identify which channels and muscles are likely to contain compensation.
   a. True
   b. False

3. Each channel follows a line of pull in a functional muscle grouping.
   a. True
   b. False

4. A local acupoint is defined as:
   a. a classic acupoint with a very specific location along one of the channels.
   b. a traditional acupoint located on any channel that is close to the area of pathology.
   c. a traditional acupoint found at the end of a channel that runs through an area of pathology.

SUMMARY

Massage in China began as a system of bone, joint, and soft tissue therapy called Tui-na. Acupressure is a subdivision of Tui-na that applies therapy to the channels and the acupoints found along them.

Acupressure began thousands of years ago. There is much speculation as to how acupressure was discovered. By 770 BCE, techniques and theory were being compiled in written works, such as the *NeiJing Internal Classic*. Throughout the Han, Sui, and Ming dynasties more information was compiled in various texts, and different schools of thought were developed. In the 1970s, U.S. President Nixon's visit to China revealed Chinese medical practices such as acupuncture to the Western world. In modern times, many researchers have investigated acupressure concepts.

The practice of acupressure stems from the traditional Chinese perspectives on the nature of the world and the body. The most important concepts influencing the practice of TCM and acupressure are the duality of Yin/Yang; the principle of constant change (the Tao); and the five elements. Understanding these concepts gives an important foundation for the use of acupressure and developing treatment plans.

The five elements (Fire, Earth, Metal, Water, and Wood) are associated with the organ systems of the body. The elements and organs both generate and control one another in order to maintain balance in the body. Understanding the generating cycle and the controlling cycle can guide the development of a treatment plan towards the balancing of the elements, channels, and myoskeletal structures of the body.

The organs and channels of the body are organized into Yin/Yang pairings which represent the balancing of opposites within the body. The channels of the body are bilateral; each one has a mirror copy on the left and right side of the body.

Each channel is associated with a particular organ and with the Yin/Yang principles of that organ. Therefore, each channel is paired with a Yin or Yang complement channel. Each serves to balance the function of the other.

Qi flows through the channels in a set sequence. The pattern of flow demonstrates how Qi flows from one body part to the next and shows how pathology can spread through the body. The channels represent chains of interconnected muscular structures. The channel pairings and the flow of Qi are very useful concepts when assessing and treating myoskeletal pathology with acupressure.

Along the channels, there are acupoints that commonly reflect pathology and are used to treat pathology. Some of these acupoints have traditional locations, and some—called Ashi acupoints—reflect local pathology. The performance of acupressure techniques requires the use of Qi to focus the mind and body.

DISCUSSION QUESTIONS

1. How does the Taoist principle of "going with the flow" apply to the application of massage and bodywork?
2. Use the generating cycle to explain how applying treatment to the Heart channel can help a client with pathology along the Spleen channel.
3. Use the controlling cycle to explain how applying treatment to the Spleen channel can help a client with inflammation of the medial ankle along the Kidney channel.
4. What methods can help a bodyworker to focus their Qi for treatment?

16 The Techniques of Acupressure Therapy

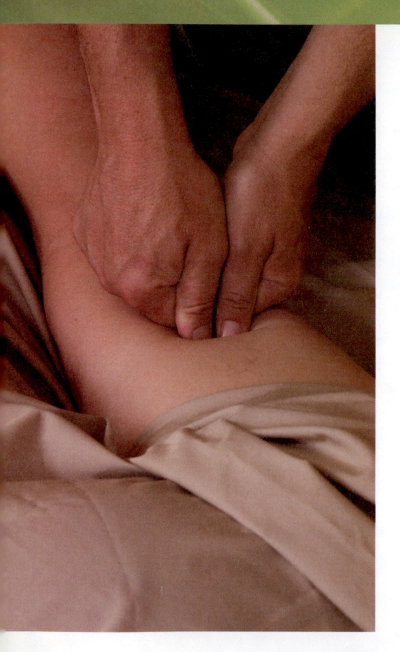

CHAPTER HIGHLIGHTS

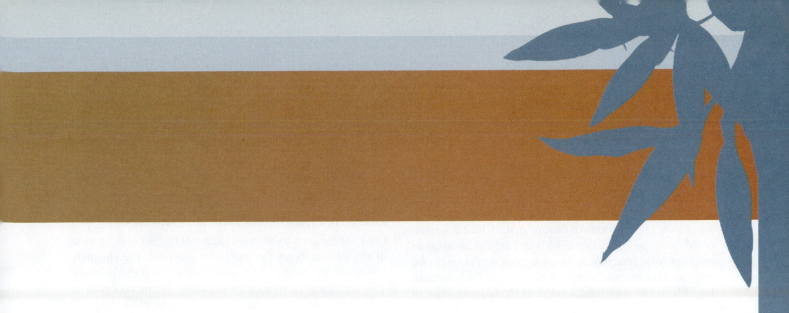

CHAPTER OBJECTIVES

- Understand assessment and planning using acupressure theory
- Consider necessary preparation for acupressure treatment
- Learn how to apply acupressure

- Investigate different approaches to working the channels
- Identify the contraindications for applying acupressure

KEY TERMS

OVERVIEW

The techniques of acupressure vary from basic applications, such as simply rubbing sore channels, to elaborate diagnoses and acupoint selection. The specific techniques a therapist chooses will depend upon what pathology they are treating, as well as other factors such as age, size, and health of the client. The tradition and school of thought under which each therapist learned their craft will also influence the treatment strategies. Acupressure, like all forms of therapy in the Chinese system, evolved over time in the households and individual hospitals throughout Asia. Therefore, there are as many ways to apply the therapy as there are practitioners performing it. Each therapist brings his or her own education, experience, and sense of artistry to the session.

For the modern day practitioner, this rich history offers many opportunities to explore a variety of techniques and traditions. Each individual should find those traditions that match up with their own ideas and experience to help develop their own personal approach.

ACUPRESSURE FOR THE BODYWORKER

Acupressure has far reaching effects, and acupoints are used to treat all types of disease in the body. The therapy can assist in treating diseases ranging from simple stomach aches, to more complicated syndromes, such as cancer. Using acupoints to treat internal disorders is a very intricate process and requires a very precise TCM diagnosis. This type of diagnosis involves the evaluation of a large number of physical, emotional, and environmental signs and symptoms. The process requires a thorough knowledge of all the principles of traditional Chinese medicine and its diagnostic system. Performing this type of diagnosis and formulating a treatment plan for internal medical conditions is out of scope for this text. Here the focus is on the use of acupressure for the bodyworker to treat the myoskeletal system. In this case, a much more simplified process for assessment and treatment is available.

In Chinese theory, when pathology is confined to the muscles, bones, and joints, the disease is understood as being "a channel disorder." It is important to remember that acupressure channels represent all the tissues, including the muscles, bones, and joints that run along its path. Therefore, tension, injury, or distortions in any of these structures are reflected in the channel system. When the focus is on treating channel disorders (i.e., myoskeletal disorders), a working knowledge of the location and trajectory of the channels and acupoints is all that is required. The selection of channels and acupoints to be treated is guided by a fairly simple method of assessment.

Assessment

The assessment allows the therapist to identify the **primary affected channels.** These are the channels that run through the main area of complaint. There are also a number of associated channels that may be affected due to compensation and other adjustments to the primary dysfunction. It is important to remember that each channel covers a specific part of the limb or torso, but is also connected to all the other channels through a network. As the injury progresses over time, the connected areas will be recruited into the process, and other channels will develop their own pathology. Assessment begins by finding the primary affected channels first, which will lead to the associated channels.

IDENTIFYING THE PRIMARY AFFECTED CHANNELS

Look for the primary affected channels by first making note of any pain or injury that the client presents. The channels closest to the pain or injury are considered the primary affected channels. In addition to noting the areas of pain, it is important to observe the client's posture. Note the position of the head, shoulders, hips, knees, and feet. Using basic postural analysis, make note of any imbalances from left to right, front to back, and top to bottom. Ideally, the body should be balanced on all sides (see Chapter 1 for more on posture analysis). Any change from side to side would suggest more or less tension on one side or the other. Tension causes muscles to shorten, thereby shortening the channel. Make note of the length of each channel and compare it to the length of the same channel on the opposite side of the body (see Figure 16.1 ■).

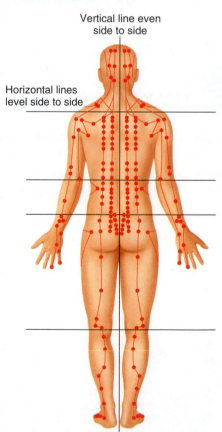

Vertical line even side to side

Horizontal lines level side to side

FIGURE 16.1

In a Balanced Posture, a Vertical Line Separates the Body into Equal Left and Right Halves. The Hips and Shoulders Align Horizontally.

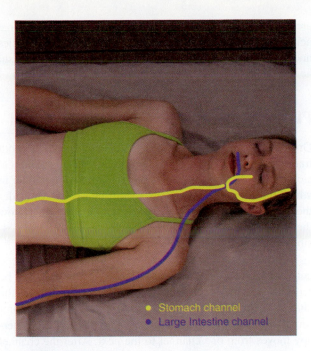

FIGURE 16.2

The Locations of the Large Intestine and Stomach Channels as They Pass Along the Neck.

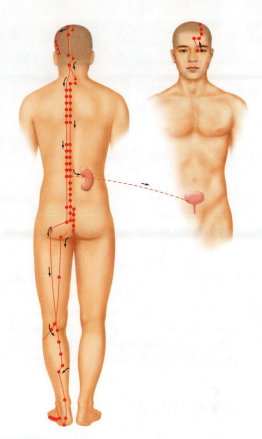

FIGURE 16.3

The Path of the Urinary Bladder Channel

An unhealthy position of any of the joints or major body parts will reveal the tension in the channels. For example, the position of the head can give insight to the relative length of the Large Intestine and Stomach channels. The Large Intestine channel runs across the anterior lateral neck, and the Stomach channel runs across the anterior medial neck (see Figure 16.2 ■). If the head is tilted to the side, it suggests tension in the Large Intestine channel. If it is tilted forward it suggests tension in the Stomach channel. If it is tilted at a 45-degree angle both channels are likely affected.

It is important to observe the entire length of all the primary channels involved. Because the channels represent lines of pull, tension at one acupoint will often cause tension somewhere else along the line. For example, if the neck portion of the Urinary Bladder channel is affected, there may be associated tension in the back, gluteals, hamstrings, and/or calf muscles. This is because this channel runs across the back all the way to the foot along the posterior leg (see Figure 16.3 ■).

IDENTIFYING ASSOCIATED CHANNELS

Once the major locations of pain and tension are noted and the primary affected channels are identified, it is important to look further for compensation and other related issues. As described in Chapters 14 and 15, there are a number of channels that balance, control, and support each major channel. When these channels become affected due to pathology in a primary channel, they are called **associated channels.** The channels that are likely to become associated channels are those which have strong functional connections with the primary channel.

- **The complementary channels (Yin/Yang pairs):** First, check the complement to the primary channel based on the traditional Yin/Yang pairing of channels. Remember, the **complementary channel (Yin/Yang pair)** is found on the other side of the limb or body from the channel in question. (Refer to Chapter 14 for a complete list of Yin/Yang pairs and diagrams of their locations.) Very often, the Yin/Yang complement will be the first to show some sort of associated pathology because it counteracts the movement of its paired channel.

- **The mirror channels (left- and right-side pairs):** Remember, the 12 primary channels are bilateral; there is an exact duplicate of each channel found on the other side of the body. Just as it is important to assess the Yin/Yang complementary channels, it is important to consider the **mirror channel (left- and right-side pair)** on the opposite side of the body. In fact, it is not unusual to have more pronounced tension on the mirror side of the primary affected channel. Often clients do not notice the tension building up on the mirror side because they are focused on the original painful side. Also, don't forget that mirror channels can be used for therapy. Just as pathology is transmitted between these channels, therapeutic effects can be transmitted as well. This is very useful in cases where the primary

TABLE 16.1	The Flow of Qi
🕐 3–5 a.m. Lung	🕐 3–5 p.m. Urinary Bladder
🕐 5–7 a.m. Large Intestine	🕐 5–7 p.m. Kidney
🕐 7–9 a.m. Stomach	🕐 7–9 p.m. Pericardium
🕐 9–11 a.m. Spleen	🕐 9–11 p.m. San Jao
🕐 11 a.m.–1 p.m. Heart	🕐 11 p.m.–1 a.m. Gall Bladder
🕐 1–3 p.m. Small Intestine	🕐 1–3 a.m. Liver

affected side is too painful to treat or is inaccessible due to a cast or other condition. Here, the therapy can be focused on the mirror channel so the client can receive healing benefits without having to receive treatment on the painful side.

- **The Flow of Qi:** Once the paired and mirror channels are assessed, the next step is to follow the chart of the flow of Qi, and check the channels that are next in line. As discussed in Chapter 15, the flow of Qi (Table 16.1 ■) is a helpful guide for following the progression of pathology as it moves through the body.

LOCATING ACTIVE ACUPOINTS

Once the primary channels are identified and the associated channels have been assessed, the next thing to do is to locate **active acupoints.** Palpate the channels, feeling for any lumps, bumps, tension, or focal points of pain. Acupoints exhibiting any of these pathologies are considered to be active acupoints. It is very common to start by palpating the traditional channel acupoints located closest to the primary area of complaint. Continue by checking the traditional acupoints along the channel until you reach its distal acupoints at both ends of the channel (beginning and end).

When all the active traditional points are located on the affected channels, it is time to palpate for active Ashi acupoints. Ashi acupoints are painful or tense spots that are not traditional, numbered acupoints. It is important to remember that drawings of TCM channels typically represent only the centerline of the channel, as this is where the traditional acupoints are found. Ashi acupoints are commonly found in the

? DID YOU KNOW

Often when palpating for traditional acupoints, you may find that the exact focal spot of tenderness is not right on the centerline of the channel, but a few millimeters to either side. It is important to remember that all individuals are different and variations are normal.

areas between the centerlines of the channels and traditional acupoints. Remember, the channels represent all the muscles and tissues next to, under, and around each centerline. Ashi acupoints can be found anywhere in these extended areas.

PLANNING THE ACUPRESSURE SESSION

Once the channels have been assessed and the active (both traditional and Ashi) acupoints are located, the treatment session can be planned. This includes planning out the order in which the channels and acupoints will be treated. Consider the flow of Qi through the channels, and make note of how the affected channels fall into sequence (Table 16.1). If possible, the channels should be treated in that sequence.

Sometimes, it is difficult to follow the flow of Qi due to considerations such as the client's ability to move and/or be repositioned. In this case, modifications to the order of the channels can be made. It is important for the client to be comfortable while still allowing access to the channels as the therapy moves from one channel to the next. After the channel sequence is selected, it is important to plan which acupoints you want to focus on. There are a number of factors that you must consider when choosing these points:

1. Select the active acupoints from both the primary and associated channels involved in the pathology.
2. Select as many of the active Ashi acupoints in the local area of pathology as possible.
3. Identify the traditional distal acupoints from each channel. These are the points at the beginning and end of the channel. They should be used whenever possible (whether active or not) as they will help move the Qi through the entire channel.
4. It is also a good idea to include "classically effective acupoints" that are traditionally established as effective for releasing the entire channel. These acupoints are very powerful and should be included whenever possible, whether they are active or not. See Table 16.2 ■ for a list of these points

Overall, try to treat as many active acupoints as possible. However, factors such as age, degree of pathology, and overall health status may prompt a change in those numbers. A client who is older or who may be weakened by chronic illness may tolerate less therapy than a younger or relatively healthier client. In this case be judicious in your choices and limit the acupoints to those that are the most active. The client's body can be taxed by the therapy and will need a fair amount of energy (Qi) to devote to healing.

Overworking a tired, older, or more severely compromised client would sap the Qi reserves and ultimately hinder the positive effects of the therapy. Balance is always the goal in Chinese therapy. Choose enough acupoints to properly treat the pathology, but not so many that the client has trouble managing the therapy.

First, choose those acupoints that are the most active. Then you may work as many of the lesser ones as the client

TABLE 16.2	"Classically Effective Acupoints" with Ability to Clear the Entire Channel		
Lung—	#1,	#5,	#7
Large Intestine—	#4,	#11,	#20
Stomach—	#9,	#36,	#41
Spleen—	#6,	#9,	#10
Heart—	#2,	#3,	#7
Small Intestine—	#5,	#11,	#18
Urinary Bladder—	#10,	#40,	#60
Kidney—	#1,	#3,	#10
Pericardium—	#2,	#3,	#6
San Jao—	#5,	#14,	#23
Gall Bladder—	#20,	#21,	#30
Liver—	#3,	#8,	#13

will tolerate well. As you develop your skill, you will be better able to distinguish the points that are most important to treat. This will allow you to focus your therapy, achieving better results.

Finally, keep in mind that if you plan to use acupressure, it is a good idea to keep reference materials handy. This may include charts on the channels and acupoints, the flow of Qi clock, and any others you find useful. There are many details to consider and there is no harm in looking things up to help formulate the best plan.

ACUPRESSURE APPLICATION

Accommodations for Acupressure

Acupressure is often performed on the floor, on a large mat, or on a low massage table. This is because a number of different body parts may be used to apply pressure, including the knees, feet, and elbows. I like to use a large mat, as it allows me to sit and/or kneel next to the client in order to use my body most effectively.

It is important for you to wear flexible clothing, as it allows freedom of movement and provides comfort throughout the therapy. It is also recommended that the client wear clothing that is not too bulky or restrictive. This allows the therapy to be applied without the client having to undress. It is better to work the client while he or she is clothed than to use a drape. Acupressure uses very little stroking techniques and often requires the client to be repositioned frequently during therapy in order to reach all the acupoints in the right sequence. Therefore, it is better if they are clothed. Furthermore, when they are clothed, you can incorporate passive stretching techniques quickly and easily without having to manage a sheet drape.

Mental Focus and Preparation

Asian forms of treatment place heavy emphasis on focusing the therapist's own Qi in order to properly perform therapy. Proper concentration is a key element in creating the most effective therapy. Focusing Qi is essentially a mind/body focus. An easy way to do this is to take a moment before approaching the client for therapy and take a few deep slow breaths. Clear the mind and focus on the rise and fall of your chest. This will help focus your mind and center your body. Set aside all personal

QUICK QUIZ #31

1. During an assessment, you should: (Circle all that apply)
   a. check the relative length of all of the channels.
   b. identify the primary affected channels.
   c. apply pressure to active acupoints in the primary affected channels for 3 to 6 seconds.
   d. look for Ashi points in the associated channels.
   e. All of the above
   f. None of the above

2. A complementary channel: (Circle all that apply)
   a. is paired with another based on traditional Yin/Yang relationships.
   b. is often found on the other side of the same limb from its complement.
   c. usually counteracts the muscular action of its complement.
   d. often shows pathology related to pathology in its complement.
   e. All of the above
   f. None of the above

3. If a channel on the right side of the body is injured, it is very unusual for its mirror channel on the left side to show any related pathology.
   a. True
   b. False

4. When planning an acupressure treatment session: (Circle all that apply)
   a. the channels must always be treated in the order of the flow of Qi.
   b. plan to treat as many active channel points as possible.
   c. always plan to treat each Ashi point in the local area of pathology.
   d. try to include acupoints that are traditionally established to clear the entire channel, even if they are not active.
   e. All of the above
   f. None of the above

HOLISTIC CONNECTION

Translated from Japanese, the word *Reiki* refers to "spiritual energy" or "sacred life force."

Reiki is an ancient alternative healing method that seeks to obtain health and energetic balance through the use of "universal life energy." Reiki practitioners use their access to this energy field to interpret and/or direct the energy field of the patient. A practitioner may pass their hands over the patient or rest their hands on or a few inches away from the patient in several specific positions.

The ideas of focusing energy in Reiki and the focusing of Qi in Chinese medicine are similar in theory, history, and practice. Much remains to be learned about the energy fields of the body and in the environment, but some evidence suggests that the application of Reiki may affect the autonomic nervous system, perception of pain, anxiety, memory, and behavior (Aetna InteliHealth Inc., 1996–2010).

---

thoughts and concerns and approach the client with an open, compassionate mind. When applying pressure, it is important to concentrate your energy on each acupoint; this will help open up the channels and clear the stagnation.

Applying Pressure

Varying rhythms, pressures, and techniques creates different styles of acupressure. Some techniques, like the Japanese form of acupressure called *Shiatsu*, are very vigorous. Shiatsu uses firm pressure applied for 3 to 5 seconds. In other forms of acupressure, acupoints are held for a minute or longer, even up to 3 minutes. Sometimes, the therapist will trace small circles or rapidly move the fingers to cause a slight vibration to the point. In some cases, the acupoints are kneaded or tapped with specific rhythms. Most of the time, acupressure is applied with a steady pressure of the thumbs, fingers, elbows, and/or knuckles.

Generally speaking, lighter pressure of a shorter duration tends to be stimulating, while deeper pressure of a longer duration tends to be more sedating. When the muscle is weak or when the client is frail, use light pressure with a short duration. When the muscle is very tense and the client is robust, use firmer pressure with a longer duration.

When applying pressure, instruct the client to use a scale of 1 to 10 to describe the amount of discomfort and/or pressure he or she is experiencing. One is very little, and ten is too much. Always allow the client to direct the amount of pressure. It is best to work in a pressure that is tolerable to the client (just below a level that causes guarding). This is usually a 6 on the scale of 1 to 10, but the number can vary.

Breathing

It is important that both you and the clients exhale as pressure is being applied. Instructing the client to exhale on the pressure is important as it relaxes her or his body, allowing the pressure to sink deeper and to facilitate a better release.

Traditional techniques instruct a practitioner to "breathe into the acupoint." Close your eyes, focus attention on the painful spot, and exhale deeply. Traditional therapists recommend that you visualize "breathing healing energy" into the area as the acupoint is held.

It is also important to always ease out of the pressure slowly and to inhale as the pressure is released. By inhaling upon the release, the torso is stabilized, allowing you to pull away from the client without stressing your lower back.

Methods of Contact

The body part used to contact the acupoint will depend on the area being worked and the relative size of the musculature. Using different contact points to apply pressure helps prevent overuse and will decrease the impact of bodywork on your body.

THUMBS

- **Physical description:** When applying thumb pressure to the acupoint, it is best to use a supported thumb position (see Figure 16.4 ■). Keep the wrist firm. The elbow should be straight, but not locked. The shoulders should be relaxed, and the back is kept straight. Resist letting your shoulders rise towards your ears. Lean into

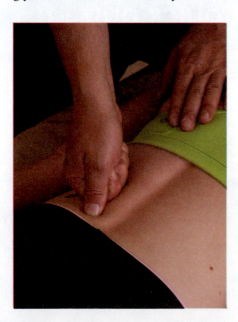

FIGURE 16.4

The Hand Position for Applying Pressure with the Thumb

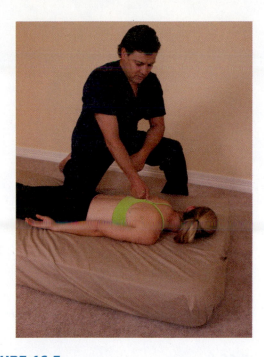

FIGURE 16.5a

The Position for Applying Pressure with the Thumb with the Client on a Mat

the acupoint. The pressure is delivered using your body weight, rather than the muscles of the forearm (see Figure 16.5a ■). Hold the position for 3 to 5 seconds, then release the pressure slowly. On larger body parts, you may use two thumbs together (see Figure 16.5b ■).

- **Common areas of use:** The thumbs can be used almost anywhere on the body. They are effective for applying both firm and gentle pressure. The thumbs

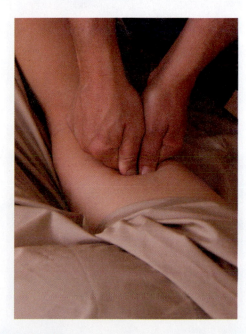

FIGURE 16.5b

The Hand Positions for Applying Pressure with the Two Thumbs Close Together

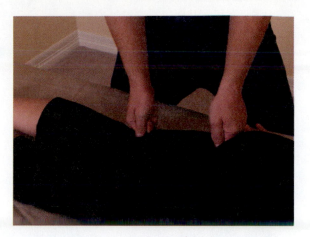

FIGURE 16.6

The Hand Positions for Applying the Thumbs to Two Acupoints at the Same Time

are commonly used when applying pressure to two acupoints simultaneously (see Figure 16.6 ■).

- **Special considerations:** The thumb is perhaps the most standard tool used in the application of acupressure. It is the strongest digit, and, when used properly, can be very durable.

FINGERS

- **Physical description:** When using the fingers, a supported two-finger technique is best. Place the second finger on top of the index finger so that the second finger supports the index finger (see Figure 16.7 ■). Each finger supports the other allowing for greater pressure. Keep the wrist firm. The elbow should be straight, but not locked. The shoulders should be relaxed, and the back is kept straight. Resist letting your shoulders rise towards your ears. Lean into the acupoint. The pressure is delivered using your body weight, rather than the muscles of the forearm (see Figures 16.8a ■ and 16.8b ■). Hold the position for 3 to 5 seconds, then release the pressure slowly.

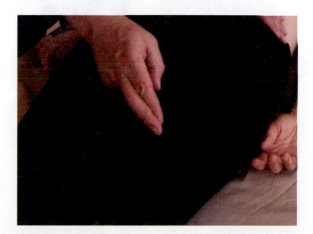

FIGURE 16.7

The Position for Applying Pressure Using a Supported Fingers Technique

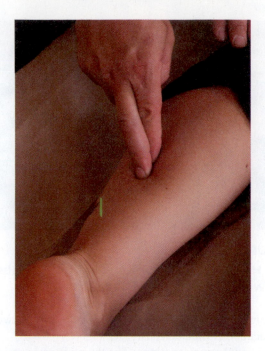

FIGURE 16.8a

The Position for Applying Pressure with the Fingers While the Client Is on a Table

- **Common areas of use:** The fingers work best when treating small muscles or delicate areas with little or no musculature. The face, neck, and the medial arms and legs are common examples.
- **Special considerations:** Be careful when using the fingers, as these are not as durable as the thumbs. Use them sparingly.

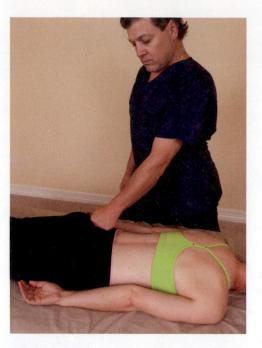

FIGURE 16.9

The Position for Applying Pressure with the Fists While the Client Is on a Table

FISTS/PALMS

- **Physical description:** Place the fists or palms on the client. Keep the elbows firm and the shoulders relaxed. Lean into the client using your body weight to apply the pressure (see Figures 16.9 ■ and 16.10 ■). Hold the position for 3 to 5 seconds, then release the pressure slowly.

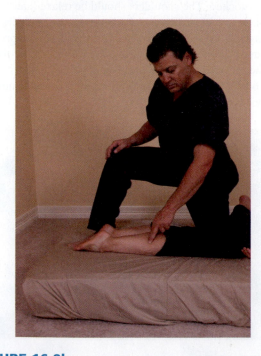

FIGURE 16.8b

The Position for Applying Pressure with the Fingers While the Client Is on a Mat

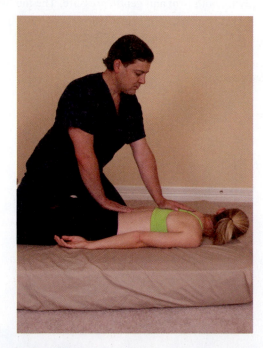

FIGURE 16.10

The Position for Applying Pressure with the Palms While the Client Is on a Mat

- **Common areas of use:** The fists and palms are used almost anywhere on the body. The fists are good for thick muscles like the back and gluteals. The palms are generally easier for the client to accept, so they are more widely used than the fist.
- **Special considerations:** Both hand positions are good for introducing pressure to the client's body during the warm-up. They are also used on acupoints when the client cannot tolerate the focused pressure of the thumbs and fingers.

ELBOW

- **Physical description:** Make sure to keep your back straight. Kneel or stand next to the client, placing the olecranon gently onto the acupoint. Keep your shoulders down and resist letting them rise towards your ears. Use your other hand to hold onto the wrist of the arm that is applying pressure. This helps stabilize your working arm. If the acupoint is too tender, you may put counterpressure on your wrist, which will soften the contact point of the elbow (see Figures 16.11a ■ and 16.11b ■). Hold the position for 3 to 5 seconds, then release the pressure slowly.
- **Common areas of use:** Using the elbow is a popular way to work acupoints in larger muscles. It is good for muscles such as the gluteals, thighs, and back. The elbow is also a good choice for larger more muscular clients.
- **Special considerations:** The elbow, and specifically the olecranon process, is much more durable than the fingers and thumbs. It also offers a leverage advantage and so generates firmer pressure. This is important because a little effort goes a long way with this technique. Be careful not to overdo the pressure.

HEEL/FOOT

- **Physical description:** When using the heels or feet for pressure, it is easiest to have the client lie on a floor mat rather than on a table. Stand next to the client, and while

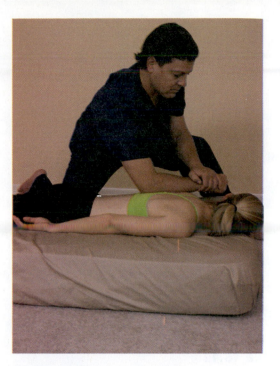

FIGURE 16.11b

The Position for Applying Pressure with the Elbow While the Client Is on a Mat

keeping one foot on the mat, push the heel, ball, or arch of the other foot into the client's body (see Figures 16.12 ■, 16.13 ■, and 16.14 ■). Instead of using the muscles of the leg, it is best to rock your body weight forward onto the leg applying the pressure. The foot can be used to

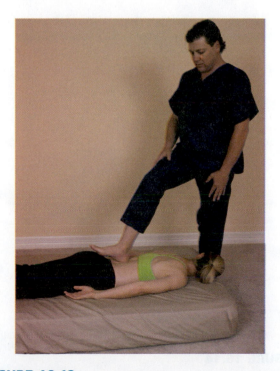

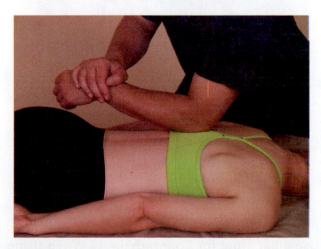

FIGURE 16.11a

The Position for Applying Pressure with the Elbow While the Client Is on a Table

FIGURE 16.12

The Position for Applying Pressure with the Heel While the Client Is on a Mat

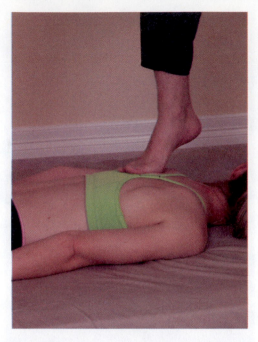

FIGURE 16.13

The Position for Applying Pressure with the Ball of the Foot While the Client Is on a Mat

knead the acupoints as well. Hold the position for 3 to 5 seconds, then release the pressure slowly.

- **Common areas of use:** The heel or ball of the foot is commonly used to work larger body parts or areas of heavy muscle. The legs are much stronger than the arms and can generate more pressure on these areas.

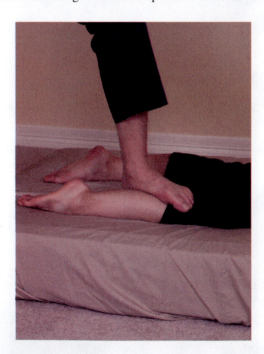

FIGURE 16.14

The Position for Applying Pressure with the Arch of the Foot While the Client Is on a Mat

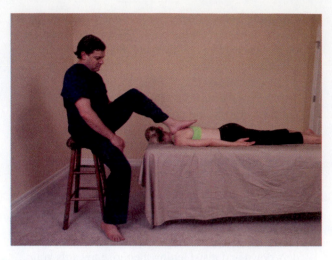

FIGURE 16.15

Sit on a Barstool in Order to Use the Foot as a Contact Point While the Client Is on a Table.

- **Special considerations:** When working with the client on a table, you can sit on a bar stool and apply pressure with the feet (see Figure 16.15 ■). Be careful when working on smaller body parts or clients. Balance is important when using your feet. When working on a mat, you can place a bar stool next to the work area for counterbalance (see Figure 16.16 ■). Therapists who work with their feet frequently will install bars along the wall or on the ceiling to use for balance.

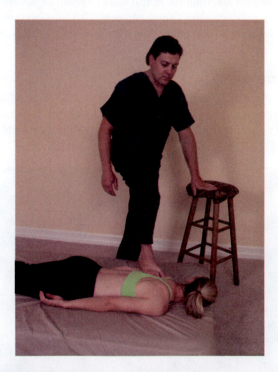

FIGURE 16.16

Use a Bar Stool for Counterbalance When Using the Foot as a Contact Point While the Client Is on a Mat.

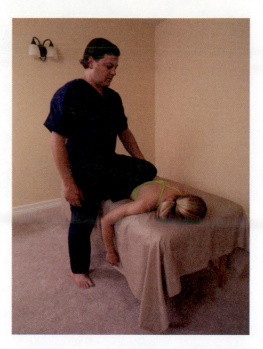

FIGURE 16.17a

The Position for Applying Pressure with One Knee While the Client Is on a Table

KNEES/SHINS

- **Physical description:** The knee and shin are used together as a contact point to help spread out your body weight so that you do not put too much pressure on the client's body. You may use either one knee/shin (see Figures 16.17a ■ and 16.17b ■) or both

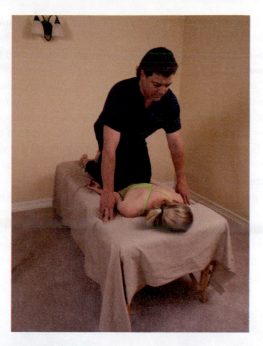

FIGURE 16.18a

The Position for Applying Pressure with Both Knees While the Client Is on a Table

knees/shins (see Figures 16.18a ■ and 16.18b ■). The choice depends on where you are working. Generally, one knee is used on smaller areas (arms, lower legs) and two knees are used on larger areas (back, hips, upper leg). Place your hands on the table/mat for support. Then place your knee(s) on top of the areas being

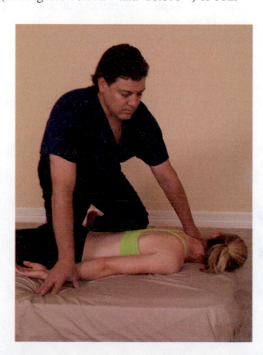

FIGURE 16.17b

The Position for Applying Pressure with One Knee While the Client Is on a Mat

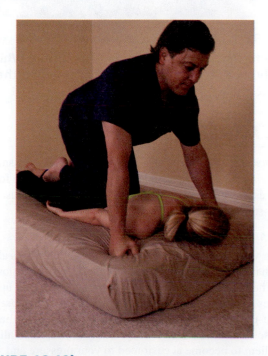

FIGURE 16.18b

The Position for Applying Pressure with Both Knees While the Client Is on a Mat

treated. Slowly rock your body weight forward into the upper shin(s) and knee(s), applying the pressure. Hold the position for 3 to 5 seconds, then release the pressure slowly.

- **Common areas of use:** The knees/shins are commonly used to work larger body parts or areas of heavy muscle, such as the back, gluteals, and upper legs. This is because when you are kneeling on the client, they are generally supporting most of your body weight. Therefore it is important to be on an area that can support the weight.
- **Special considerations:** Be careful when working on smaller body parts or clients. Balance is important when using your knees. If you are using a table instead of the floor or a mat, you can place a bar stool next to the work area to expand the space to place your hands (see Figure 16.19 ■).

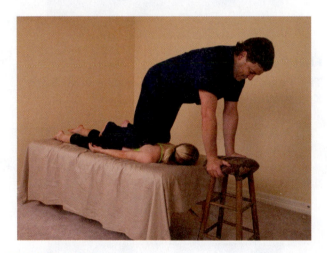

FIGURE 16.19

How to Use a Barstool for Extra Support While Applying Pressure with Both Knees While the Client Is on a Table

THE ACUPRESSURE ROUTINE

Acupressure treatment begins with a thorough assessment, preparing the space, and focusing the Qi. The routine for an acupressure treatment session itself is best applied using a three-step process.

STEP 1. WARM-UP

Using your palms, begin slow rhythmic compressions along the channels. Work the channels in the order of the flow of Qi. The gentle rhythmic palm pressure helps warm up the tissues and prepare them for the work to follow. Use the warm-up to assess the client's tissues and to familiarize yourself with the client's body. The warm-up also allows the client to become accustomed to your pressure and your personal Qi. During the warm-up, encourage the client to practice along with you in breathing out with the pressure and breathing in upon the release.

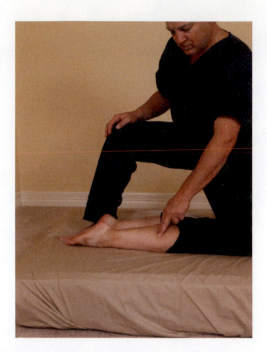

FIGURE 16.20a

Treating One Acupoint at a Time

STEP 2. TREAT THE ACUPOINTS

There are two basic methods for approaching the treatment of points along the channels. Each has its own advantages depending on the specific pathology and the overall treatment plan.

Treat from beginning to end: This is a very simple approach where you work each active point, starting from the beginning of the channel, progressing through the injury site to the end of the channel. You then move on to the next channel as determined by the flow of Qi or the treatment plan, and move through the points in the same way. The acupoints are treated either one at a time (see Figure 16.20a ■), or in some cases two acupoints can be worked simultaneously (see Figure 16.20b ■). When working two points at a

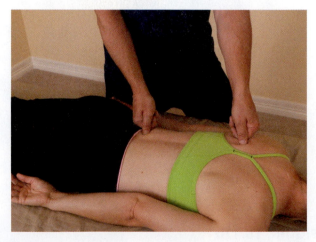

FIGURE 16.20b

Treating Two Points Together

time, you will treat those points that are right next to each other in line along the channel. For example, along the Spleen channel, you may treat Sp 1 and Sp 2 simultaneously, then Sp 4 and Sp 5, and so on.

The amount and duration of pressure required depends on a variety of circumstances:

- If the muscle is weak or very painful, apply light pressure and hold for 6 to10 seconds. This may be repeated on the same spot two to three times.
- If an area is very tight, knotted, or if the muscle is well developed, a deeper pressure is often required. Use moderate to deep pressure and hold the acupoint for 30 seconds or longer. This can be repeated on the same acupoint two to three times. Always use the client's tolerance to guide the level of pressure that you apply.

As you work the channel, it is important to treat any Ashi acupoints along the way. After reaching the end of one channel, move along to the next channel in the order of Qi flow. Continue until all channels in need of therapy have been treated.

Treat from the ends toward the middle: Another technique is to work acupoints on both ends of the channels or on both sides of the pathology simultaneously. Often the points located at the ends of the channels are considered the most influential on the flow of Qi. Therefore, placing pressure on these points at the same time may help move the stubborn, stagnated Qi that is causing pain and persistent pathology. The idea is to cause the Qi from both ends of the channel to move together and act on both sides of the blockage.

This is an excellent treatment for very painful or hard to treat areas, such as the groin or around joints. Pressure can be applied on both sides of the pathology, allowing you to avoid placing pressure directly on painful or complicated areas, while still achieving a strong healing effect.

To perform the technique, start by working the first and last active points along the affected channel. Place pressure on both points evenly and at the same time. Hold for 5 to 30 seconds, then gently release. Move to the next two points in from the ends of the channel and apply pressure. These points will be the second and second-to-last acupoints along the channel. Continue on to the next two points in from the ends, and repeat until you reach the middle or the points closest to the injury site.

Some channels, such as the Stomach channel, are very long, and working both ends is impossible. In such cases, work as far apart as you can, and proceed from there. For example, if the pain is in the lateral knee along the Stomach channel, instead of pressing on St 1, which is located in the face (and is a long reach from the foot), the treatment may begin on St 31, which is the first point on the leg, and St 41 which is another active point on the ankle/foot (see Figure 16.21 ■, which shows the Stomach points on the leg). Figure 16.22a ■ shows a second position for pressure on the Stomach channel for treating a lateral knee injury (St 32 and St 40). Figure 16.22b ■ shows the closest position for treating pain on the Stomach channel at the knee (St 34 and St 36). These will be the last acupoints treated using this method.

STEP 3. COOL DOWN AND CONCLUDE THE THERAPY

The cool down is similar to the warm-up. The palms are used to press each acupoint along the channel in the order of the flow of Qi. In this way, circulation of blood, fluids, and Qi is encouraged through all the areas. The cool down may also

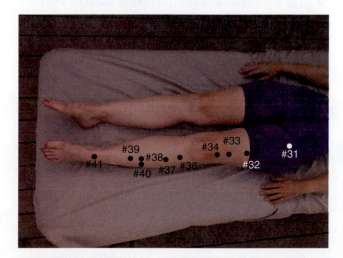

FIGURE 16.21

The Points on the Stomach Channel Along the Leg

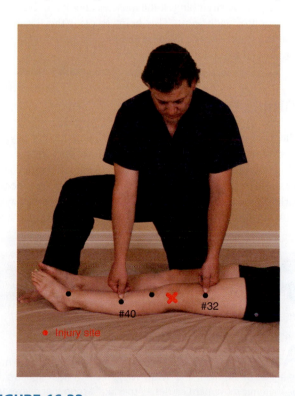

FIGURE 16.22a

Treating Two Distant Acupoints on the Stomach Channel When There Is Pathology at the Knee

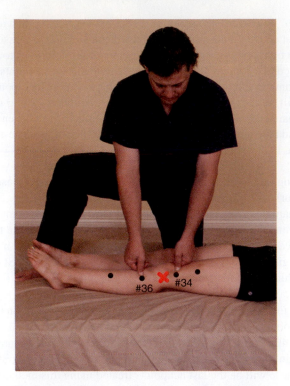

FIGURE 16.22b

Treating Two Close-Together Acupoints on the Stomach Channel When There Is Pathology at the Knee

include passive stretching of the muscles and/or passive range of motion of each joint. This helps to clear the tissues by pumping wastes out of the area and into the lymph system to be removed from the body.

COURSE OF TREATMENT

Whenever possible, acupressure is performed every day for a period of two weeks. It is important to reapply the therapy before the old unbalanced positions and Qi patterns are able to establish themselves again. However, in today's hectic world it may only be practical to treat the client three days a week or even as little as once a week. It is important to note

that the longer the duration between the treatments, the slower the progress will be. However, even though longer intervals between sessions may cause more treatments in the long run, it is still possible to get good results.

It is essential to re-evaluate the client before each subsequent treatment. Every day is different, and the new circumstance will create new conditions in the client's body. Also, as the therapy progresses, the client's body will change as it heals. It is important to address these new changes in the client's body to keep up with the healing process. This requires that you do a thorough assessment each time the client comes in for therapy. Tailor the treatment to each new expression as well as any old patterns that still exist.

CAUTIONS

- It is important to apply pressure slowly to enable the layers of tissue to relax and allow the depth. Never press an area in an abrupt, forceful, or jarring way. This just causes resistance and is counterproductive.
- When treating the abdomen, use only light pressure and focus your attention and Qi. The abdomen is considered to be the *Hara*, or center of the body's Qi; therefore special care is applied when working there.
- To prevent any adverse reactions to the therapy, have the client wait at least 1 hour after a heavy meal before receiving treatment.
- Finally, areas with a high concentration of lymph nodes, such as the armpit (axilla) and back of the knee (*popliteal fossa*), should be worked carefully and gently. Heavy pressure directly on a lymph node is not recommended.

CONTRAINDICATIONS

- **Acute illness**—It is difficult for the client to heal when she or he is already fighting an infection. Have the client rest and focus on fighting the illness before taxing the client's body further with therapy.
- **Pregnancy**—Generally, most healthy pregnancies will tolerate light acupressure. However, it is not advisable to work the inner ankle, especially the Kidney channel, and specifically the acupoint Large Intestine #4 (on the hand), as these acupoints can cause uterine contractions.
- **Areas of acute injury**—If the tissue is torn, limit the work to the distal acupoints on the affected channels. If the injury is severe, the therapy can be focused on the channel on the other side of the body (the mirror channel). For example, if the Lung channel on the right arm is severely affected or too painful, the therapy can be focused on the Lung channel on the left arm instead.
- **Common contraindications**—If a particular condition is contraindicated for general relaxation massage, it is probably contraindicated for acupressure as well.

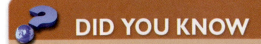

DID YOU KNOW

A traditional technique to close an acupressure session is to hold the ankles of the client and gently swing the legs from side to side. The rhythmic movement causes a "snaking" action that relaxes the knees and hips and impacts the entire spine. The technique will help relax the back, neck, and shoulders.

QUICK QUIZ #32

1. It is easiest to perform acupressure while the client is dressed because: (Circle all that apply)
   a. the client may be repositioned frequently to treat each point in the correct order.
   b. the treatment room will be kept at a cool temperature.
   c. it is easier to incorporate stretching techniques into the session.
   d. it is easier and more efficient to not have to manage a drape.
   e. All of the above
   f. None of the above

2. When a muscle is more tense, deeper pressure of longer duration is generally recommended because it has a more sedating effect on the tissues.
   a. True
   b. False

3. The fingertips are the most standard tool used for acupressure and are the most durable digits used as a contact point.
   a. True
   b. False

4. Acupressure can be performed effectively by: (Circle all that apply)
   a. applying pressure to all active points, in order from one end of the channel to the other.
   b. applying pressure to only two points, one in the local area of injury and one at the distal end of the channel.
   c. reassessing the client before each new treatment session.
   d. applying treatment once per week.
   e. All of the above
   f. None of the above

SUMMARY

There are a variety of techniques and traditions of acupressure therapy. Acupressure can treat a range of diseases from internal disorders to pathology found in the myoskeletal system. Treating disease of the internal organs requires complicated skills; however, treating the muscles, bones, and joints is quite simple.

Before therapy, an assessment must take place. The assessment includes an observation of the posture and the relative length of the channels. First, the primary affected channels should be identified. The Yin/Yang pairs, mirror channels, and the channels that follow the flow of Qi must all be checked for compensatory pathology. The active acupoints along the channels and the Ashi acupoints must be noted by palpating the channels.

Acupressure therapy is applied while the client is in comfortable clothing and lying on a large mat, on the floor, or on a suitable low table. It is important to properly focus the mind before applying pressure. Help the client to focus her or his Qi during the treatment by having the client breathe with you. Exhale with the application of pressure and inhale upon the release of pressure.

There are a variety of methods used to apply pressure. The duration and depth of pressure may vary. The pressure may be constant, or it may be applied with some movement, such as tapping, vibrating, or circular motion.

The heels, elbows, thumbs, and fingers are commonly used as contact points. Each has its own relative benefits for use on different areas or circumstances. The routine consists of a warm-up, treatment of acupoints, and then a cool down.

Treatment of the acupoints may be done working each acupoint in the order of Qi flow or by treating points at both ends simultaneously and working towards the middle. Acupressure should be performed daily or as often as possible through the course of treatment. It is important to be aware of the general cautions and the contraindications of applying pressure.

DISCUSSION QUESTIONS

1. Explain three methods of identifying associated channels.
2. Explain the importance of understanding Yin/Yang complements when performing an assessment and formulating a treatment plan.
3. Describe the type and duration of pressure you might use to apply pressure to acupoints on a robust client with very tense muscles.

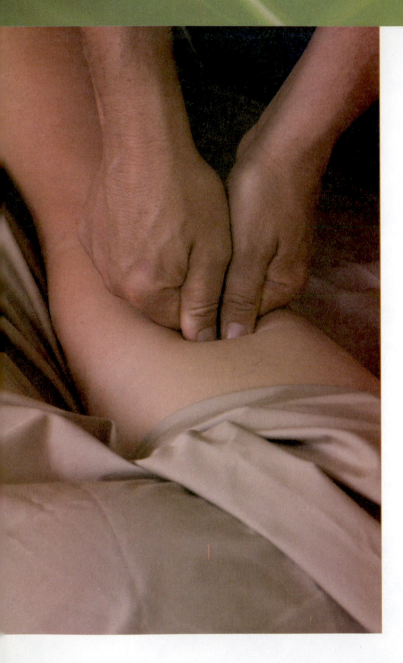

17 Sample Protocols for Acupressure Therapy

 CHAPTER HIGHLIGHTS

Chapter Objectives

Key Terms

Application of the Techniques

Summary

Discussion Questions

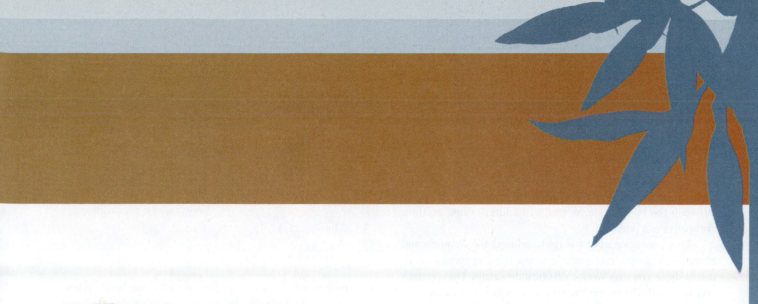

CHAPTER OBJECTIVES

- Understand how to apply the techniques of acupressure
- Explore a sample acupressure protocol following the channels through the body
- Practice acupressure techniques

KEY TERMS

Channel *336*

Flow of Qi *336*

Classically effective
  acupoints *336*

Traditional acupoint *338*

Local acupoint *339*

Distant acupoint *339*

APPLICATION OF THE TECHNIQUES

Acupressure has a wide variety of uses and applications. It may be used to treat specific areas of pathology and compensation, or it can be used to treat the whole body for general wellness.

Treating all the **channels** of the body is an excellent tool for maintaining general myoskeletal health. A whole body acupressure treatment will help to ensure balance between the body systems and will address most existing compensation patterns.

There are a variety of ways to address the channels and acupoints. You may treat multiple channels and acupoints simultaneously, or you may work each one individually. The approach you take will depend on the size and relative musculature of your client, as well as other factors such as time constraints. Treating multiple points and/or channels simultaneously saves time, but it may not be practical on larger clients or may not be desirable depending upon the issues being treated.

The protocols highlighted here can be combined into a full body protocol; therefore, the order in which the body parts are presented here produces a protocol which flows according to acupressure theory. The protocols may also be

TABLE 17.1	Classically Effective Acupoints with Ability to Clear the Entire Channel
Lung 1, 5, 7	Urinary Bladder 10, 40, 60
Large Intestine 4, 11, 20	Kidney 1, 3, 10
Stomach 9, 36, 41	Pericardium 2, 3, 6
Spleen 6, 9, 10	San Jao 5, 14, 23
Heart 2, 3, 7	Gall Bladder 20, 21, 30
Small Intestine 5, 11, 18	Liver 3, 8, 13

used individually to treat specific areas of the body. When treating specific pathologies, refer to the treatment protocol detailed in Chapter 16 and use the simple point prescriptions for each area.

Whether you are performing a full body session or treating a specific pathology, there are a few key concepts to consider when formulating your acupressure protocol.

1. Know all the muscles in the area that will be treated.
2. Know the channels being treated and their relationships to other channels.
3. Know the direction of the **flow of Qi** for each channel.
4. Know the acupoints along the affected channels.
5. Know the **classically effective acupoints** that help clear the channel (Table 17.1 ■).

A suitable protocol will be easy to prepare if you combine your knowledge of the channels and acupoints with the selection of appropriate contact points. Table 17.2 ■ provides a quick reference to the contact points and their common uses.

Remember that acupressure is usually applied with a steady pressure that is held for three counts or longer.

DID YOU KNOW

Before Every Acupressure Treatment

Remember to obtain a proper client history and perform a thorough assessment. This is important in order to develop a good plan and to rule out any techniques that may be contraindicated.

TABLE 17.2	Contact Points for Acupressure Techniques	
Contact Point	Description	Common Uses
Fingers	The lightest contact point	Best for shallow areas, smaller muscles, and more sensitive tissues
Thumbs	Provides deeper pressure than fingers. Thumbs are stronger and more durable	Best for thicker muscles and more durable tissues
Fists/palms	Provides deep penetration into tissues, but less invasive due to broad contact point	Good for large and/or robust muscles
Elbows/forearms	Provides deep penetration and strong pressure with less work. Adjusting contact from olecranon process to flatter surfaces of forearm will adjust penetration	Good for larger muscles and larger, more robust clients
Heels/feet	Has the capacity to generate great pressure due to the strength of the legs behind the contact point. The heel is more invasive than the broader contact of the foot	Best used on the largest and most robust muscles
Knees/shins	Provides strong pressure, but is less invasive than the heels due to broad contact point. Adjusting contact from knee to the flatter surfaces of the shin will adjust penetration	Best for large muscles that are sensitive

Generally speaking, lighter pressure of a shorter duration tends to be stimulating. Deeper pressure of a longer duration tends to be more sedating. When the muscle is weak or the client is frail, use light pressure with a short duration. When the muscle is very tense and the client is robust, use firmer pressure with a longer duration.

Also, depending on the size of your client, the individual techniques may be combined to treat multiple channels and multiple points simultaneously. This is done to simplify treatment in areas where channels are too close together or on small bodies. In larger areas where the channels are more spread out, points and channels are treated individually.

SAMPLE PROTOCOL

Myoskeletal Wellness Protocol

This protocol begins with an overall warm-up of each area. The warm-up prepares the client's body for therapy, and allows you to focus your Qi. Once the warm-up is complete, there are two options for performing specific acupoint work. Your choice depends on the needs of the client and the time frame in which you have to work. The first choice requires more time and is more thorough. This is because you are treating all active acupoints, including the classically effective points for the channel(s). The second choice is a simple point prescription that can be used to treat each area. The point prescription includes a combination of points based on local and distant principles. The local acupoints presented are typically very effective in treatment and may be selected for treatment based on their proximity to the area of pathology. The distant acupoints presented in the tables are strong in treatments and are chosen because of their position towards the ends of the channel(s) or away from the local area. Since only a few points are chosen, this is more time efficient. It is effective when there is less time to work or in cases where you want to decrease the intensity of treatment.

Conveniently, the warm-ups for each area can be combined together into a gentle whole-body treatment when applied without including the specific acupoint work for each area.

This protocol begins by treating the Yang channels first. This is recommended because according to Chinese theory, the Yang channels are usually more tense as they support more of the body's posture and therefore carry the most Qi.

THE THREE YANG CHANNELS OF THE ARM

There are three Yang channels that run from the hand to the head (see Figure 17.1 ■):

- Large Intestine channel (posterior/lateral section—index side)
- San Jao channel (posterior/central section—middle)
- Small Intestine channel (posterior medial section—pinky side)

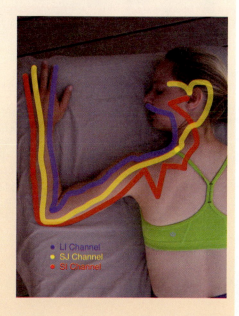

FIGURE 17.1

The Three Yang Channels of the Arm/Hand. The Large Intestine Channel (Blue), the San Jao Channel (Yellow), and the Small Intestine Channel (Red)

The Posterior Forearm and Hand

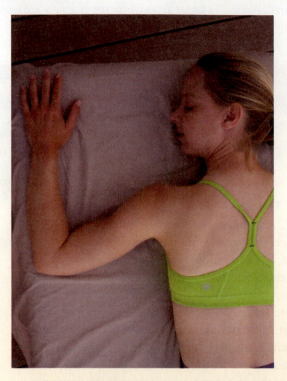

Because the Yang channels are located along the posterior side of the body, begin with the client in the prone position with the arms positioned out to the sides of the head (see Figure 17.2 ■). In the hand and forearm, the three Yang channels are close together so they are most often warmed up simultaneously. In other cases (large hands/arms) warm them up individually.

☑ Review the muscles and channels of the hand and forearm (see Table 17.3 ■ and Figure 17.3 ■).

☑ Review the **traditional acupoints** of each channel (Chapter 14).

☑ Choose contact points that are appropriate for the client's hand and forearm (Table 17.2).

FIGURE 17.2

The Positioning of the Client for Beginning the Acupressure Sequence

TABLE 17.3	Channels and Muscles of the Posterior Forearm and Hand	
Acupressure Channel	Location of Muscles	Name of Muscle
Large Intestine channel	Lateral edge of posterior forearm	*Supinator*
		Abductor pollicis longus
		Extensor pollicis brevis
		Abductor pollicis longus
		Extensor indicis
		Dorsal interossei
		Extensor pollicis longus
		Anconeus
		Brachioradialis
San Jao channel	Middle of posterior forearm	*Dorsal interossei*
		Extensor digitorum communis
		Extensor digitorum communis
Small Intestine channel	Medial edge of posterior forearm	*Extensor carpi ulnaris*
		Dorsal interossei
		Extensor digiti minimi

FIGURE 17.3

The Major Muscles of the Posterior Forearm and Hand

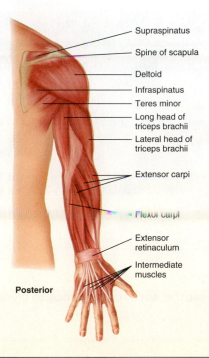

- Supraspinatus
- Spine of scapula
- Deltoid
- Infraspinatus
- Teres minor
- Long head of triceps brachii
- Lateral head of triceps brachii
- Extensor carpi
- Flexor carpi
- Extensor retinaculum
- Intermediate muscles

Posterior

WARM-UP

1. Take a deep breath and while breathing out, begin to apply pressure to the back of the client's hand. Hold firm pressure on the hand for 3 counts, then release the pressure.

2. Move to the area of the hand or wrist that is just proximal to where you first applied pressure (i.e., the next few acupoints). Breathe out and apply pressure for 3 counts, then release the pressure.

3. Move along the channels just proximal to your last area of pressure (i.e., the next few acupoints). Breathe out and apply pressure for 3 counts, then release the pressure.

4. Continue breathing out and applying pressure for 3 seconds to successively more proximal acupoints along the channels of the forearm until you reach the elbow.

5. Breathe out and apply pressure to the lateral elbow for 3 counts, then release the pressure.

TREAT THE SPECIFIC ACUPOINTS (CHOOSE ONE OF THE FOLLOWING APPROACHES)

- Treat all active Ashi and traditional acupoints located during assessment of the area. Include the classically effective points for each channel.
  - Large Intestine channel: 4, 11, and 20
  - San Jao channel: 5, 14, and 23
  - Small Intestine channel: 5, 11, and 18
- Use the simple point prescription to treat the forearm and hand (Figure 17.4 ■ and Table 17.4 ■) Choose one or more of the recommended **local acupoints,** and place pressure on it while simultaneously placing pressure on a **distant acupoint** for each body region.

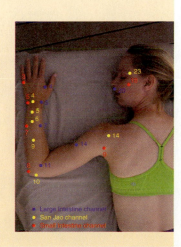

FIGURE 17.4

The Location of Acupoints for the Simple Point Prescription to Treat the Posterior Forearm and Hand

TABLE 17.4 **Simple Point Prescription for the Posterior Hand and Forearm**

Body Region	Local Acupoints	Distant Acupoints
Posterior/lateral forearm and hand	LI 4—treats thumb and first finger LI 5—treats lateral wrist LI 7—treats lateral forearm	LI 14, LI 11
Posterior/center forearm and hand	SJ 4—treats hand and fingers SJ 6—treats posterior wrist SJ 9—treats posterior forearm	SJ 14, SJ 10
Posterior/medial forearm and hand	SI 3—treats medial hand and ring and little fingers SI 5—treats medial wrist SI 7—treats medial forearm	SI 9, SI 8

CLOSE
Repeat the warm-up sequence to close the area.

The Upper Back, Posterior Shoulder, and Upper Arm

ELBOW AND UPPER ARM
Most of the time, the three Yang channels are close together in the upper arm so they can be warmed up simultaneously. In cases where the client is larger, work the channels and points separately. Start treating each channel at the elbow and work along its course until you reach the shoulder.

- ☑ Review the muscles and channels of the elbow and upper arm (see Table 17.5 ■ and Figure 17.5 ■).
- ☑ Review the traditional acupoints of each channel (Chapter 14).
- ☑ Choose contact points that are appropriate for the client's elbow and upper arm (Table 17.2).

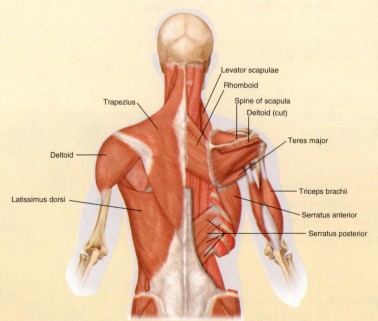

FIGURE 17.5

The Major Muscles of the Upper Back, Posterior Shoulder, and Posterior Upper Arm

Levator scapulae, Rhomboid, Spine of scapula, Deltoid (cut), Trapezius, Teres major, Deltoid, Latissimus dorsi, Triceps brachii, Serratus anterior, Serratus posterior

TABLE 17.5 **Channels and Muscles of the Upper Back, Posterior Shoulder, and Upper Arm**

Acupressure Channel	Location of Muscles	Name of Muscle	
Small Intestine channel	Medial and posterior edges of the upper arm and shoulder	*Trapezius* *Latissimus dorsi* *Levator scapulae* *Teres minor* *Teres major* *Triceps brachii* *Infraspinatus*	
		Assistant muscles to SI channel	*Rhomboid major* *Rhomboid minor*
San Jao channel	Middle of upper arm superior shoulder	*Trapezius* *Triceps brachii* *Supraspinatus*	
Large Intestine channel	Lateral and posterior edges of the upper arm and shoulder	*Triceps brachii* *Supraspinatus* *Deltoid*	
Urinary Bladder channel	Upper back and posterior neck	*Trapezius* *Latissimus dorsi* *Levator scapulae* *Rhomboid major* *Rhomboid minor*	
Gall Bladder channel	Lateral neck and (sides) of upper back	*Latissimus dorsi* *Teres minor* *Teres major* *Serratus anterior*	

WARM-UP

1. Take a deep breath and while breathing out, apply pressure just proximal to the elbow on the upper arm for 3 counts, then release the pressure.

2. Move along the channels just proximal to your last area of pressure (i.e., the next few acupoints). Breathe out and apply pressure for 3 counts, then release the pressure.

3. Continue breathing out and applying pressure for 3 seconds to successively more proximal acupoints along the channels of the upper arm until you reach the shoulder.

TREAT THE SPECIFIC ACUPOINTS (CHOOSE ONE OF THE FOLLOWING APPROACHES)

- Treat all active Ashi and traditional acupoints located during assessment of the area. Include the classically effective points for each channel:
  ◦ Large Intestine channel: 4, 11, and 20
  ◦ San Jao channel: 5, 14, and 23
  ◦ Small Intestine channel: 5, 11, and 18

TABLE 17.6	Simple Point Prescription for the Elbow and Upper Arm	
Body Region	Local Acupoints	Distant Acupoints
Posterior/lateral elbow and upper arm	LI 10—treats area distal to elbow LI 11—treats lateral elbow LI 14—treats lateral upper arm	LI 18, LI 17
Posterior/center elbow and upper arm	SJ 9—treats area distal to elbow SJ 10—treats posterior elbow SJ 13—treats upper arm	SJ 16, SJ 15
Posterior/medial elbow and upper arm	SI 8—treats medial elbow and upper arm	SI 11, SI 9

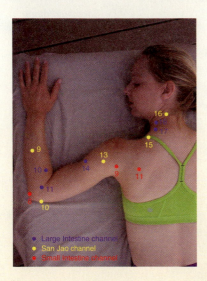

- Use the simple point prescription to treat the elbow and upper arm (see Figure 17.6 ■ and Table 17.6 ■). Choose one or more of the recommended local acupoints and place pressure on it while simultaneously placing pressure on a distant acupoint for each body region.

FIGURE 17.6

The Location of Acupoints for the Simple Point Prescription to Treat the Elbow and Upper Arm

CLOSE

Repeat the warm-up sequence to close the area.

POSTERIOR SHOULDER AND LATERAL NECK

At the shoulder, the three Yang channels spread out. The Large Intestine channel and the San Jao channel continue along the superior shoulder, while the Small Intestine channel continues along the posterior scapula. Sometimes in smaller clients, these three may be warmed up simultaneously; however, in most clients you will warm them individually. Work each channel from the lateral shoulder to the neck, ending on the lateral side of the head.

☑ Review the muscles and channels of the shoulder and lateral neck (Table 17.5 and Figure 17.5).

☑ Review the traditional acupoints of each channel (Chapter 14).

☑ Choose contact points that are appropriate for the client's shoulder (Table 17.2).

WARM-UP

1. Breathe out and apply pressure to the lateral shoulder for 3 counts, then release the pressure.

2. Move along the channels just proximal to your last area of pressure (i.e., the next few acupoints). Breathe out and apply pressure for 3 counts, then release the pressure.

3. Continue breathing out and applying pressure for 3 seconds to successively more proximal acupoints along the channels of the shoulder until you reach the neck.

4. Breathe out and apply pressure to the lateral/posterior neck for 3 seconds and then release the pressure.

TREAT THE SPECIFIC ACUPOINTS (CHOOSE ONE OF THE FOLLOWING APPROACHES)

- Treat all active Ashi and traditional acupoints located during assessment of the area. Include the classically effective acupoints for each channel:
  - Large Intestine channel: 4, 11, and 20
  - San Jao channel: 5, 14, and 23
  - Small Intestine channel: 5, 11, and 18
- Use the simple point prescription to treat the shoulder and lateral neck (see Figure 17.7 ■ and Table 17.7 ■). Choose one or more of the recommended local acupoints and place pressure on it while simultaneously placing pressure on a distant acupoint for each body region.

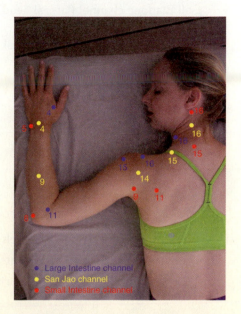

FIGURE 17.7

The Location of Acupoints for the Simple Point Prescription to Treat the Posterior Shoulder

TABLE 17.7	Simple Point Prescription for the Posterior Shoulder and Lateral Neck	
Body Region	**Local Acupoints**	**Distant Acupoints**
Posterior/superior shoulder and lateral neck	LI 15—treats superior shoulder LI 16—treats base of neck LI 18—treats lateral neck	LI 4, LI 11
Posterior shoulder and lateral neck	SJ 14—treats posterior shoulder SJ 15—treats posterior upper shoulder SJ 16—treats lateral neck	SJ 4, SJ 9
Posterior/inferior shoulder and lateral neck	SI 9—treats posterior axilla SI 11—treats scapular region SI 15—treats base of neck SI 17—treats lateral neck	SI 5, SI 8

CLOSE

Repeat the warm-up sequence to close the area.

THE THREE YANG CHANNELS OF THE LEG

There are three Yang channels that run from the head to the foot (see Figure 17.8 ■). They cover the posterior and lateral sides of the body, neck, and head:

- Urinary Bladder channel (posterior head, torso, legs, and feet)
- Gall Bladder channel (lateral head, torso, legs, and feet)
- Stomach channel (anterior/lateral head, torso, legs, and feet)

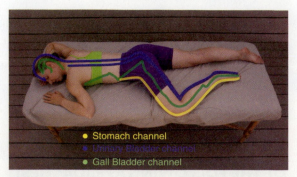

● Stomach channel
● Urinary Bladder channel
● Gall Bladder channel

FIGURE 17.8

The Three Yang Channels of the Leg/Foot. The Gall Bladder Channel (Green), the Urinary Bladder Channel (Blue), and the Stomach Channel (Yellow)

The Posterior Head and Neck

The emphasis here is the posterior head and neck where the Urinary Bladder channel is located (see Figure 17.9 ■). This portion of the protocol is designed to work the Urinary Bladder channel individually.

☑ Review the muscles and channels of the posterior head and neck (see Table 17.8 ■ and Figure 17.10 ■).

☑ Review the traditional acupoints of each channel (Chapter 14).

☑ Choose contact points appropriate for the head and/or neck (Table 17.2).

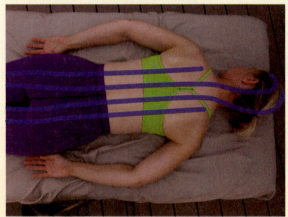

FIGURE 17.9

The Location of the Urinary Bladder Channel on the Head, Neck, and Posterior Torso

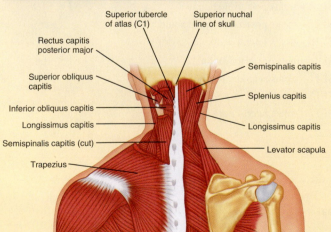

FIGURE 17.10

The Major Muscles of the Posterior Neck

TABLE 17.8	Channels and Muscles of the Posterior Neck	
Acupressure Channel	Location of Muscles	Name of Muscle
Urinary Bladder channel	Attaching to vertebra, scapula, and clavicle	*Trapezius*
	Cervical vertebral	*Splenius capitus*
		Splenius cervicis
	Erector spinae	*Iliocostalis cervicis*
		Longissimus capitis
		Longissimus cervicis
		Spinalis capitis
		Spinalis cervicis
	Transversospinalis	*Semispinalis capitis*
		Semispinalis cervicis
	Suboccipital neck muscles	*Rectus capitis posterior major*
		Rectus capitis posterior minor
		Obliquus capitis inferior
		Obliquus capitis superior
	Vertebral muscles	*Multifidi*
		Rotatores
		Interspinales
	Intertransversarii	*Intertransversarii posteriores*
Du channel	Vertebral muscles	*Multifidis*
		Rotatores
		Interspinalis
	Intertransversarii	*Intertransversarii poteriores*

WARM-UP

1. Breathe out and apply pressure to the anterior/lateral forehead for 3 counts, then release the pressure.

2. Move along the Urinary Bladder channel just superior to your last area of pressure (i.e., the next few acupoints). Breathe out and apply pressure for 3 counts, then release the pressure.

3. Continue breathing out and applying pressure for 3 seconds to successive acupoints along the Urinary Bladder channel until you reach the neck.

4. Breathe out and apply pressure to the posterior neck for 3 seconds and then release the pressure.

TREAT THE SPECIFIC ACUPOINTS (CHOOSE ONE OF THE FOLLOWING APPROACHES)

- Treat all active Ashi and traditional acupoints located during assessment of the area. Include the classically effective acupoints for the Urinary Bladder channel: 10, 40, and 60.
- Use the simple point prescription to treat the posterior head and neck (see Figure 17.11 ■ and Table 17.9 ■). Choose one or more of the recommended local acupoints and place pressure on it while simultaneously placing pressure on a distant acupoint for each body region.

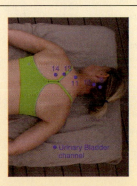

FIGURE 17.11

The Location of Acupoints for the Simple Point Prescription to Treat the Posterior Neck

TABLE 17.9	Simple Point Prescription for the Posterior Head and Neck	
Body Region	Local Acupoints	Distant Acupoints
Posterior head and neck	UB 9—treats head UB 10—treats superior neck UB 11—treats base of neck	UB 14, UB 13

CLOSE

Repeat the warm-up sequence to close the area.

The Posterior Torso (Back and Sacrum)

This portion of the protocol continues to work on the single Urinary Bladder channel. The Urinary Bladder channel has a unique feature in that it splits into two sections along the posterior torso. One section runs along the erector spinae just lateral to the vertebral column. The other one runs just lateral to the first (Figure 17.9). On larger clients you may need to work these individually, or you may use the knees/shins and forearms to help cover the larger area.

☑ Review the muscles and channels of the posterior torso (see Table 17.10 ■ and Figure 17.12 ■).

☑ Review the traditional acupoints of each channel (Chapter 14).

☑ Choose appropriate contact points for the posterior torso (Table 17.2). You may want to use an assortment of contact points for the back.

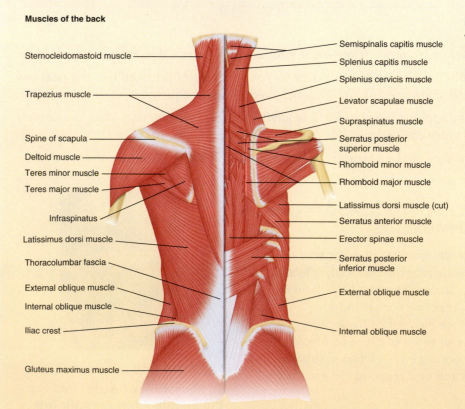

Muscles of the back

- Sternocleidomastoid muscle
- Trapezius muscle
- Spine of scapula
- Deltoid muscle
- Teres minor muscle
- Teres major muscle
- Infraspinatus
- Latissimus dorsi muscle
- Thoracolumbar fascia
- External oblique muscle
- Internal oblique muscle
- Iliac crest
- Gluteus maximus muscle

- Semispinalis capitis muscle
- Splenius capitis muscle
- Splenius cervicis muscle
- Levator scapulae muscle
- Supraspinatus muscle
- Serratus posterior superior muscle
- Rhomboid minor muscle
- Rhomboid major muscle
- Latissimus dorsi muscle (cut)
- Serratus anterior muscle
- Erector spinae muscle
- Serratus posterior inferior muscle
- External oblique muscle
- Internal oblique muscle

FIGURE 17.12

The Major Muscles of the Posterior Torso, Back, and Sacrum

TABLE 17.10	Channels and Muscles of the Posterior/Lateral Torso (Back and Sacrum)	
Acupressure Channel	Location of Muscles	Name of Muscle
Urinary Bladder channel	Posterior aspect of the torso	*Trapezius*
		Latissimus dorsi
		Iliocostalis thoracis
		Iliocostalis lumborum
		Longissimus thoracis
		Spinalis thoracis
		Semispinalis thoracis
		Serratus posterior inferior
		Serratus posterior superior
		Multifidi
		Rotatores
		Interspinales
		Intertransversarii posteriores
		Intertransversarii lateralus
		Intertransversarii mediales
		Quadratus lumborum
Gall Bladder channel	Lateral aspect of the torso	*Latissimus dorsi*
Du channel	Along the vertebral column	*Multifidi*
		Rotatores
		Interspinales

WARM-UP

1. Breathe out and apply pressure to the posterior upper back (at the base of the neck) for 3 counts, then release the pressure.

2. Move along the Urinary Bladder channel just inferior to your last area of pressure (i.e., the next few acupoints). Breathe out and apply pressure for 3 counts, then release the pressure.

3. Continue breathing out and applying pressure for 3 seconds to successively move inferior acupoints along the Urinary Bladder channel until you reach the sacrum.

4. Breathe out and apply pressure to the sacrum for 3 seconds, then release the pressure.

TREAT THE SPECIFIC ACUPOINTS (CHOOSE ONE OF THE FOLLOWING APPROACHES)

- Treat all active Ashi and traditional acupoints located during assessment of the area. Include the classically effective acupoints for the Urinary Bladder channel: 10, 40, 60.
- Use the simple point prescription to treat the back (see Figure 17.13 ■ and Table 17.11 ■). Choose one or more of the recommended local acupoints and place pressure on it while simultaneously placing pressure on a distant acupoint for each body region.

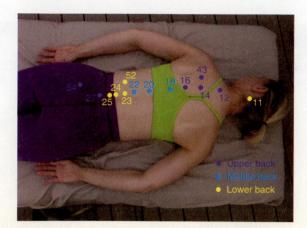

FIGURE 17.13

The Location of Acupoints for the Simple Point Prescription to Treat the Posterior Torso, Back, and Sacrum

TABLE 17.11	Simple Point Prescription for the Posterior Torso	
Body Region	Local Acupoints	Distant Acupoints
Upper back	UB 12—treats superior portion UB 14—treats middle portion UB 16—treats inferior portion UB 43—treats middle/lateral portion	UB 54, UB 27
Middle back	UB 18—treats superior portion UB 20—treats middle portion UB 22—treats inferior portion	UB 54, UB 27
Lower back	UB 23—treats superior portion UB 24—treats middle portion UB 25—treats inferior portion UB 52—treats middle lateral portion	UB 12, UB 11

CLOSE

Repeat the warm-up sequence to close the area.

The Posterior Hip and Thigh

The Urinary Bladder channel takes two paths along the gluteals. One runs just lateral to the *saggital groove*, and the other one runs laterally toward the greater trochanter. When the client is larger, you may need to warm up these lines separately. In smaller clients, you may be able to work these simultaneously. Both lines run from the buttocks along the posterior upper thigh and join together in the posterior knee. They can often be treated simultaneously when using broader contact points, such as the shins and knees (see Figure 17.14 ■).

☑ Review the muscles and channels of the posterior hip and upper thigh (see Table 17.12 ■ and Figure 17.15 ■).

☑ Review the traditional acupoints of each channel (Chapter 14).

☑ Choose contact points for the posterior hip and upper thigh (Table 17.2). You may want to use an assortment of contact points for this area.

FIGURE 17.14

The Location of the Urinary Bladder Channel
on the Hip and Thigh

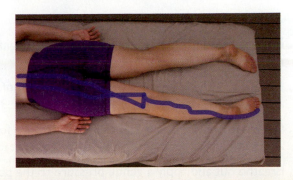

TABLE 17.12	Channels and Muscles of the Posterior/Lateral Hip and Thigh	
Acupressure Channel	Location of Muscles	Name of Muscle
Urinary Bladder channel	Posterior aspect of the hip and thigh	*Gluteus maximus*
		Biceps femoris
		Semitendinosus
		Semimembranosus
		Gluteus medius
		Piriformis
		Obturator internus
		Gemellus superior
		Gemellus inferior
		Obturator externus
		Quadratus femoris
		Gluteus minimus
Gall Bladder channel	Lateral aspect of the hip and thigh	*Gluteus maximus*
		Gluteus medius
		Piriformis
		Gemellus superior
		Gemellus inferior
		Biceps femoris

FIGURE 17.15

The Major Muscles of the Posterior Hip and Thigh

Muscles of the posterior left hip and thigh

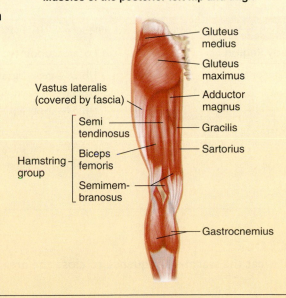

WARM-UP

1. Breathe out and apply pressure to the upper gluteals (just adjacent to the sacrum) for 3 counts, then release the pressure.

2. Move along the Urinary Bladder channel just inferior to your last area of pressure (i.e., the next few acupoints). Breathe out and apply pressure for 3 counts, then release the pressure.

3. Continue breathing out and applying pressure for 3 seconds to successively more inferior acupoints along the Urinary Bladder channel until you reach the posterior knee.

4. Breathe out and apply a gentle pressure to the posterior knee for 3 seconds, then release the pressure.

TREAT THE SPECIFIC ACUPOINTS (CHOOSE ONE OF THE FOLLOWING APPROACHES)

- Treat all active Ashi and traditional acupoints located during assessment of the area. Include the classically effective acupoints for the Urinary Bladder channel: 10, 40, 60.
- Use the simple point prescription to treat the hip and thigh (see Figure 17.16 ■ and Table 17.13 ■). Choose one or more of the recommended local acupoints and place pressure on it while simultaneously placing pressure on a distant acupoint for each body region.

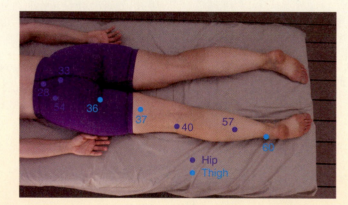

FIGURE 17.16

The Location of Acupoints for the Simple Point Prescription to Treat the Posterior Hip and Thigh

TABLE 17.13	Simple Point Prescription for Posterior Hip and Upper Thigh	
Body Region	Local Acupoints	Distant Acupoints
Posterior hip	UB 28—treats sacral area UB 33—treats coccix area UB 54—treats hip	UB 57, UB 40
Posterior upper thigh	UB 36—treats superior thigh and lower glutes UB 37—treats thigh UB 40—treats posterior knee	UB 60, UB 57

CLOSE
Repeat the warm-up sequence to close the area.

The Posterior Lower Leg

In the lower leg, the branches of the Urinary Bladder channel join to form a single line that runs down the calf and into the lateral foot. However, it is important to warm the entire calf and not just the midline, as the channel spreads into the lateral areas.

☑ Review the muscles and channels of the posterior lower leg (see Table 17.14 ■ and Figure 17.17 ■).

☑ Review the traditional acupoints (Chapter 14).

☑ Choose appropriate contact points for the lower leg (Table 17.2).

TABLE 17.14	Channels and Muscles of the Posterior/Lateral Lower Leg and Foot	
Acupressure Channel	Location of Muscles	Name of Muscle
Urinary Bladder channel	Posterior aspect of lower leg and plantar aspect of foot	*Gastrocnemius*
		Flexor digitorum brevis
		Soleus
		Plantaris
		Quadratus plantae
		Lumbricales
		Adductor hallucis
		Popliteus
		Flexor hallucis longus
		Flexor digitorum longus
		Tibialis posterior
		Dorsal interossei
		Plantar interossei
Gall Bladder channel	Lateral aspect of lower leg and foot	*Abductor digiti minimi*
		Flexor digiti minimi brevis
		Gastrocnemius
		Soleus

FIGURE 17.17

The Major Muscles of the Posterior Lower Leg and Foot

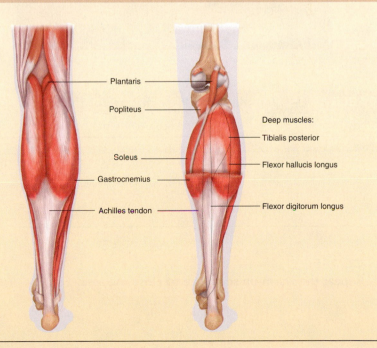

Plantaris

Popliteus

Deep muscles:

Tibialis posterior

Soleus

Flexor hallucis longus

Gastrocnemius

Achilles tendon

Flexor digitorum longus

WARM-UP

1. Breathe out and apply pressure to the proximal calf (just below the knee) for 3 counts, then release the pressure.

2. Move along the Urinary Bladder channel just inferior to your last area of pressure (i.e., the next few acupoints). Breathe out and apply pressure for 3 counts, then release the pressure.

3. Continue breathing out and applying pressure for 3 seconds to successively more inferior acupoints along the Urinary Bladder channel until you reach the ankle.

4. Breathe out and apply a gentle pressure to the lateral ankle and foot for 3 seconds, then release the pressure.

TREAT THE SPECIFIC ACUPOINTS (CHOOSE ONE OF THE FOLLOWING APPROACHES)

- Treat all active Ashi and traditional acupoints located during assessment of the area. Include the classically effective acupoints for the Urinary Bladder channel: 10, 40, and 60.
- Use the simple point prescription to treat the lower leg (see Figure 17.18 ■ and Table 17.15 ■). Choose one or more of the recommended local acupoints and place pressure on it while simultaneously placing pressure on a distant acupoint for each body region.

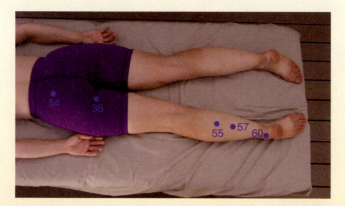

FIGURE 17.18

The Location of Acupoints for the Simple Point Prescription to Treat the Posterior Lower Leg

TABLE 17.15	Simple Point Prescription for the Posterior Lower Leg	
Body Region	Local Acupoints	Distant Acupoints
Posterior lower leg	UB 55—treats superior lower leg	UB 54, UB 36
	UB 57—treats lower leg	
	UB 60—treats ankle	

CLOSE
Repeat the warm-up sequence to close the area.

The Plantar Surface of the Foot

You will need to rotate the foot so that the plantar surface is up. This will allow better access to this area.

☑ Review the muscles and channels of the foot (Table 17.14 and Figure 17.17).

☑ Review the traditional acupoints (Chapter 14).

☑ Choose a contact point for the foot (Table 17.2).

WARM-UP

1. Breathe out and apply pressure to the heel of the foot for 3 counts, then release the pressure.

2. Move along the plantar surface just inferior to your last area of pressure. Breathe out and apply pressure for 3 counts, then release the pressure.

3. Continue breathing out and applying pressure for 3 seconds to successively more inferior acupoints along the plantar surface until you reach the toes.

4. Breathe out and apply a gentle pressure to each toe for 3 seconds, then release the pressure.

TREAT THE SPECIFIC ACUPOINTS (CHOOSE ONE OF THE FOLLOWING APPROACHES)

- Treat all active Ashi and traditional acupoints located during assessment of the area. Include the classically effective acupoints for the Urinary Bladder channel: 10, 40, 60.
- Use the simple point prescription to treat the foot (see Figure 17.19 ■ and Table 17.16 ■). Choose one or more of the recommended local acupoints and place pressure on it while simultaneously placing pressure on a distant acupoint for each body region.

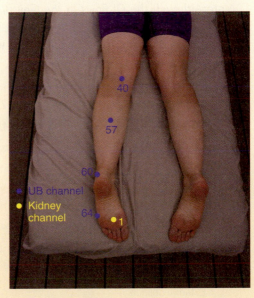

FIGURE 17.19

The Location of Acupoints for the Simple Point Prescription to Treat the Foot

TABLE 17.16	Simple Point Prescription for the Plantar Surface of the Foot	
Body Region	**Local Acupoints**	**Distant Acupoints**
Plantar and lateral surface of foot	K 1—treats plantar surface UB 60—treats heel UB 64—treats lateral foot and toes	UB 57, UB 40

CLOSE

Repeat the warm-up sequence to close the area.

The Lateral Leg, Hip, and Torso

The lateral leg contains the Gall Bladder channel, which runs along the sides of the body and on to the lateral head. This portion of the protocol will address that channel individually. Assist the client in slightly raising the knee and bending out at the hip. This will place the leg into a "frog leg" position, which gives access to the lateral leg and hip (see Figure 17.20 ■).

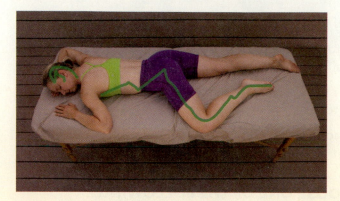

FIGURE 17.20

The Location of the Gall Bladder Channel Along the Leg, Hip, and Torso

Note: Although the Qi flows in the Gall Bladder channel from head to foot, this channel can be treated starting at the foot and working toward the head. This helps maintain a smooth flow of the bodywork for this protocol. In some cases you may choose to work the channel from head to foot to maintain the integrity of the Qi flow.

- ☑ Review the muscles and channels and of the lateral leg, hip, and torso (Tables 17.10, 17.12, 17.14, 17.21, 17.23, 17.25 and Figures 17.12, 17.15, 17.17, 17.21 ■).
- ☑ Review the traditional acupoints of the channel (Chapter 14).
- ☑ Choose contact points for the lateral leg (Table 17.2).

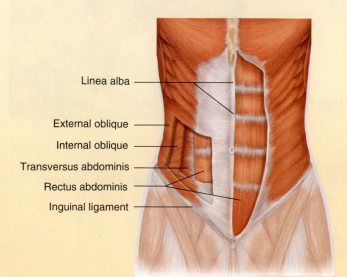

FIGURE 17.21

The Major Muscles of the Anterior Torso

Linea alba

External oblique

Internal oblique

Transversus abdominis

Rectus abdominis

Inguinal ligament

WARM-UP

1. Breathe out and apply pressure to the lateral ankle for 3 counts, then release the pressure.

2. Move along the Gall Bladder channel to the points just superior to your last area of pressure. Breathe out and apply pressure for 3 counts, then release the pressure.

3. Continue breathing out and applying pressure for 3 seconds to successively more superior acupoints along the lateral leg until you reach the hip.

4. Breathe out and apply a gentle pressure to the hip for 3 seconds, then release the pressure.

5. Continue past the hip applying pressure for 3 seconds to successively more superior points of the Gall Bladder channel until you reach the *axilla*.

6. Breathe out and apply a gentle pressure to the axilla for 3 seconds, then release the pressure.

7. Apply pressure to the side of the neck and work successively up to the side of the head and treat its lateral aspect.

TREAT THE SPECIFIC ACUPOINTS (CHOOSE ONE OF THE FOLLOWING APPROACHES)

- Treat all active Ashi and traditional acupoints located during assessment of the area. Include the classically effective acupoints for the Gall Bladder channel: 20, 21, and 30 .
- Use the simple point prescription to treat the lateral leg, hip, and torso (see Figure 17.22 ■)and Table 17.17 ■). Choose one or more of the recommended local acupoints and place pressure on it while simultaneously placing pressure on a distant acupoint for each body region.

FIGURE 17.22

The Location of Acupoints for the Simple Point Prescription to Treat the Lateral Leg, Hip, and Torso

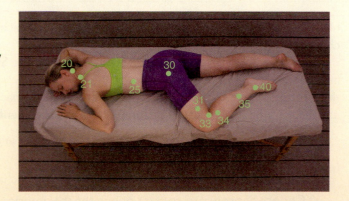

TABLE 17.17	Simple Point Prescription for the Lateral Leg, Hip, and Torso	
Body Region	**Local Acupoints**	**Distant Acupoints**
Lateral lower leg	GB 40—treats lateral ankle	GB 31, GB 30
	GB 35—treats lateral lower leg	
	GB 34—treats lateral knee	
Lateral thigh	GB 33—treats superior knee	GB 31, GB 30
	GB 31—treats lateral thigh	
	GB 30—treats hip and superior thigh	
Lateral torso	GB 25—treats lower lateral ribs	GB 30, GB 20
	GB 21—treats lateral upper ribs and shoulder	

CLOSE

Repeat the warm-up sequence to close the area.

QUICK QUIZ #33

1. A whole-body acupressure protocol: (Circle all that apply)
   a. is beneficial for overall myoskeletal health.
   b. helps to bring balance among all body systems.
   c. can be broken down for more specific treatments.
   d. includes an excellent whole-body warm-up protocol.
   e. All of the above
   f. None of the above

2. Which of the following contact points would be suitable for treating the Urinary Bladder channel along the posterior torso? (Circle all that apply)
   a. Fist/palms
   b. Elbow/forearm
   c. Heel/foot
   d. Knee/shin
   e. All of the above
   f. None of the above

3. The Urinary Bladder channel is the only channel which runs through the gastrocnemius muscle.
   a. True
   b. False

4. In most cases the Large Intestine, San Jao, and Small Intestine channels in the forearm and hand are too far apart to warm up simultaneously.
   a. True
   b. False

5. On which body part(s) would you find the classically effective acupoints of the Heart channel?
   a. Lateral elbow, upper arm, and wrist
   b. Medial elbow, upper arm, and wrist
   c. Posterior elbow, upper arm, and wrist

The Face and Anterior Neck

Have the client turn over into the supine position to finish the Yang channels and treat the last leg Yang channel.

This is the Stomach channel (see Figure 17.23 ■). The Stomach channel begins below the eye and includes most of the major muscles of the face. When working on the neck, keep your contact point on the lateral portion of the neck (over the sternocleidomastoid). This will minimize the pressure on the esophagus, which is generally uncomfortable for the client.

☑ Review the muscles and channels of the face and anterior neck (see Table 17.18 ■, Table 17.19 ■, Figure 17.24 ■, and Figure 17.25 ■).

☑ Review the traditional acupoints of the Stomach channel (Chapter 14).

☑ Choose appropriate contact points for the anterior neck and face (Table 17.2).

FIGURE 17.23

The Location of the Stomach Channel Along the Face, Neck, and Chest

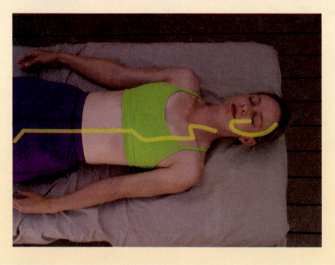

TABLE 17.18	Channels and Muscles of the Head and Facel		
Acupressure Channel	Location of Muscles	Name of Muscle	
Stomach channel	Anterior and lateral head and face	*Plantar interossei*	
		Temporalis	
		Masseter	
		Depressor labii inferioris	
		Depressor anguli oris	
		Levator anguli oris	
		Zygomaticus major	
		Zygomaticus minor	
		Buccinator	
		Risorius	
Urinary Bladder channel	Anterior and superior head and face	*Plantar interossei*	
		Levator palpebrae superioris	
		Corrugator supercilii	
		Epicranius	*occipitalis*
			frontalis
Gall Bladder channel	Lateral head and face	*Plantar interossei*	
		Temporalis	
		Masseter	
		Temporoparietalis	
		Auricularis anterior	
		Auricularis posterior	
		Auricularis superior	
San Jao channel	Lateral head and face	*Plantar interossei*	
		Temporalis	
		Masseter	
		Temporoparietalis	
		Auricularis anterior	
		Auricularis posterior	
		Auricularis superior	
Du channel	Central head and face	*Corrugator supercilii*	
		Procerus	
		Depressor septi	
		Nasalis	
		Mentalis	
Small Intestine channel	Lateral head and face	*Medial pterygoid*	
		Lateral pterygoid	
		Zygomaticus major	
		Zygomaticus minor	
Large Intestine channel		*Orbicularis oris*	
		Levator labii superioris	*Angular head*
			Infraorbital head

TABLE 17.19	Channels and Muscles of the Anterior/Lateral Neck	
Acupressure Channel	Location of Muscles	Name of Muscle
Stomach channel	Anterior neck	*Platysma*
		Digastricus
		Stylohyoid
		Mylohyoid
		Geniohyoid
		Sternohyoid
		Sternothyroid
		Thyrohyoid
		Longus colli
		Longus capitis
		Rectus capitus anterior
		Rectus capitus lateralis
		Intertransversarii anteriores
Large Intestine channel	Anterior/lateral neck	*Platysma*
		Sternocleidomastoid
		Rectus capitus anterior
		Rectus capitus lateralis
		Scalenus anterior
San Jao channel	Lateral neck	*Sternocleidomastoid*
		Scalenus medius
Small Intestine channel	Posterior/lateral	*Scalenus posterior*

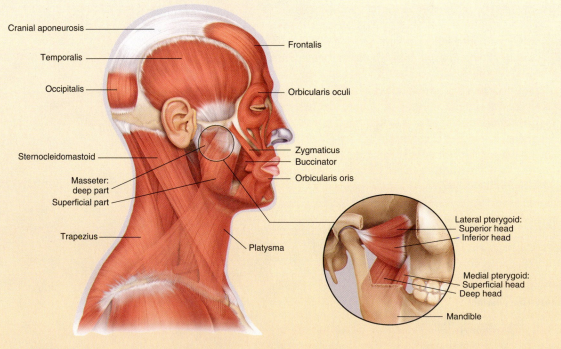

FIGURE 17.24

The Major Muscles of the Head and Face

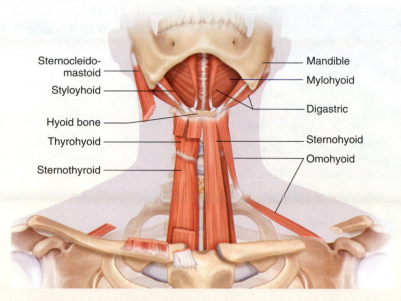

FIGURE 17.25
The Major Muscles of the Anterior Neck

WARM-UP

1. Breathe out and apply pressure to the cheek and the area just below the eye for 3 counts, then release the pressure.

2. Move along the Stomach channel to the points just inferior to your last area of pressure. Breathe out and apply pressure for 3 counts, then release the pressure.

3. Continue breathing out and applying pressure for 3 seconds to successively more inferior acupoints along the face until you reach the anterior neck.

4. Breathe out and apply a gentle pressure to the anterior neck for 3 seconds, then release the pressure.

5. Continue breathing out and applying pressure for 3 seconds to successively more inferior acupoints along the neck until you reach the clavicle.

6. Breathe out and apply a gentle pressure to the clavicle for 3 seconds, then release the pressure.

TREAT THE SPECIFIC ACUPOINTS (CHOOSE ONE OF THE FOLLOWING APPROACHES)

- Treat all active Ashi and traditional acupoints located during assessment of the area. Include the classically effective acupoints for the Stomach channel: 9, 36, and 41.
- Use the simple point prescription to treat the face and neck (see Figure 17.26 ■ and Table 17.20 ■). Choose one or more of the recommended local acupoints and place pressure on it while simultaneously placing pressure on a distant acupoint for each body region.

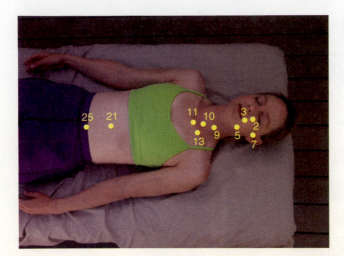

FIGURE 17.26

The Location of Acupoints for the Simple Point Prescription to Treat the Head, Face, and Anterior Neck

TABLE 17.20	Simple Point Prescription for the Face and Anterior Neck	
Body Region	Local Acupoints	Distant Acupoints
Face	ST 2—treats inferior eye and upper sinuses	ST 13, ST 9
	ST 3—treats superior/lateral mouth (upper jaw)	
	ST 5—treats lower jaw and masseter	
	ST 7—treats temporomandibular joint	
Anterior Neck	ST 9—treats superior neck	ST 25, ST 21
	ST 10—treats middle neck	
	ST 11—treats inferior neck	

CLOSE

Repeat the warm-up sequence to close the area.

The Anterior Chest and Torso

Here we are continuing to work the Stomach channel along the chest and abdominal region. The rib area is often sensitive and/or ticklish. Use a broad contact point to help minimize this. When working on female clients, just work superior and inferior to the breasts.

☑ Review the muscles and channels of the anterior torso (see Table 17.21 ■ and Figure 17.21).

☑ Review the traditional acupoints (Chapter 14).

☑ Choose an appropriate contact point for the anterior chest and torso (Table 17.2).

TABLE 17.21	Channels and Muscles of the Anterior/Lateral Torso (Abdomen)	
Stomach channel	Anterior torso	*Obliquus externus abdominis*
		Rectus abdominis
		Intercostales externi
		Intercostales interni
		Subcostales
		Diaphragm
		Transverses abdominis
Gall Bladder channel	Lateral torso	*Obliquus externus abdominis*
		Intercostales externi
		Obliquus internus
		Intercostales interni
		Subcostales
		Diaphragm
		Transverses abdominis

WARM-UP

1. Breathe out and apply pressure to the points on the upper chest for 3 counts, then release the pressure.

2. Move along the Stomach channel to the points just inferior to your last area of pressure (i.e., the next few acupoints). Breathe out and apply pressure for 3 counts, then release the pressure.

3. Continue breathing out and applying pressure for 3 seconds to successively more inferior acupoints along the anterior torso until you reach the anterior hip.

4. Breathe out and apply a gentle pressure to the anterior hip for 3 seconds, then release the pressure.

TREAT THE SPECIFIC ACUPOINTS (CHOOSE ONE OF THE FOLLOWING APPROACHES)

- Treat all active Ashi and traditional acupoints located during assessment of the area. Include the classically effective acupoints for the Stomach channel: 9, 36, and 41.
- Use the simple point prescription to treat the anterior chest and torso (see Figure 17.27 ■ and Table 17.22 ■). Choose one or more of the recommended local acupoints and place pressure on it while simultaneously placing pressure on a distant acupoint for each body region.

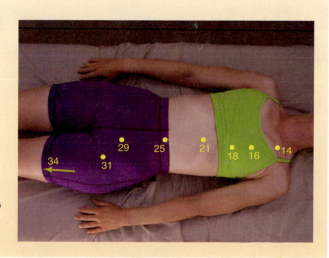

FIGURE 17.27

The Location of Acupoints for the Simple Point Prescription to Treat the Anterior Torso (Arrow Indicates Location of Acupoint on the Distal Thigh)

TABLE 17.22	Simple Point Prescription for the Anterior Chest and Torso	
Body Region	Local Acupoints	Distant Acupoints
Anterior chest	ST 14—treats superior chest ST 16—treats middle chest ST 18—treats inferior chest	ST 29, ST 25
Anterior abdomen	ST 21—treats superior abdomen ST 25—treats middle abdomen ST 29—treats inferior abdomen	ST 34, ST 31

CLOSE
Repeat the warm-up sequence to close the area.

The Anterior/Lateral Hip and Thigh

This portion of the protocol continues along the Stomach channel to treat the lateral sweep of the quadriceps muscle (see Figure 17.28 ■).

☑ Review the muscles and channels of the anterior/lateral hip and thigh (see Table 17.23 ■ and Figure 17.29 ■).

☑ Review the traditional acupoints of the Stomach channel (Chapter 14).

☑ Choose a contact point for the anterior/lateral hip and thigh (Table 17.2).

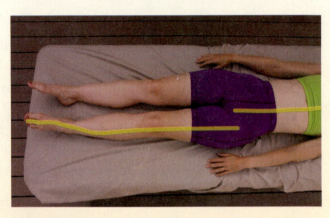

FIGURE 17.28

The Location of the Stomach Channel on the Thigh and Hip

TABLE 17.23	Channels and Muscles of the Anterior/Lateral Hip and Thigh		
Acupressure Channel	Location of Muscles	Name of Muscle	
Stomach channel	Anterior/lateral hip and thigh	*Tensor fascia latae*	
		Quadriceps femorus	*rectus femorus* *vastus lateralis* *vastus intermedius*
		Psoas major	
		Iliacus	
Gall Bladder channel	Lateral hip and thigh	*Quadriceps femorus*	*vastus lateralis*
		Iliacus	
		Tensor fascia latae	

FIGURE 17.29

The Major Muscles of the Anterior Hip and Thigh

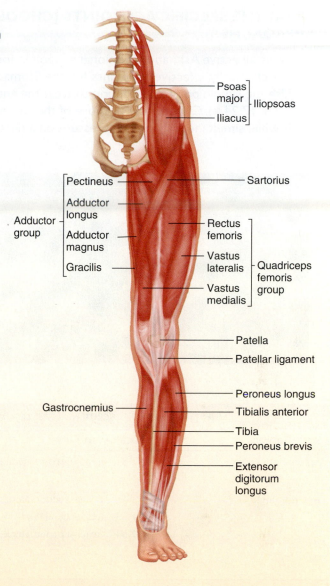

Psoas major ⎤
Iliacus ⎦ Iliopsoas

Pectineus

Adductor longus

Adductor group

Adductor magnus

Gracilis

Sartorius

Rectus femoris

Vastus lateralis

Vastus medialis

Quadriceps femoris group

Patella

Patellar ligament

Peroneus longus

Gastrocnemius

Tibialis anterior

Tibia

Peroneus brevis

Extensor digitorum longus

WARM-UP

1. Breathe out and apply pressure to the Stomach channel at the anterior/lateral hip for 3 counts, then release the pressure.

2. Move along the Stomach channel to the points just inferior to your last area of pressure (i.e., the next few acupoints). Breathe out and apply pressure for 3 counts, then release the pressure.

3. Continue breathing out and applying pressure for 3 seconds to successively more inferior acupoints along the upper leg until you reach the knee.

4. Breathe out and apply a gentle pressure to the knee for 3 seconds, then release.

TREAT THE SPECIFIC ACUPOINTS (CHOOSE ONE OF THE FOLLOWING APPROACHES)

- Treat all active Ashi and traditional acupoints located during assessment of the area. Include the classically effective acupoints for the Stomach channel: 9, 36, and 41.
- Use the simple point prescription to treat the anterior/lateral hip and thigh (see Figure 17.30 ■ and Table 17.24 ■). Choose one or more of the recommended local acupoints and place pressure on it while simultaneously placing pressure on a distant acupoint for each body region.

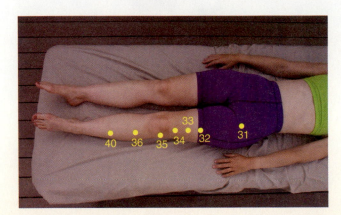

FIGURE 17.30

The Location of Acupoints for the Simple Point Prescription to Treat the Anterior/Lateral Hip and Thigh

TABLE 17.24	Simple Point Prescription for the Anterior/Lateral Hip and Thigh	
Body Region	Local Acupoints	Distant Acupoints
Anterior hip	ST 31—treats anterior/lateral hip	ST 36, ST 35
Anterior thigh	ST 32—treats superior/lateral thigh ST 33—treats lateral thigh ST 34—treats superior/lateral knee	ST 40, ST 36

CLOSE

Repeat the warm-up sequence to close the area.

The Anterior/Lateral Lower Leg

- ☑ Review the muscles and channels of the anterior/lateral lower leg (see Table 17.25 ■ and Figure 17.31 ■).
- ☑ Review the traditional acupoints of Stomach channel (Chapter 14).
- ☑ Choose a contact point for the anterior/lateral lower leg (Table 17.2).

TABLE 17.25	Channels and Muscles of the Anterior/Lateral Lower Leg and Foot	
Acupressure Channel	Location of Muscles	Name of Muscle
Stomach channel	Anterior aspect of lower leg	*Tibialis anterior*
		Peroneus longus
		Extensor digitorum brevis
		Extensor hallicus longus
		Peroneus brevis
		Peroneus tertius
		Extensor digitorum longus
Gall Bladder channel	Lateral aspect of lower leg	*Peroneus longus*
		Peroneus brevis
		Peroneus tertius

FIGURE 17.31

The Major Muscles of the Anterior/Lateral Lower Leg and Foot

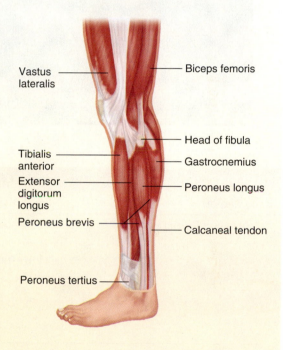

Vastus lateralis

Biceps femoris

Head of fibula

Tibialis anterior

Gastrocnemius

Extensor digitorum longus

Peroneus longus

Peroneus brevis

Calcaneal tendon

Peroneus tertius

WARM-UP

1. Breathe out and apply pressure to the Stomach channel at the anterior/lateral lower leg (just below the knee) for 3 counts, then release the pressure.

2. Move along the Stomach channel to the points just inferior to your last area of pressure (i.e., the next few acupoints). Breathe out and apply pressure for 3 counts, then release the pressure.

3. Continue breathing out and applying pressure for 3 seconds to successively more inferior acupoints along the shin until you reach the top of the foot.

4. Breathe out and apply a gentle pressure to the top of the foot for 3 seconds, then release.

TREAT THE SPECIFIC ACUPOINTS (CHOOSE ONE OF THE FOLLOWING APPROACHES)

- Treat all active Ashi and traditional acupoints located during assessment of the area. Include the classically effective acupoints for Stomach channel: 9, 36, and 41.
- Use the simple point prescription to treat the anterior lateral lower leg (see Figure 17.32 ■ and Table 17.26 ■). Choose one or more of the recommended local acupoints and place pressure on it while simultaneously placing pressure on a distant acupoint for each body region.

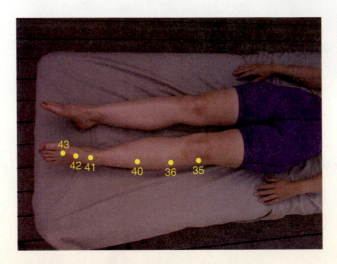

FIGURE 17.32

The Location of Acupoints for the Simple Point Prescription to Treat the Anterior/ Lateral Lower Leg and Foot

TABLE 17.26	Simple Point Prescription for the Anterior/Lateral Lower Leg	
Body Region	Local Acupoints	Distant Acupoints
Anterior lower leg and ankle	ST 36—treats inferior knee and shin ST 40—treats lower leg ST 41—treats anterior ankle	ST 42, ST 41
Anterior foot	ST 42—treats center foot (metatarsals) ST 43—treats first and second toes	ST 35, ST 36

CLOSE

Repeat the warm-up sequence to close the area.

THE THREE YIN CHANNELS OF THE LEG

The Yin channels include the anterior muscles and some of the softer and more sensitive areas of the body. There are three Yin channels that flow from the feet to the chest (see Figure 17.33 ■).

- Spleen channel
- Liver channel
- Kidney channel

FIGURE 17.33

The Three Yin Channels of the Leg/Foot: the Spleen Channel (Yellow), the Liver Channel (Green), and the Kidney Channel (Blue)

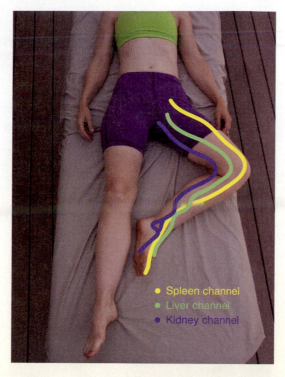

● Spleen channel
● Liver channel
● Kidney channel

The Anterior/Medial Lower Leg

Assist the client in slightly raising the knee and bending out at the hip. This will place the leg into a "frog leg" position, which gives access to the medial leg and hip (see Figure 17.33). The medial leg contains all three Yin channels, and they are very close together so they are most often warmed up simultaneously.

☑ Review the muscles and channels of the anterior/medial lower leg (see Table 17.27 ■ and Figure 17.31).

☑ Review the traditional acupoints of each channel (Chapter 14).

☑ Choose contact points suitable for the anterior/medial lower leg (Table 17.2).

TABLE 17.27	Channels and Muscles of the Anterior and Medial Lower Leg and Foot	
Acupressure Channel	Location of Muscles	Name of Muscle
Spleen channel	Anterior/medial lower leg and foot	*Abductor hallucis*
		Gastrocnemius
		Soleus
Liver channel	Middle/medial lower leg and foot	*Gastrocnemius*
		Soleus
Kidney channel	Posterior/medial lower leg and foot	*Flexor hallucis longus*
		Flexor digitorum longus
		Flexor hallucis brevis
		Gastrocnemius
		Soleus

WARM-UP

1. Breathe out and apply pressure to the *instep* of the foot for 3 counts, then release the pressure.

2. Move along the channels to the medial ankle. Breathe out and apply pressure for 3 counts, then release the pressure.

3. Continue breathing out and applying pressure for 3 seconds to successively more superior acupoints along the medial lower leg until you reach the knee.

4. Breathe out and apply a gentle pressure to the medial knee for 3 seconds, then release.

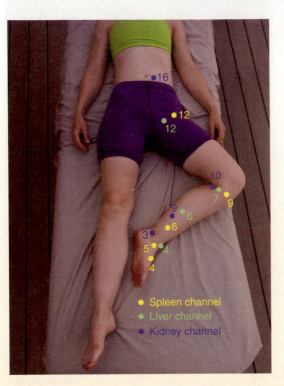

● Spleen channel
● Liver channel
● Kidney channel

TREAT THE SPECIFIC ACUPOINTS (CHOOSE ONE OF THE FOLLOWING APPROACHES)

- Treat all active Ashi and traditional acupoints located during assessment of the area. Include the classically effective acupoints for each channel.
  ○ Spleen channel: 6, 9, 10
  ○ Liver channel: 3, 8, 13
  ○ Kidney channel: 1, 3, 10
- Use the simple point prescription to treat the anterior/medial lower leg (see Figure 17.34 ■ and Table 17.28 ■). Choose one or more of the recommended local acupoints and place pressure on it while simultaneously placing pressure on a distant acupoint for each body region.

FIGURE 17.34

The Location of Acupoints for the Simple Point Prescription to Treat the Anterior/Medial Lower Leg

TABLE 17.28	Simple Point Prescription for the Anterior/Medial Lower Leg	
Body Region	Local Acupoints	Distant Acupoints
Anterior/medial lower leg	SP 5—treats anterior/medial ankle SP 6—treats anterior/medial lower leg SP 9—treats anterior medial/inferior knee	SP 4, SP 12
Middle/medial lower leg	LV 4—treats medial ankle LV 6—treats lower leg LV 7—treats inferior knee	LV 4, LV 12
Posterior/medial lower leg	K 3—treats posterior/medial ankle K 9—treats posterior/medial lower leg K 10—treats posterior medial knee	K 3, K 16

CLOSE

Repeat the warm-up sequence to close the area.

The Anterior/Medial Thigh

Often the three Yin channels in this portion of the leg are close enough to warm up simultaneously. In the case of larger clients, one or more of these channels may be warmed up individually. The anterior/medial thigh leg can be quite sensitive, so it is important to be careful and remember to communicate with the client.

☑ Review the muscles and channels of the anterior/medial thigh (see Table 17.29 ■ and Figure 17.29).

☑ Review the traditional acupoints of each channel (Chapter 14).

☑ Choose contact points suitable for the anterior/medial thigh (Table 17.2).

TABLE 17.29	Channels and Muscles of the Anterior and Medial Hip and Thigh	
Acupressure Channel	Location of Muscles	Name of Muscle
Spleen channel	Anterior/medial aspect of thigh	Sartorius
		Quadriceps femoris vastus medialis
		Psoas major
		Iliacus
		Pectineus
Liver channel	Medial aspect of thigh	Gracilis
		Adductor longus
		Adductor magnus
		Pectineus
		Adductor brevis
Kidney channel	Posterior/medial aspect of thigh	Gracilis
		Adductor longus
		Adductor magnus
		Psoas major
		Adductor brevis

WARM-UP

1. Breathe out and apply pressure to the channels at the anterior medial thigh (just superior to the knee) for 3 counts, then release the pressure.

2. Move along the channels to the points just superior to your last area of pressure. Breathe out and apply pressure for 3 counts, then release the pressure.

3. Continue breathing out and applying pressure for 3 seconds to successively more superior acupoints along the upper leg until you reach the groin.

4. Breathe out and apply a gentle pressure to the lower groin for 3 seconds, then release.

TREAT THE SPECIFIC ACUPOINTS (CHOOSE ONE OF THE FOLLOWING APPROACHES)

- Treat all active Ashi and traditional acupoints located during assessment of the area. Include the classically effective acupoints for each channel.
  - Spleen channel: 6, 9, 10
  - Liver channel: 3, 8, 13
  - Kidney channel: 1, 3, 10
- Use the simple point prescription to treat the anterior/medial thigh (see Figure 17.35 ■ and Table 17.30 ■). Choose one or more of the recommended local acupoints and place pressure on it while simultaneously placing pressure on a distant acupoint for each body region.

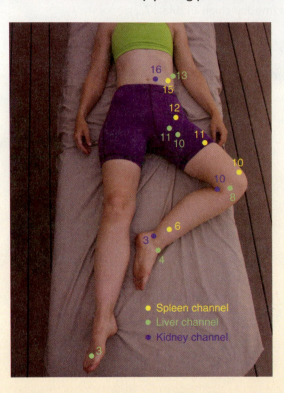

FIGURE 17.35

The Location of Acupoints for the Simple Point Prescription to Treat the Anterior Medial Thigh

TABLE 17.30	Simple Point Prescription for the Anterior/Medial Thigh	
Body Region	Local Acupoints	Distant Acupoints
Anterior/medial thigh	SP 10—treats anterior/medial superior knee SP 11—treats anterior/medial thigh SP 12—treats anterior/medial superior thigh (inguinal area)	SP 15, SP 6
Center/medial thigh	LV 8—treats the medial knee LV 10—treats medial thigh LV 11—treats medial superior thigh	LV 13, LV 4
Posterior/medial thigh	K 10—treats entire length of posterior/medial thigh	K 16, K 3

CLOSE

Repeat the warm-up sequence to close the area.

The Anterior Torso

Most of the time, the three Yin channels are close together in the anterior torso, so they are warmed up simultaneously (see Figure 17.36 ■). In cases where the client is larger and you are unable to cover them simultaneously, you may work the channels separately.

☑ Review the muscles, channels, and acupoints of the anterior torso (see Table 17.31 ■ and Figure 17.21).

☑ Review the traditional acupoints of each channel (Chapter 14).

☑ Choose contact points suitable for the anterior torso (Table 17.2).

FIGURE 17.36

The Three Yin Channels on the Torso: The Spleen Channel (Yellow), the Liver Channel (Green), and the Kidney Channel (Blue)

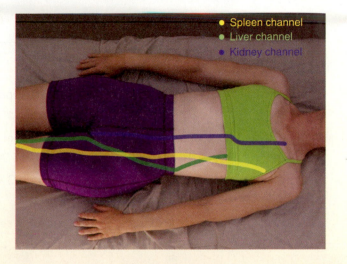

- Spleen channel
- Liver channel
- Kidney channel

TABLE 17.31	Channels and Muscles of the Anterior/Medial Torso (Abdomen)	
Acupressure Channel	Location of Muscles	Name of Muscle
Spleen channel	Anterior torso	*Obliquus externus abdominis*
		Rectus abdominis
		Intercostales externi
		Obliquus internus
		Intercostales interni
		Subcostales
		Diaphragm
		Transverses abdominis
		Cremaster
Kidney channel	Anterior/medial torso	*Obliquus externus abdominis*
		Rectus abdominis
		Intercostales externi
		Obliquus internus
		Intercostales interni
		Subcostales
		Transverses thoracis
		Diaphragm
		Transverses abdominis

(Continued)

TABLE 17.31	Continued	
Acupressure Channel	Location of Muscles	Name of Muscle
Liver channel	Anterior/lateral torso	*Obliquus externus abdominis*
		Rectus abdominis
		Intercostales externi
		Obliquus internus
		Intercostales interni
		Subcostales
		Diaphragm
		Transverses abdominis

WARM-UP

1. Breathe out and apply pressure to the channels superior to the pubis for 3 counts, then release the pressure.

2. Move along the channels to the acupoints just superior to your last area of pressure. Breathe out and apply pressure for 3 counts, then release the pressure.

3. Continue breathing out and applying pressure for 3 seconds to successively more superior acupoints along the torso until you reach the chest.

4. Breathe out and apply pressure to the chest for 3 seconds, then release.

TREAT THE SPECIFIC ACUPOINTS (CHOOSE ONE OF THE FOLLOWING APPROACHES)

- Treat all active Ashi and traditional acupoints located during assessment of the area. Include the classically effective acupoints for each channel.
  - Spleen channel: 6, 9, 10
  - Liver channel: 3, 8, 13
  - Kidney channel: 1, 3, 10
- Use the simple point prescription to treat the anterior torso (see Figure 17.37 ■ and Table 17.32 ■). Choose one or more of the recommended local acupoints and place pressure on it while simultaneously placing pressure on a distant acupoint for each body region.

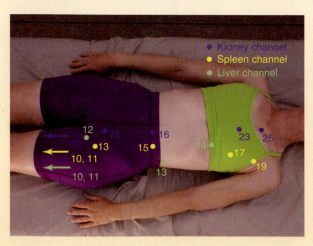

FIGURE 17.37

The Location of Acupoints for the Simple Point Prescription to Treat the Anterior Torso (Arrows Indicate the Location of Acupoints on the Distal Thigh)

TABLE 17.32	Simple Point Prescription for the Anterior Torso	
Body Region	**Local Acupoints**	**Distant Acupoints**
Anterior torso	SP 13—treats anterior lower abdomen (suprapubic area)	SP 11, SP 10
	SP 15—treats anterior abdomen	
	SP 17—treats anterior lower rib cage	
	SP 19—treats anterior upper rib cage	
Anterior /lateral torso	LV 12—treats anterior/lateral lower abdomen (suprapubic area)	LV 11, LV 10
	LV 13—treats anterior/lateral torso (end of 12th rib)	
	LV 14—treats anterior/lateral lower rib cage	
Medial torso	K 12—treats lower abdomen (suprapubic area)	K 10
	K 16—treats middle of abdomen	
	K 23—treats lower rib cage	
	K 25—treats upper rib cage	

CLOSE

Repeat the warm-up sequence to close the area.

THE THREE YIN CHANNELS OF THE ARM

There are three Yin channels that flow from the chest to the hands (see Figure 17.38 ■).

- The Heart channel
- The Pericardium channel
- The Lung channel

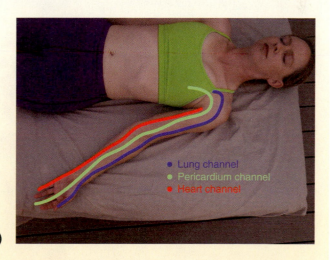

FIGURE 17.38

The Three Yin Channels of the Arm/Hand: The Heart Channel (Red), the Pericardium Channel (Green), and the Lung Channel (Blue)

The Anterior Chest and Upper Arm

Most of the time, the three Yin channels are close together in the chest and upper arm so they are warmed up simultaneously. In cases where the client is larger and you are unable to cover them simultaneously, you may work the channels separately starting each at the chest and working along its course until you reach the elbow.

☑ Review the muscles, channels, and acupoints of the anterior chest and upper arm (see Table 17.33 ■ and Figures 17.39 ■ and 17.41).

☑ Review the traditional acupoints of each channel (Chapter 14).

☑ Choose contact points suitable for the anterior chest and upper arm (Table 17.2).

TABLE 17.33   Channels and Muscles of the Anterior Shoulder and Upper Arm

Acupressure Channel	Location of Muscles	Name of Muscle
Lung channel	Anterior/lateral chest and upper arm	*Deltoid*
		Biceps brachii
		Pectoralis minor
		Pectoralis major
Pericardium channel	Anterior chest and upper arm	*Pectoralis major*
		Biceps brachii
		Pectoralis minor
Heart channel	Anterior and medial chest and upper arm	*Coracobrachialis*
		Biceps brachii
Kidney channel	Anterior medial chest	*Pectoralis major*
		Subclavius
Stomach channel	Anterior chest	*Pectoralis major*
		Subclavius
Spleen channel	Anterior/lateral chest	*Pectoralis major*

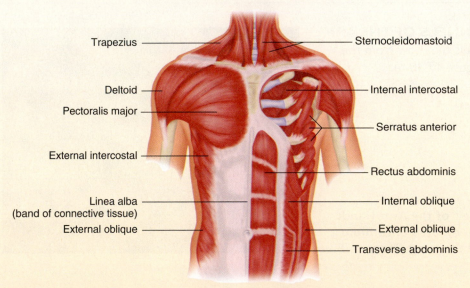

FIGURE 17.39

The Major Muscles of the Anterior Chest and Upper Arm

Trapezius
Sternocleidomastoid
Deltoid
Internal intercostal
Pectoralis major
Serratus anterior
External intercostal
Rectus abdominis
Linea alba (band of connective tissue)
Internal oblique
External oblique
External oblique
Transverse abdominis

WARM-UP

1. Breathe out and apply pressure just proximal to the axilla on the anterior chest for 3 counts, then release the pressure.

2. Move along the channels just distal to your last area of pressure (i.e., the next few acupoints). Breathe out and apply pressure for 3 counts, then release the pressure.

3. Continue breathing out and applying pressure for 3 seconds to successively more distal acupoints along the channels of the upper arm until you reach the elbow.

4. Breathe out and apply a gentle pressure to the elbow for 3 seconds, then release the pressure.

TREAT THE SPECIFIC ACUPOINTS (CHOOSE ONE OF THE FOLLOWING APPROACHES)

- Treat all active Ashi and traditional acupoints located during assessment of the area. Include the classically effective acupoints for each channel.
  - Lung channel: 1, 5, 7
  - Pericardium channel: 2, 3, 6
  - Heart channel: 2, 3, 7
- Use the simple point prescription to treat the chest and upper arm (see Figure 17.40 ■ and Table 17.34 ■). Choose one or more of the recommended local acupoints and place pressure on it while simultaneously placing pressure on a distant acupoint for each body region.

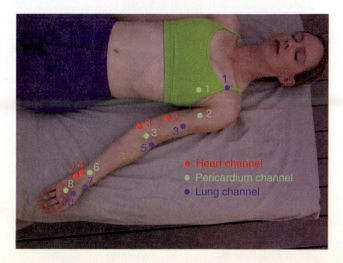

FIGURE 17.40

The Location of Acupoints for the Simple Point Prescription to Treat the Anterior Chest and Upper Arm

TABLE 17.34	Simple Point Prescription for the Anterior Chest and Upper Arm	
Body Region	**Local Acupoints**	**Distant Acupoints**
Anterior/superior chest and upper arm	L 1—treats superior lateral chest L 3—treats anterior/lateral biceps L 5—treats anterior/lateral elbow	L 10, L 7
Anterior chest and center of upper arm	P 1—treats inferior lateral chest P 2—treats proximal upper arm P 3—treats middle of elbow	P 8, P 6
Anterior/inferior chest and upper arm	H 2—treats proximal medial upper arm H 3—treats anterior/medial elbow	H 7, H 4

CLOSE

Repeat the warm-up sequence to close the area.

The Anterior Forearm and Hand

In the hand and forearm the three Yin arm channels are close together, so they are most often warmed up simultaneously.

- ☑ Review the muscles, channels, and acupoints of the forearm and hand (see Table 17.35 ■ and Figure 17.41 ■).
- ☑ Review the traditional acupoints of each channel (Chapter 14).
- ☑ Choose contact points that are appropriate for the client's forearm and hand (Table 17.2).

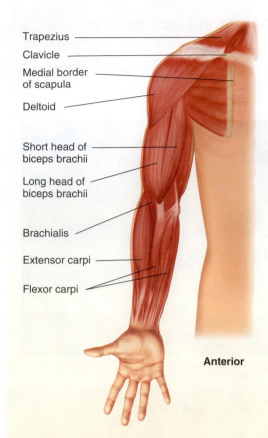

Trapezius

Clavicle

Medial border of scapula

Deltoid

Short head of biceps brachii

Long head of biceps brachii

Brachialis

Extensor carpi

Flexor carpi

Anterior

FIGURE 17.41

The Major Muscles of the Anterior Forearm and Hand

TABLE 17.35	Channels and Muscles of the Anterior and Medial Forearm and Hand	
Acupressure Channel	Location of Muscles	Name of Muscle
Heart channel	Anterior/medial forearm and hand	*Pronator teres*
		Flexor carpi ulnaris
		Palmaris longus
		Palmaris brevis
		Flexor digitorum profundus
		Abductor digiti minimi
		Flexor digiti minimi brevis
		Opponens digiti minimi
		Pronator quadratus
		Palmar interossei
		Lumbricales
Pericardium channel	Anterior/middle forearm and hand	*Pronator teres*
		Flexor carpi radialis
		Palmaris brevis
		Flexor digitorum superficialis
		Flexor digitorum profundus
		Pronator quadratus
		Palmar interossei
		Lumbricales

TABLE 17.35   **Continued**

Acupressure Channel	Location of Muscles	Name of Muscle
Lung channel	Anterior/lateral forearm and hand	*Abductor pollicis brevis*
		Flexor pollicis brevis
		Opponens pollicis
		Adductor pollicis
		Flexor pollicis longus
		Pronator quadratus
		Palmar interossei
		Lumbricules
		Flexor carpi radialis

WARM-UP

1. Take a deep breath, and while breathing out begin to apply pressure to the area just distal to the elbow. Hold firm pressure for 3 counts, then release the pressure.

2. Move to the area of the forearm that is just distal to where you first applied pressure (i.e., the next few acupoints). Breathe out and apply pressure for 3 counts, then release the pressure.

3. Move along the channels just distal to your last area of pressure (i.e., the next few acupoints). Breathe out and apply pressure for 3 counts, then release the pressure.

4. Continue breathing out and applying pressure for 3 seconds to successively more distal acupoints along the channels of the forearm until you reach the hand.

5. Breathe out and apply pressure to the hand for 3 counts, then release the pressure.

TREAT THE SPECIFIC ACUPOINTS (CHOOSE ONE OF THE FOLLOWING APPROACHES)

• Treat all active Ashi and traditional acupoints located during assessment of the area. Include the classically effective acupoints for each channel.
  ◦ Lung channel: 1, 5, 7
  ◦ Pericardium channel: 2, 3, 6
  ◦ Heart channel: 2, 3, 7

• Use the simple point prescription to treat the forearm (see Figure 17.42 ■ and Table 17.36 ■). Choose one or more of the recommended local acupoints and place pressure on it while simultaneously placing pressure on a distant acupoint for each body region.

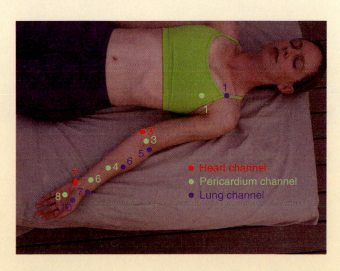

FIGURE 17.42

The Location of Acupoints for the Simple Point Prescription to Treat the Anterior Forearm and Hand

TABLE 17.36	Simple Point Prescription for the Anterior Forearm and Hand	
Body Region	**Local Acupoints**	**Distant Acupoints**
Anterior/lateral forearm and hand	L 6—treats middle of anterior-lateral forearm L 7—treats lateral wrist L 10—treats anterior base of the thumb	L 5, L 1
Anterior/center forearm and hand	P 4—treats middle of forearm P 6—treats distal forearm/wrist P 8—treats center of palm/fingers	P 3, P 1
Anterior/medial forearm and hand	H 7—treats medial wrist H 8—treats medial palm and fingers	H 2, H 3

CLOSE

Repeat the warm-up sequence to close the area.

QUICK QUIZ #34

1. The elbow is the best contact point to use on the point ST 2.
   a. True
   b. False

2. Which of the following contact points are best suited to use in the rib area? (Circle all that apply)
   a. Thumb
   b. Elbow
   c. Fist
   d. Palm
   e. All of the above
   f. None of the above

3. The Yin leg channels include: (Circle all that apply)
   a. Heart channel
   b. Kidney channel

   c. Spleen channel
   d. Stomach channel
   e. Liver channel

4. Which points would be suitable to treat when working the Stomach channel along the anterior lower leg on a client with a primary complaint in the tibialis anterior?
   a. ST 36 & ST 41
   b. ST 36 & ST 35
   c. ST 43 & ST 35
   d. ST 9
   e. All of the above
   f. None of the above

HOLISTIC CONNECTION

Psychiatrist and neurologist Dr. Johannes Schultz developed a complementary modality called *autogenic therapy. Autogenic* means "self-originating." This therapy is similar to meditation, self-hypnosis, and biofeedback. With the use of visual imagery and body awareness-focusing techniques, a client is able to achieve deep relaxation and "passive concentration."

Autogenic therapy is thought to enhance healing and recuperation. Some evidence suggests that it may be beneficial for anxiety, stress, athletic performance, and phantom limb pain (Aetna InteliHealth Inc., 1996–2010). Explore incorporating autogenic therapy or other relaxation techniques into your massage protocols to further the benefits of your massage.

SUMMARY

When applying your acupressure protocol, remember the basic principles of this approach. The selection of acupoints to be treated should be laid out based on the assessment, the flow of Qi, etc. Since this can be complex, feel free to prepare a reminder or keep your SOAP notes close by for reference.

Be aware of your body mechanics. If you will be treating the client on a floor mat, your body mechanics should be adjusted accordingly. Always use proper leverage to provide the correct pressure and to maintain your energy and posture.

Determine ahead of time if you will need any additional tools or supplies, such as an extra blanket, bolsters, a heat source, etc. Adjust any furniture or objects in the room to accommodate for techniques you may be performing on a floor mat.

Remember to focus your thoughts and your Qi and help the client to do so as well. Communicate with the client throughout the protocol.

As you become more practiced and comfortable with applying acupressure, you will develop more creative protocols. You may combine the acupressure protocols for any body part or set of body parts with other methods, such as deep tissue therapy, neuromuscular therapy, myofascial therapy, and more.

DISCUSSION QUESTIONS

1. Explain which contact points and which acupoints you might choose for treating the posterior torso in a client who is very thin and fairly sensitive to deep pressure.

2. The warm up sequences may be used together, in order, as a whole body treatment. How does this differ from a whole body Swedish massage?

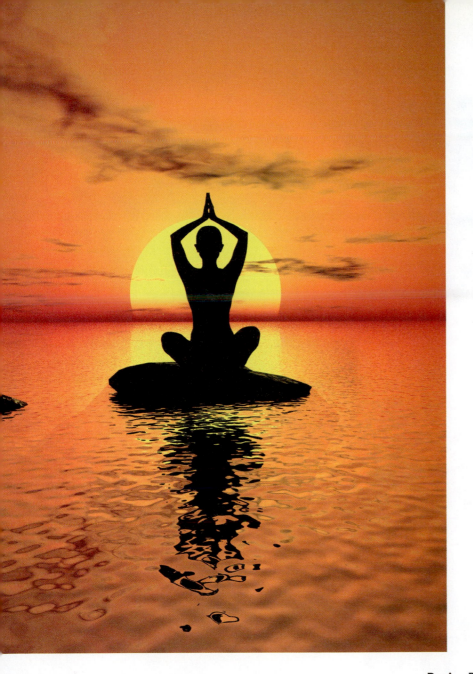

PART

6

The Holistic Approach

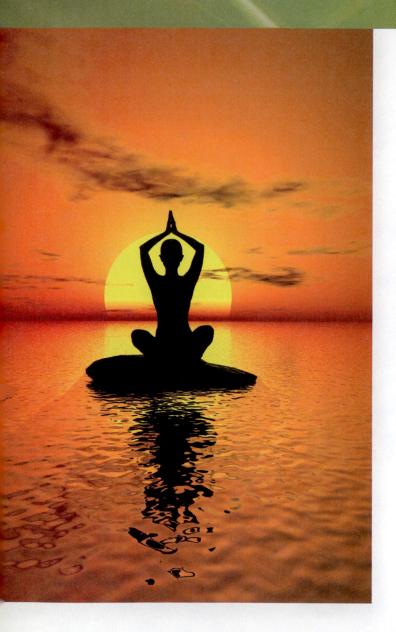

18 Putting It All Together

CHAPTER HIGHLIGHTS

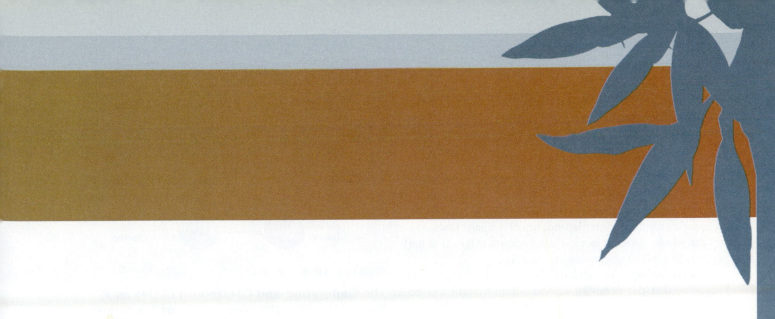

 ## CHAPTER OBJECTIVES

- Understand principles of holism and holistic bodywork
- Understand how the four therapeutic approaches fit together
- Explore a framework for combining the techniques
- Practice creating holistic treatment plans

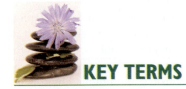 ## KEY TERMS

A BRIEF HISTORY OF HOLISM

As early as the fourth century BCE, Aristotle discussed the notion that "the whole is greater than the sum of its parts." The term **holism** was coined by J. C. Smuts, a South African statesman and general, in 1926. The word *holism* comes from the Greek word *holos* meaning "whole" or "complete." Holism is a worldview or philosophical perspective that emphasizes the understanding of whole systems. A holistic perspective is concerned with the interdependence of the parts that make up the whole. The perspective also acknowledges that the system as a whole affects each of its parts.

A **reductionist,** or **mechanistic,** viewpoint, by contrast, suggests that the behavior of the whole system can be explained solely by the behavior of its parts. With more recent discoveries in quantum physics and other fields of study, the mechanistic scientific view has begun to seem limited. The holistic view has emerged as a valuable and inclusive way of explaining the nature of things.

The philosophy of holism is the basis behind the holistic approach in health and medicine (Benking & van Meurs, 1997). A holistic medical viewpoint recognizes that the whole body is made from a collection of parts (i.e., tissues, organs, cells, etc.), and it is the interaction and cooperation of the parts that contribute to the behavior of the whole body. However, it is also understood that the body as a whole influences each of its parts. The parts cannot function by themselves. They need the information from the whole system in order to perform their individual functions correctly. In other words, the whole determines the behavior of the parts and at the same time is dependent upon each part and the interactions between them.

This view is akin to the traditional Chinese medical concepts of Yin/Yang and the five elements. These two concepts exemplify holistic theory. Yin/Yang represent the dynamic interaction and interdependence of the two halves of a whole. The whole does not exist without each half, and each half cannot exist without the whole. The five elements represent holistic theory by explaining the interactions of the many aspects of nature and the body through the generating and controlling cycles. These cycles show how all aspects of life

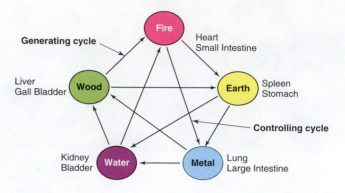

FIGURE 18.1

The Generating and Controlling Cycles as Part of the Five Element Theory of Traditional Chinese Medicine

operate within a continuous circle of interaction (see Figure 18.1 ■). Each element generates and controls the others while they all contribute to the whole.

A HOLISTIC APPROACH TO BODYWORK

A holistic approach to bodywork includes a few different levels of understanding. First, it means being inclusive of a variety of modalities and techniques. A holistic approach to bodywork also means taking a holistic view of our individual clients. It is important to consider the unique emotional, cultural, spiritual, and physical attributes that make each client whole. Finally we must take a holistic view of each client's body. This means seeing the body of each individual client as a whole functioning system with intricately connected parts working in unison.

Understanding that many factors contribute to a client's particular condition is an important element of holistic thinking. Then we must consider the impact these factors have on the musculoskeletal system. The four therapeutic approaches presented in this book provide a solid foundation for understanding the structure and function of the body as well as the impact pathology has on the musculoskeletal system. Each approach includes techniques that analyze pathology from a certain viewpoint. Basically, the four therapeutic approaches represent different sides of a balanced and well-rounded knowledge of the body. When combined, they create the whole picture (see Figure 18.2 ■). Together, the deep tissue, neuromuscular, myofascial, and acupressure approaches provide a diverse set of tools for addressing pathology. Bringing these theories and strategies together will allow you to combine techniques to address the whole musculoskeletal system.

How the Four Therapeutic Approaches Complement Each Other

Each of the four therapeutic approaches has a unique history and distinct tradition. Each has a different focus and a clear perspective about the nature of and causes of pathology.

DID YOU KNOW

According to holistic thought, a whole system is like a pixilated picture. When looking up close, you can see that each pixel occupies its own space and helps to define the whole. When you step back to observe the whole image, each pixel is no longer distinct, but the whole image is complete. The view of the whole image brings a new definition to each of its parts.

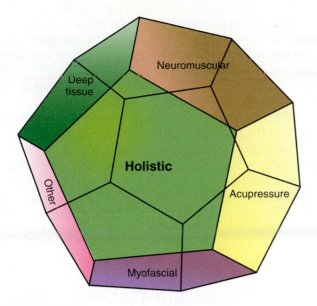

FIGURE 18.2

The Four Major Therapeutic Approaches Compose Different Sides of the Whole Realm of Holistic Bodywork

While the four approaches have clear differences, it is important to note how much they overlap (see Figure 18.3 ■). Each of them supports, balances, and complements the others. There are many examples throughout the text where each approach explains observations about the body and its pathology in ways that are consistent with the others. One of the most profound ways in which the approaches complement each other is in their agreement on the interconnectedness of all parts of the body.

Start by considering the channel theory of the acupressure approach. The channels are represented by lines on the skin, which identify the underlying muscles, fascia, organs, vessels, and bones. The channels follow the pathways of nerves and blood vessels as well as functional groupings of muscles, which work together to hold up and move the body.

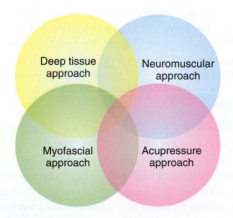

FIGURE 18.3

The Four Major Approaches Overlap in Theory and Technique

There are 12 major (Jing) acupressure channels and are all connected to each other through a series of smaller channels called the Luo. All channels and the corresponding body parts are integrated structurally and functionally through the Jing and the Luo.

Upon close examination, there is a strong parallel between the acupressure channels and the myofascial meridians, or the "anatomy trains" as described by Thomas Myers. According to Thomas Myers, the myofascial meridians represent functional groupings of muscles and fascia, which cooperate to support and move the body.

Furthermore, the myofascial system is described as a net or a web of connective tissue that runs throughout the body. All major myofascial structures are structurally and functionally connected to each other (and even to the internal organs) by smaller extensions of the fascial web. Like the Jing and the Luo of the acupressure approach, the myofascial approach also has major meridians and smaller netlike extensions.

The interconnectedness of the body is also highlighted in the deep tissue approach through the concept of compensation and the layering of muscles. The muscles are arranged so that they support and stabilize each other. This creates a series of cross layering that connects the body parts together into structural and functional groupings. This arrangement influences the entire balance of the body and explains how an imbalance in one area will affect many different areas through the process of compensation.

Neuromuscular theories help to further explain and support the concept of interconnected body systems and compensation. Pfluger's laws of symmetry, radiation, and generalization explain how pain and pathology progress through the body via the neurological structures and the pain reflex cycle. Pathology may begin in one area, but over time will affect new areas via the nerves and spinal cord. This process may continue until the whole body expresses pathology.

Here we see how the theories and perspectives of the different approaches support the theories of the others. Though each has value on its own, when combined these four approaches create a more complete picture of the physiology, pathology, and treatment of the body. The important thing to remember is that whenever you use any of the approaches to apply treatment to a particular component of the client's whole body, you will always have an effect on all of the other components. For example, as you are treating the myofascia with the torquing technique, you will simultaneously treat the nerves, vessels, and layers of muscles. No matter what approach you take, you will affect the whole. As the client's whole body responds to the bodywork therapy, each of its components will be affected in turn.

Ultimately, the theories and techniques of the different approaches are used together to perform treatments that are in many cases stronger than using a single approach. Understanding each approach fully allows you to see the many connections between them and to create new combinations of therapies. This will allow you to be more flexible to address the infinite varieties of pathology that a client may present.

Combining the Approaches

There are many ways to combine the approaches. In the clinic setting, you will draw from all of your knowledge and therapeutic techniques to address a client's condition. You will combine the useful elements of each method with your personal experience to create a cohesive approach that addresses the client's specific concerns. This allows you to eventually create your own unique combinations that fit your style and body type.

In addition, the client often presents with an assortment of pathology. Their condition may involve multiple structures such as muscles, joints, ligaments, and tendons as well and nerves, lymph, and blood vessels. Pathology is also often complicated by emotions and mental resistance brought on by the pain and circumstances surrounding the injury. Therefore, each client will require a unique treatment specialized to suit their specific pathology, personal preferences, and emotional state.

Creating a treatment plan to address all of these circumstances is not as complicated as it sounds. Learning massage therapy is similar to learning to cook. Cooking requires a strong foundation of technical skill that is drawn from a variety of cultures, traditions, and individual approaches. Those skills, techniques, and approaches can be combined in a vast number of ways.

Also, a chef must always consider who the meal is being prepared for and will tailor the preparation to the guest. The combinations are determined by the proficiency, knowledge, skill, and creativity of the chef.

Just like cooking, in massage you must first learn the basic skills, techniques, and traditions. You begin studying individual approaches and their techniques separately. You will even apply techniques by following step-by-step plans similar to cooking recipes. Understanding the basics of each therapeutic approach gives you the ability to work like a chef. You will be able to see the best ways to combine the theories and techniques so that you can tailor your treatments to the needs of your client. The huge variety in your clients' needs and their unique conditions will help to inspire you toward a creative use of your skills.

With all the possibilities of pathology and all the possibilities for treatment available to you, making a plan can seem daunting. However, putting together a holistic treatment plan is like any other massage skill—it takes practice to become confident and proficient. Practice making treatment plans to

experiment with combining techniques just as you practice your massage skills. This can be done in the classroom or on your own by making up case studies and then assessing them and creating a plan. As you play with these ideas outside of the clinic setting, you will become more comfortable and the planning process will become more intuitive.

Whenever you come across an unusual or challenging case, don't be afraid to review your reference materials or consult with fellow professionals. This will help you to be creative and generate new ideas. The following outline for holistic planning will help you as you begin to practice creating holistic treatments. (Additional tools for practicing this type of planning will be presented later in this chapter.) As you become more proficient, you will become more creative and find new ways to combine the theories and treatment techniques.

A PLAN FOR HOLISTIC TREATMENT (SOAP)

Any treatment plan must begin with a proper assessment. We recommend using the SOAP note format for developing your assessment and your plan for treatment. (A complete discussion of the contents and structure of the SOAP note is presented in Chapter 1.) The following discussion of the SOAP process is simplified to emphasize a holistic perspective. Review the details of the SOAP method, including postural analysis (Chapter 1), and then include these additional holistic concepts into your analysis, planning, and treatment.

Subjective

The first step in the planning process is taking the client history. Along with your questions about the nature of the client's physical complaints, you should also take into account the variety of circumstances that may be contributing to the pathology. When taking a holistic view of the client, you will need to consider the many factors that influence the client's body and mind. Factors such as dietary habits, exercise habits, living arrangements, jobs, relationships, etc., all have an impact on the client's health and ability to manage illness.

It is important to avoid being too intrusive with personal questions, and performing a detailed analysis of the client's life is out of the scope of our practice as bodyworkers. However, asking some general questions about these matters is appropriate and will open the door for the client to present information that may be relevant to their treatment.

Objective
OBSERVATION

Begin by using basic postural analysis and, if needed, use the passive and resisted techniques discussed in Chapter 1. Note the position of the head, shoulders, hips, knees, and feet relative to each other. Remember to compare both sides of the body to each other instead of comparing the client to an ideal.

A holistic analysis can seem quite cumbersome when attempting to observe the body and keep track of the compensations and muscle structures involved. However, using the acupressure approach offers a simplified and holistic

---

? DID YOU KNOW

In the martial arts there is a saying that white belts have the same basic knowledge as the black belts; it's just that the black belts know the basics inside and out. The impressive skill of the black belts comes from their ability to apply creative new combinations of the basic techniques.

assessment technique. The simple 12-channel system can help you keep track of the areas of pathology rather than keeping track of many individual muscles and bones (see Figure 18.4 ■). Use the 12 channels and the flow of Qi clock (see Figure 18.5 ■) to guide your observation of the client.

Note which channels have pain or discomfort as well as which ones are harboring tension. Then, follow the length of the channel looking for compensation. When you reach the end of the channel, look to the next channel along the flow of Qi for further compensation. Also take a look at the other associated channels (i.e., mirror channels, Yin/Yang complements). Using this system as a starting point will provide a good sound knowledge of where the client is holding tension or other pathology. This makes a complex analysis of the client's overall posture and compensation patterns quick and simple. Review Chapter 16 for more on the acupressure approach to assessment.

PALPATION

The acupressure approach is also easy to use when performing the palpation portion of the assessment. Following the pathways of the channels and the flow of Qi will help you systematically work through the body. Palpate the channels looking for trigger points, knots, adhesions, hypertonicity, etc.. It's important to note that any of the pathological conditions that

are discussed throughout the four therapeutic approaches may be present. The channels extend to all muscles from superficial to deep. Therefore, when palpating the channels, it is important to feel for all of the layers of muscles, especially the deeper stabilizing layers. Remember that the deep layers often harbor the most chronic pathology. Also keep in mind the continuity of the network of fascia. The fascial system extends through all layers of tissue and connects the body from head to toe. This will help remind you to look for compensation in distant areas from the pathology.

Assessment

The formula for assessment is S + O = A. Forming a holistic assessment from the information in the subjective and objective sections includes taking into account many factors, then figuring out how they fit together. In order to stand back and look at the information as a whole, it is helpful to ask questions about the pathology from the viewpoint of each of the four therapeutic approaches.

DEEP TISSUE APPROACH

☑ Which muscles are affected?

☑ In which layer are the affected muscles found?

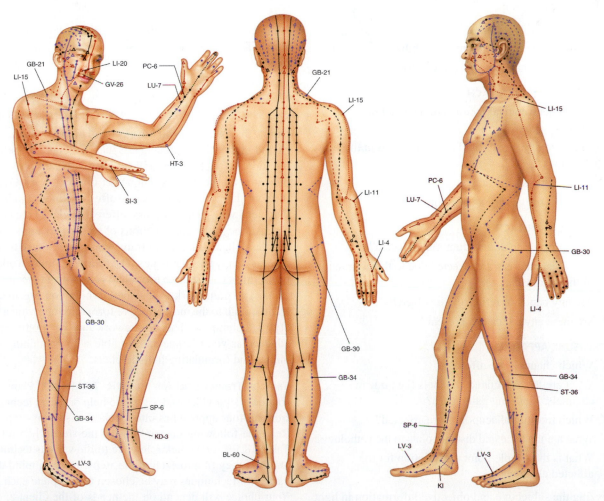

FIGURE 18.4
The Locations of the 12 Major Channels on the Body

FIGURE 18.5

The Flow of Qi Clock

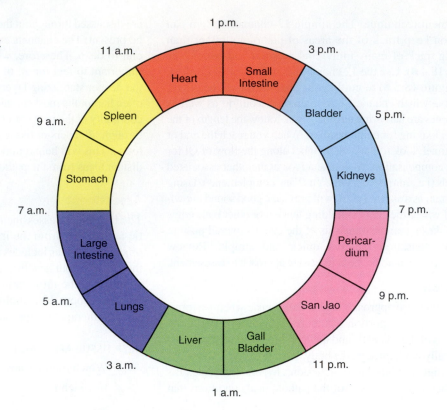

☑ What role do those muscles play in the function of the area (i.e., prime mover, stabilizer, synergist)?

☑ What compensations exist throughout the body?

NEUROMUSCULAR APPROACH

☑ Which neurological factors are involved in this pathology?

☑ Are there any emotional factors involved in the pathology?

☑ Which reflexes are activated?

☑ Are there trigger points present?

MYOFASCIAL APPROACH

☑ Which myofascial meridian(s) is affected?

☑ What distant areas are affected due to the continuity of the myofascial net?

☑ Are any bands of retinacula involved?

☑ Are there any adhesions present?

ACUPRESSURE APPROACH

☑ Which channels are affected?

☑ What are the associated channels (i.e., mirror channels, Yin/Yang pairs, etc.)?

☑ Which traditional acupoints are affected?

☑ What are the local and distant points to the pathology?

☑ What is the simple point prescription for the affected channels?

Analyzing the subjective and objective information in light of the four therapeutic approaches will give you a fairly complete picture of the client's condition. You will then be able to formulate a holistic assessment as well as a plan for treatment.

Plan

CHOOSING TECHNIQUES FOR HOLISTIC TREATMENT SESSIONS

During treatment you will use any or all of the techniques discussed in the four approaches. Specific techniques or combinations of techniques will be chosen based on what is indicated by the client's unique set of conditions. Overall, the four therapeutic approaches offer treatment modalities that blend very well to address different angles of the pathology. Although the combinations of techniques are virtually limitless, there is a general framework you can use to organize and apply the techniques. The following framework will be useful as you begin to formulate your holistic therapy sessions. The framework is designed to help you organize the techniques into the most effective format for applying a variety of techniques. This framework can be modified and adjusted as you become comfortable with combining techniques and formulating holistic plans.

Sample Framework for Holistic Treatment Plan   The framework provided is designed to help organize techniques from all four approaches into a cohesive step-by-step plan. Read the following descriptions of the steps, then refer to Table 18.1 ■ for a quick reference to the various techniques and how they fit into each of the steps. Keep in mind that a variety of techniques may be chosen to complete each step. Your choice will depend on the needs of the client and the circumstances of the session.

STEP ONE: WARM-UP

- **The goal:** The main goal of the warm-up is to prepare the tissues for the work to follow. It is important to encourage circulation to the area as it warms the myofascia and makes it more receptive to deep work. Another goal of this phase is to verify the trigger points, tender spots, active acupoints, and other myofascial adhesions and restrictions discovered during the assessment.

- **The techniques:** Compression and petrissage and jostling are excellent techniques to use for the warm-up. These three are effective because they can be performed gently and are good for introducing your pressure to the client's body. They are also well suited for the first step because they do not require lubricant. This is important as the next step uses myofascial techniques, which require dry skin for their proper application.

In addition to compression and petrissage, it is very common and useful to use a selection of basic warm-up techniques, such as rocking, effleurage, and tapotement.

DID YOU KNOW

Before any technique can be applied, it is important to remember some important principles:

Proper body mechanics—Working deeper with less effort by using leverage is important to all applications.

Slow deliberate rate/rhythm—This is important to prevent guarding and to allow the client to better receive the therapy.

Use very little lubrication—It is important to achieve a good grip for the application of all four approaches. In some cases, such as during the myofascial techniques, no lubrication is used. Be prepared to use a sheet or towel to wipe the area before attempting those techniques.

TABLE 18.1	Guide to Use of Techniques for a Holistic Massage Routine		
Step	Goal	Approach	Techniques
Warm-up	Prepare and assess the tissues	Acupressure	Compression
		Swedish massage	Jostling, rocking, petrissage, effleurage
Address Superficial Layers	Release the superficial layers	Myofascial therapy	**Indirect methods:**
			Standard release
			Torquing
			Skin pushing
			Skin dragging
			Fascial lift
			Skin rolling
Address Deeper Layers	Separate the muscle fibers to work deep into muscles	Deep tissue therapy	**Separation phase techniques:**
			Long strokes applied first with the grain, then against the grain of the muscle using thumbs, fingers, knuckles, and elbows
Treat Specific Pathologies	Resolve the trigger points and adhesions and treat the acupoints	Neuromuscular therapy	**NMT direct methods:**
			Trigger point pressure release, stripping strokes
		Myofascial therapy	**MFT direct methods:**
			Direct stretch, deep fiber friction
		Acupressure therapy	Pressure to the active acupoints or on the acupoints of the simple acupoint prescription for the affected channels
Integrate and Close	Bring the muscle fibers back into alignment and encourage circulation to the area	Deep tissue therapy	**Reorganization phase techniques:**
			Long strokes applied along the grain using forearms, palms, and flat fists
		Acupressure	Compression
		Swedish massage	Petrissage, effleurage, and tapotement
Stretch and Re-educate	Lengthen the muscles and teach a new resting length	Neuromuscular therapy	**NMT indirect methods:**
			Facilitated stretching:
			Postisometric relaxation, reciprocal inhibition, and positional release

STEP TWO: ADDRESS THE SUPERFICIAL LAYER

- **The goal:** The goal of this step is to release the superficial fascia and to encourage circulation to the deeper tissues. It is important to release the superficial layer to allow for the deeper work to follow.

- **The techniques:** The techniques best suited to this step are drawn from the myofascial approach, as the main goal is to release the fascia. Any of the indirect myofascial techniques can be selected depending upon the body part being treated. Table 18.1 presents the best techniques to use during this step of treatment.

STEP THREE: ADDRESS THE DEEPER LAYERS

- **The goal:** The goal of this step is to work deeper into the muscular layers by effectively separating the muscle fibers and allowing deeper penetration. Separating the fibers helps expose the pathology and opens up the muscles to allow for the specific work to follow.

- **The techniques:** The most suitable techniques to use here come from the separation phase of the deep tissue approach. This is because they are the best suited for systematically working deep into the muscle. Table 18.1 presents the best techniques to use during this step of treatment.

STEP FOUR: TREAT THE SPECIFIC PATHOLOGY

- **The goal:** The goal of this step is to address the acute or primary pathology. It is during this step that specific myofascial pathologies (i.e., trigger points, adhesions, and restrictions) should be addressed with the proper technique. Address as many pathologies as possible given the comfort level of the client and the circumstances of the treatment session. This is also the time to treat any active acupoints, or you may use the simple acupoint prescriptions and classically active acupoints at this time.

- **The techniques:** This step has the potential for using the greatest variety of techniques. This is where the artistry of combining the techniques is exercised the most. Depending on the pathology presented, you may use techniques from any of the four approaches. Use the techniques that are most effective for the pathology and that are most appropriate for the client. Table 18.1 presents the best techniques to use during this step of treatment.

STEP FIVE: INTEGRATE AND CLOSE

- **The goal:** The main goal of this step is to bring the muscle fibers back into alignment after they have been worked over by the previous two steps. Another is to flush the tissues by encouraging circulation.

- **The techniques:** The techniques of the realignment phase of DTM are the best suited for bringing the muscle fibers back into alignment. DTM is especially effective for integrating body parts because of its use of long continuous strokes. The best techniques for encouraging circulation are the basic Swedish strokes. Table 18.1 presents the best techniques to use during this step of treatment.

STEP SIX: STRETCH AND RE-EDUCATE

- **The goal:** The goal of this step is to lengthen the muscles and teach them new, longer resting lengths. This is important because even though the pathology has been alleviated within the muscle, it may still need encouragement to lengthen to its full capacity.

- **The techniques:** The techniques used here come from the neuromuscular approach. Facilitated stretching is used to re-educate the muscles. Table 18.1 presents the best techniques to use during this step of treatment.

QUICK QUIZ #35

1. A reductionist view point is one where:
   a. all things are reduced to a single common denominator.
   b. the behavior of the whole is explained only by the behavior of its parts.
   c. the behavior of the parts is affected by the behavior of the whole.
   d. None of the above

2. Which statement is most true?
   a. The four therapeutic approaches represent completely opposing views.
   b. The four therapeutic approaches overlap in their analysis and treatment.
   c. The four therapeutic approaches should be used separately.
   d. None of the above

3. Which therapeutic approach is most used during the assessment?
   a. Deep tissue massage
   b. Neuromuscular therapy
   c. Myofascial therapy
   d. Acupressure therapy

4. What techniques are recommended for use in the third step in the sample framework for holistic therapy?
   a. The indirect NMT techniques
   b. The indirect MFT techniques
   c. The separation phase of DTM
   d. Acupressure

CASE STUDIES FOR CUSTOMIZING HOLISTIC PROTOCOLS

As mentioned earlier, planning a massage protocol is an important skill to practice. The more you practice being flexible and creative, the more easily it will come to you when you are faced with real clients who always present with a variety of pathologies. Using case studies is an excellent way to rehearse and develop your planning skills.

The following case studies present two similar sets of pathologies in two different clients. Although the injuries are similar, the techniques chosen for each will vary greatly. Read through the assessment, and think about the plan you might use to treat each client. Tables 18.2 ■ and 18.3 ■ each present a possible customized holistic protocol for the two scenarios.

Case Study #1

Andrew has a large frame and is a heavily muscled offensive lineman for a college football team.

SUBJECTIVE

Andrew's chief complaint is a dull achy pain that runs across his lower back "like a belt." This pain also radiates into the hip and thigh. Andrew injured the lateral ligament of his right ankle about six months prior to the onset of the low back pain.

TABLE 18.2	Holistic Protocol for Case Study #1			
Step/Goal	Common Approaches	Suitable Techniques	Techniques Chosen	Notes
Warm-up Prepare and assess the tissues	Acupressure Swedish massage	Compression Petrissage Effleurage Rocking Tapotement	✓ ✓ ✓	Gentle techniques good for any body type
Address the superficial layer Release the superficial layers	Myofascial therapy (indirect techniques)	Standard release Torquing Skin pushing Skin drag Fascial lift Skin rolling	✓ ✓ ✓	Standard release is a good starting point and good for across the hip; skin pushing is deep so it is good for bigger clients.
Address the deeper layers Separate the muscle fibers	Deep tissue therapy (separation phase)	Four fingers Supported fingers Supported thumb Knuckle stroke Elbow stroke Muscle rolling	 ✓ ✓	These two are deeper techniques, so they are good for a more heavily muscled client.
Treat the specific pathologies Address trigger points and adhesions	Neuromuscular therapy (direct techniques) Myofascial therapy (direct techniques) Acupressure therapy	TrP pressure release Stripping strokes Direct stretch Deep fiber friction Pressure	✓ ✓ ✓	TrP pressure release for the softer, superficial trigger points and stripping strokes for the deeper ones; the simple acupoint prescription for the Urinary Bladder and Gall Bladder channels is also included.
Integrate and close Bring the fibers into alignment	Deep tissue massage (reorganization phase)	Straight-line forearm Straight-line flat fist Palm press Limb stroke Supported palms One two	✓ ✓ ✓	These techniques cover larger areas and are deeper; therefore they are best for this client.
Stretch and re-educate Lengthen muscles	Neuromuscular therapy (facilitated stretching)	Postisometric relaxation Reciprocal inhibition Positional release	✓	Stretching is powerful for lengthening the muscles.

In the course of playing football at his position, Andrew frequently stands in a forward bent posture and receives a lot of blows, which cause strain to his entire frame.

OBJECTIVE

Observation Postural analysis reveals a slight anterior tilt to the pelvis and an elevated illium on the right side. The Urinary Bladder channel along the back is shortened as well as the Gall Bladder channel along the right side of the body (see Figures 18.6 ■ and 18.7 ■).

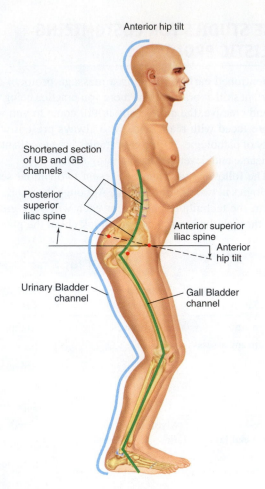

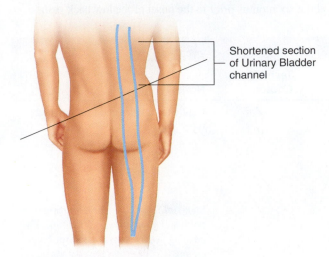

FIGURE 18.6

The Right Hip of the Client Is Elevated, Which Shortens the Muscles and Therefore the Urinary Bladder Channel on That Side

FIGURE 18.7

An Anterior Tilt in the Pelvis Causes the Urinary Bladder Channel to Be Shortened on the Back

Palpation Palpation reveals hypertonus and trigger points in the muscles of the Urinary Bladder channels (quadratus lumborum and erector spinae) in the low back. The right side is worse than the left. The Urinary Bladder channel in the hip (gluteals) is also hypertonic with a considerable amount of trigger points located close to the sacroiliac joint (S.I. joint) and crest of the illium.

ASSESSMENT (S + O = A)

History of the right ankle injury offset the right hip because the client compensated by lifting the hip to walk (called a "hip hike"). This caused extra stress to the Urinary Bladder channel of the lower back, which caused the muscles (i.e., quadratus lumborum, erector spinae) on the right side to become hypertonic and eventually form trigger points.

Over time, the tension in the right back muscles caused compensation in the muscles of the left lower back, affecting the Urinary Bladder channel on that side. The imbalance in the muscles on the right versus the left side caused stress to the sacroiliac joint.

The tension in the low back caused the anterior pelvic tilt, as the low back muscles pulled the posterior illium up.

The official assessment is **lumbago** (low back pain) due to stress to the sacroiliac joint and trigger points in the local muscles along the Urinary Bladder channel.

PLAN

Relax the hypertonic muscles and release the trigger points to take the stress off of the S.I. joint by addressing the Urinary Bladder and Gall Bladder channels on both sides of the back, hips, and thighs. The channels are addressed using the simple point prescriptions. Figure 18.1 shows the techniques chosen for this client.

GENERAL OVERVIEW

Since Andrew is a large man with an athletic build, most of the techniques chosen are of the deeper variety. The thickness of his muscles requires much deeper work.

Case Study #2

Jen is a 45-year-old executive. Her favorite pastime is barrel racing her prized horse. She has a small frame with a very lean and wiry build.

TABLE 18.3	Holistic Protocol for Case Study #2			
Step	**Common Approaches**	**Suitable Available Techniques**	**Techniques Chosen**	**Notes**
1. Warm-up To prepare and assess the tissues	Acupressure Swedish massage	Compression Petrissage Effleurage Rocking Tapotement	✓ ✓ ✓	Gentle techniques good for any body type
2. Address the superficial layer Release the superficial layers	Myofascial therapy (indirect techniques)	Standard release Torquing Skin push Skin drag Fascial lift Skin rolling	✓ ✓ ✓	Gentler techniques are chosen since the client is in pain and has a less muscular build. The fascial lift technique was chosen to help release the adhesions.
3. Address the deeper layers To separate the muscle fibers	Deep tissue therapy (separation phase)	Four fingers Supported fingers Supported thumb Knuckle stroke Elbow stroke Muscle rolling	✓ ✓	Gentler techniques are chosen since the client is in pain and has a less muscular build.
4. Treat the specific pathologies Address trigger points and adhesions	Neuromuscular therapy (direct techniques) Myofascial therapy (direct techniques) Acupressure therapy	TrP pressure release Stripping strokes Direct stretch Deep fiber friction Pressure	✓ ✓ ✓	This condition requires trigger point release and the breakdown of the adhesions, so both NMT and MFT are utilized. The classically effective acupoints for the Urinary Bladder and Gall Bladder channels are also included. Fewer acupoints are chosen, as this client is more sensitive.
5. Integrate and close Bring the fibers in alignment	Deep tissue massage (reorganization phase)	Straight-line forearm Straight-line flat fist Palm press Limb stroke Supported palms One-two	✓ ✓	Gentler techniques are chosen since the client is in pain and has a less muscular build.
6. Stretch and re-educate Lengthen muscles	Neuromuscular therapy (facilitated stretching)	Postisometric relaxation Reciprocal inhibition Positional release	✓	Since this client is in pain, reciprocal inhibition is used rather than postisometric relaxation.

SUBJECTIVE

Jen's chief complaint is consistent lower back pain that can sometimes spike into a stabbing pain, radiating into her hip and lower leg. About 11 months prior to the onset of the low back pain, Jen sustained an injury to her right hip and knee from a fall off her horse.

In the course of her hobby of riding, Jen frequently sits in a dynamic forward bent posture. She must constantly adjust to the repetitive motion of the horse she rides, which causes strain to her low back as well as her knees and hips.

OBJECTIVE

Observation   Postural analysis reveals a slight anterior tilt to the pelvis and an elevated illium on the right side. Both the Gall Bladder channel and the Urinary Bladder channel are shortened (see Figures 18.6 and 18.7).

Palpation   Palpation reveals hypertonus and trigger points in the muscles of the Urinary Bladder channel (quadratus lumborum and erector spinae) in the low back. The right side is worse than the left. The Urinary Bladder channel in the hip (gluteals) and the Gall Bladder channel along the lateral thigh are also hypertonic. Upon further inspection, adhesions were found close to the S.I. joint and out along the greater trochanter of the right hip (i.e., both the Gall Bladder and Urinary Bladder channels).

ASSESSMENT (S + O = A)

The history of the right knee and hip injury caused the adhesions to form along the S.I. joint and greater trochanter. The restrictions in the muscle caused by the adhesions caused extra stress to the Urinary Bladder channel of the lower back on the right side, making the muscles hypertonic and eventually forming trigger points.

Over time, the tension in the right back muscles caused compensation in the muscles of the left lower back (quadratus lumborum, erector spinae) affecting the Urinary Bladder channel on that side. The imbalance in the muscles on the right versus the left side caused stress to the sacroiliac joint. This may be causing tension in the underlying piriformis muscle, which is impinging on the sciatic nerve and causing pain to radiate down the leg.

The tension in the low back along the Urinary Bladder channels of both sides caused the anterior pelvic tilt as the low back muscles pulled the posterior illium up.

The official assessment is lumbago and possible **sciatica** due to stress to the sacroiliac joint, with adhesions and trigger points in the muscles of the Urinary Bladder and Gall Bladder channels of the hip and lower back.

PLAN

Relax the hypertonic muscles, release the trigger points, and break up the adhesions along the Urinary Bladder and Gall Bladder channels on both sides of the back, hips, and thighs. The classically active points for each channel are also chosen in this case. This will take the stress off of the

S.I. joint, relaxing the deeper muscles and taking stress off of the nerves. Table 18.2 shows the techniques chosen for this client.

GENERAL OVERVIEW

Since Jen has a much smaller build, the techniques chosen for her were of the lighter variety. Her wiry frame would not tolerate the deeper techniques that were chosen for Andrew. Jen also presented with adhesions that require specific techniques to resolve them.

Though both of these clients have a similar injury and assessment, the actual plan for each is considerably different because of the discrepancy in the size and musculature of the clients. The difference in the thickness and size of the muscles determines the use of different techniques and contact points.

In addition to the two plans presented above, there are many different options for treating each of these two cases. You might make different technique selections based on your available time, relative stature, and therapeutic setting. Of course you will also consider the client's expectations, past experience, and comfort level. Use Table 18.4 ■ to practice formulating your own plan for these fictional case studies. It can also be used to make practice plans on your fellow students. Appendix C provides Table 18.4 as a sample form that can be copied for use in practice. As you practice planning with a variety of techniques in a variety of situations, this thought process will flow more naturally.

You may choose to use this framework or create your own format for developing creative holistic treatment plans for your own clients. As you become comfortable combining the techniques detailed in this book, you will likely want to include techniques from other modalities as well. Being creative and open to new ideas will make your career more fun and rewarding. Taking the time to consider and plan the best ways of incorporating new techniques will make your therapies even stronger.

CHOOSING THE RIGHT THERAPEUTIC METHODS FOR YOU AND YOUR CLIENTS

As a bodyworker and health care practitioner, it is important to balance open-mindedness with **critical evaluation.** There are many forms of complementary and alternative therapies out there. For the sake of your career and the well-being of your clients, it is important to find a style that suits you and to find therapies you believe in.

Some modalities have little or no scientific supporting evidence. This does not mean that they should automatically be discounted. It can be difficult to get support and funding for scientifically rigorous studies, and many alternative therapies are simply understudied. Some topics are well studied, but not well publicized. They may be discounted through the court of public opinion rather than an evaluation of facts.

TABLE 18.4   Holistic Protocol

Step	Goal	Approaches Used	Indications	Techniques	✓
Step 1 Warm-up	Prepare and assess the tissues	Swedish	General warm-up	Rocking, effleurage, petrissage, jostling	
		Acupressure	Before myofascial techniques	Compression	
Step 2 Address Superficial Layer	Release the superficial layers	Myofascial therapy (Indirect methods)	**Very gentle** Sensitive, painful areas, esp. across joints	Standard release	
			Gentle Sensitive or more robust areas Anywhere	Torquing	
			Deep Robust areas/clients	Drag and push	
			Mild to severe tension More sensitive tissues/clients	Myofascial lift	
			Mild to severe tension More robust tissues/clients	Skin rolling	
Step 3 Address Deeper Layers	Separate the muscle fibers to work deep into muscles	Deep tissue therapy (Separation phase)	**Very gentle** Sensitive, painful areas Anywhere, esp. broad areas	Four fingers	
			Gentle Sensitive or more robust areas Anywhere	Supported fingers	
			Deep Robust areas/clients	Supported thumb	
			Deep Robust areas/clients	Knuckle stroke	
			Deep Robust areas/clients	Elbow stroke	
			Gentle to deep Sensitive or more robust areas	Muscle rolling	
Step 4 Treat Specific Pathologies	Resolve the trigger points and adhesions	Neuromuscular (Direct methods)	All trigger points	Trigger point pressure release	
			Harder, myogelotic trigger points	Stripping strokes	
		Myofascial (Direct methods)	Adhesions in more sensitive areas or clients	Direct stretch	
			Harder, firmer adhesions or more robust muscles and clients	Deep fiber friction	
		Acupressure	Active acupoints, primary and associated channels	Fingers, thumbs, fists, palms, elbow, forearm, heel, foot, knee, shin	
			Ashi acupoints	Fingers, thumbs, fists, palms, elbow, forearm, heel, foot, knee, shin	
			Local and distal acupoints	Fingers, thumbs, fists, palms, elbow, forearm, heel, foot, knee, shin	
			Simple acupoint prescription	Fingers, thumbs, fists, palms, elbow, forearm, heel, foot, knee, shin	
			Classically effective acupoints	Fingers, thumbs, fists, palms, elbow, forearm, heel, foot, knee, shin	

(Continued)

TABLE 18.4 *(Continued)*

Step	Goal	Approaches Used	Indications	Techniques	✓
Step 5 Integrate and Close	Bring the muscle fibers back into alignment	Deep tissue (Realignment phase)	Large areas	Straight-line forearm	
			Anywhere	Palm press	
			More robust muscles or clients	Straight-line flat fist	
			Large areas and more robust muscles and clients	Supported palms	
			Limbs	Limb stroke	
			Limbs	One-two	
	Encourage circulation	Swedish	**Gentle** Can be used anywhere	Rocking, effleurage, petrissage, jostling	
		Acupressure	**Gentle** Can be used anywhere	Compression	
Step 6 Stretch and Re-educate	Lengthen the muscles and teach a new resting length	Neuromuscular (Indirect techniques)	Muscular tension	Postisometric relaxation	
			Muscular tension, esp. spasm	Reciprocal inhibition	
			Very sensitive pathology, areas of focused tenderness	Positional release	

It is equally important to be skeptical and look for good support and evidence for any therapies you may try or recommend to a client. When doing your own investigations, ask yourself questions like these:

- Is this a credible source?
- Whose interests may or may not be served by what is being said?
- Does this source provide documentation for its claims?
- Does this source provide clear details about the information?

- Is this information presented in broad, sweeping statements or narrow and clearly defined statements?
- What assumptions are made in support of this information?

Remember to confer with others in your field about their experiences with complementary and alternative care. Above all else, listen to what makes sense to you when evaluating any information. The goals are to be open, continue learning, provide the best possible treatments for your clients, and, above all, enjoy your career in the field of holistic bodywork.

QUICK QUIZ #36

1. The main affected channels in both case studies were:
   a. Heart and Lung channels.
   b. Gall Bladder and Liver channels.
   c. Gall Bladder and Urinary Bladder channels.
   d. Spleen and Stomach channels.

2. Which pathology did Jen have that Andrew did not? (Circle all that apply)
   a. Trigger points

   b. Adhesions
   c. Lumbago
   d. Sciatica

3. Critical evaluation means:
   a. criticize all and therefore don't believe anything.
   b. believe all you read.
   c. scrutinize data and look for other confirmation.
   d. None of the above

SUMMARY

Holism is a worldview that emphasizes the understanding of whole systems. A holistic approach to bodywork means taking a broad view of the entire field. It also means keeping a holistic perspective on our clients as people and seeing the body of each individual client as a whole functioning system.

Performing holistic massage requires a creative combination of knowledge of the basics of theory and technique. In the clinic, you will combine the theories of massage with all the different perspectives of physiology to form a cohesive approach to treatment. All therapies and theories can be mixed and matched according to the needs of the client.

Clients present with complex patterns of pathology that include issues in focused areas and effects in distant areas of the body. Therefore, they should be approached by a combination or holistic perspective. This should include a thorough understanding of how the physiology of each of the four therapeutic approaches overlap and how they diverge. It is also crucial to understand how to use and combine each theory to complement the others.

A framework for developing holistic therapy involves looking at the client's health from a broad perspective. Begin by taking a holistic approach to the assessment. The acupressure channels provide a good starting point for a holistic evaluation of the client's condition.

Use six steps as a basic framework for practicing a holistic treatment protocol. Remember that each step contains a goal, which is designed to support the others.

It is important that you stay abreast of new information and keep your knowledge and interest fresh. When selecting from many bodywork approaches, it is important to balance open-mindedness with critical evaluation.

Finally, remember that massage is a client-centered therapeutic modality. Always make the client the center of your focus.

DISCUSSION QUESTIONS

1. Explain the relationships between a whole system and its parts from a holistic perspective.
2. Give another example of how two or more modalities support and complement each other.
3. Use Table 18.4 to create an additional sample protocol for one the case studies presented in the chapter.
4. Explain three important principles for critically evaluating information about alternative therapies.

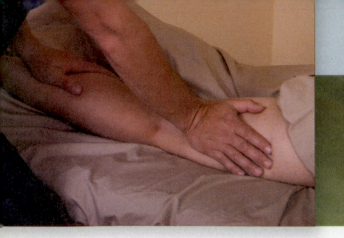

S O A P Notes

Client name: _____ Date_____

SUBJECTIVE INFORMATION (HEALTH SURVEY)—PAST & PRESENT

Exercise/activity

Nutrition/diet

Injuries/illnesses

Current medical care
  Physician's name and contact information

  Medications

OBJECTIVE INFORMATION (PHYSICAL EXAMINATION)

Posture & movement observations

Tissue palpation notes

Range of Motion (ROM) tests—passive, active, resisted
  Non-affected side

  Affected side

ASSESSMENT (S + O = A)

Primary affected area

Secondary areas

Possible syndromes/conditions

PLAN

Muscles to treat (in order of priority)

Modalities/techniques to be used

Projected treatment/appointment schedule

Client home care

SESSION NOTES

Any newly discovered pathology

Any significant myoskeletal release

Comments for next session

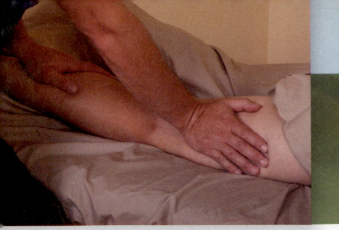

Common Referral Patterns

Referral Area	Common Source Muscles for Referred Sensation
Temporal head	Posterior suboccipitals, Sternocleidomastoid (SCM), Splenius Cervicis, Occipitalis, Temporalis, Trapezius
Forehead	Posterior suboccipitals, SCM, Zygomaticus major, Masseter, Frontalis
Posterior head	Posterior suboccipitals, SCM, Splenius cervicis, Temporalis, Occipitalis, Trapezius, Digastricus
Top of the head	SCM, Splenius capitis
Area around eyes	Posterior Suboccipitals, SCM, Zygomaticus major, Orbicularis oculi, Splenius cervicis, Temporalis, Occipitalis, Frontalis, Trapezius, Masseter
Area around mouth	Digastricus, Masseter, Trapezius, Temporalis, Orbicularis oculi, Zygomaticus major, SCM, Anterior suboccipitals
Area around ear	Masseter, SCM, Anterior suboccipitals, Posterior suboccipitals, Longus colli, Longus capitis
Posterior neck	Trapezius, Multifidus, Longus colli, Longus capitis, Levator scapulae, Anterior suboccipitals
Anterior neck	Digastricus, Longus colli, Longus capitis, SCM, Anterior suboccipitals
Upper back	Scalenes, Levator scapulae, Supraspinatus, Trapezius, Multifidi, Rhomboids, Splenius cervicis, Triceps brachii, Biceps brachii, Anconeus, Interspinales, Erector spinae
Mid back	Scalenes, Levator scapulae, Trapezius, Multifidi, Rhomboids, Latissimus dorsi, Iliocostalis thoracis, Serratus posterior superior, Infraspinatus, Serratus anterior, Erector spinae
Low back	Multifidi, Latissimus dorsi, Iliocostalis lumborum, Serratus posterior inferior, Erector spinae, Quadratus lumborum, Psoas major, Iliacus, Rectus abdominis, Diaphragm, Rotatores, Interspinales
Anterior chest	Pectoralis major and minor, Scalenes, SCM, Iliocostalis cervicis, Subclavius, External abdominal oblique, Serratus posterior superior, Serratus anterior
Side of chest	Serratus anterior, Latissimus dorsi, Serratus posterior inferior, Quadratus lumborum, Diaphragm, Erector spinae, Rectus abdominis
Abdominal area	Adductor magnus, Psoas major, Iliacus, External and internal obliques, Rectus abdominis, Erector spinae, Multifidi, Rotatores
Anterior shoulder	Infraspinatus, Subscapularis, Sternalis, Subclavius, Teres major, Scalenes, Deltoid, Brachialis, Supraspinatus, Pectoralis major and minor, Biceps brachii, Coracobrachialis, Serratus anterior, Serratus posterior superior, Latissimus dorsi
Posterior shoulder	Infraspinatus, Subscapularis, Teres major and minor, Scalenes, Deltoid, Supraspinatus, Pectoralis major and minor, Biceps brachii, Coracobrachialis, Serratus anterior, Serratus posterior superior, Latissimus dorsi, Levator scapulae, Triceps brachii, Trapezius, Iliocostalis thoracis, Rhomboids major and minor, Anconeus, Erector spinae
Anterior upper arm	Infraspinatus, Subscapularis, Scalenes, Deltoid, Supraspinatus, Pectoralis major and minor, Biceps brachii, Coracobrachialis, Serratus anterior, Serratus posterior superior, Latissimus dorsi, Brachialis, Sternalis, Subclavius
Posterior upper arm	Infraspinatus, Subscapularis, Teres major and minor, Scalenes, Deltoid, Supraspinatus, Coracobrachialis, Serratus posterior superior, Latissimus dorsi, Triceps brachii, Anconeus, Brachialis
Ulnar anterior forearm	Flexor carpi ulnaris, Pronator teres, Palmaris longus, Supinator
Ulnar posterior forearm	Supinator, Extensor digitorum, Extensor carpi ulnaris, Anconeus

Referral Area	Common Source Muscles for Referred Sensation
Radial anterior forearm	Pronator teres, Flexor carpi radialis, Brachioradialis, Supinator, Biceps brachaii
Radial posterior forearm	Brachioradialis, Extensor carpi radialis longus and brevis, Anconeus, Pronator teres, Extensor digitorum
Anterior hand	Pronator teres, Palmaris longus, Flexor digitorum superficialis, Flexor carpi radialis, Interossei, Flexor carpi ulnaris, Flexor pollicus brevis, Opponens pollicis, Adductor pollicis
Posterior hand	Extensor digitorum, Extensor indicis, Extensor carpi ulnaris, Extensor carpi radialis brevis, Interossei, Abductor digiti minimi, interossei, Extensor carpi radialis longus, Adductor pollicis
Gluteal and posterior upper leg	Quadratus lumborum, Tensor fascia latae, Adductor magnus, Lateral hip rotators, Lumbar ligaments, Gluteus maximus-medius and minimus, Psoas major, Iliacus, Rectus abdominus, Piriformis, Erector spinae, Multifidi, Interspinales
Anterior upper leg	Quadriceps, Adductor longus and brevis, Adductor magnus, Tensor fascia latae, Lateral hip rotators, Gluteus minimus, Psoas major, Iliacus, Internal and external oblique, Rectus abdominis, Pectineus, Gracilis
Anterior lower leg	Plantaris, Tibialis posterior and anterior, Peroneus longus and brevis, Extensor digitorum longus, Extensor hallucis longus
Posterior lower leg	Hamstrings, Popliteus, Plantaris, Tibialis posterior, Flexor digitorum longus, Flexor hallucis longus, Peroneus longus and brevis, Soleus, Gastrocnemius
Anterior ankle and dorsal foot	Peroneus longus and brevis, Interossei, Tibialis anterior, Extensor digitorum longus, Extensor hallucis longus
Posterior ankle and plantar foot	Peroneus longus and brevis, Interossei, Flexor digitorum longus and brevis, Flexor hallucis longus, Adductor hallucis, Abductor hallucis, Soleus, Gastrocnemius

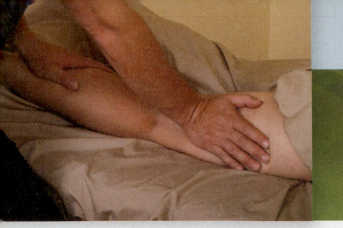

Holistic Protocol

Step	Goal	Approaches Used	Indications	Techniques	✓
Step 1 Warm-up	Prepare and assess the tissues	Swedish	General warm-up	Rocking, effleurage, petrissage, jostling	
		Acupressure	Before myofascial techniques	Compression	
Step 2 Address Superficial Layer	Release the superficial layers	Myofascial therapy (Indirect methods)	**Very gentle** Sensitive, painful areas, esp. across joints	Standard release	
			Gentle Sensitive or more robust areas Anywhere	Torquing	
			Deep Robust areas/clients	Drag and push	
			Mild to severe tension More sensitive tissues/clients	Myofascial lift	
			Mild to severe tension More robust tissues/clients	Skin rolling	
Step 3 Address Deeper Layers	Separate the muscle fibers to work deep into muscles	Deep tissue therapy (Separation phase)	**Very gentle** Sensitive, painful areas Anywhere, esp. broad areas	Four fingers	
			Gentle Sensitive or more robust areas Anywhere	Supported fingers	
			Deep Robust areas/clients	Supported thumb	
			Deep Robust areas/clients	Knuckle stroke	
			Deep Robust areas/clients	Elbow stroke	
			Gentle to deep Sensitive or more robust areas	Muscle rolling	

Step	Goal	Approaches Used	Indications	Techniques	✓
Step 4 Treat Specific Pathologies	Resolve the trigger points and adhesions	Neuromuscular (Direct methods)	All trigger points	Trigger point pressure release	
			Harder, myogelotic trigger points	Stripping strokes	
		Myofascial (Direct methods)	Adhesions in more sensitive areas or clients	Direct stretch	
			Harder, firmer adhesions or more robust muscles and clients	Deep fiber friction	
		Acupressure	Active acupoints, primary and associated channels	Fingers, thumbs, fists, palms, elbow, forearm, heel, foot, knee, shin	
			Ashi acupoints	Fingers, thumbs, fists, palms, elbow, forearm, heel, foot, knee, shin	
			Local and distal acupoints	Fingers, thumbs, fists, palms, elbow, forearm, heel, foot, knee, shin	
			Simple acupoint prescription	Fingers, thumbs, fists, palms, elbow, forearm, heel, foot, knee, shin	
			Classically effective acupoints	Fingers, thumbs, fists, palms, elbow, forearm, heel, foot, knee, shin	
Step 5 Integrate and Close	Bring the muscle fibers back into alignment	Deep tissue (Realignment phase)	Large areas	Straight-line forearm	
			Anywhere	Palm press	
			More robust muscles or clients	Straight-line flat fist	
			Large areas and more robust muscles and clients	Supported palms	
			Limbs	Limb stroke	
			Limbs	One-two	
	Encourage circulation	Swedish	**Gentle** Can be used anywhere	Rocking, effleurage, petrissage, jostling	
		Acupressure	**Gentle** Can be used anywhere	Compression	
Step 6 Stretch and Re-educate	Lengthen the muscles and teach a new resting length	Neuromuscular (Indirect techniques)	Muscular tension	Postisometric relaxation	
			Muscular tension, esp. spasm	Reciprocal inhibition	
			Very sensitive pathology, areas of focused tenderness	Positional release	

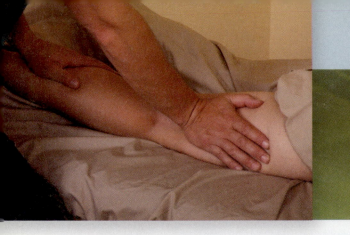

Answer Key

CHAPTER 1

Quick Quiz #1 Answers

1. b
2. a, b, c
3. a
4. e
5. a

Quick Quiz #2 Answers

1. a
2. d
3. b, c, e
4. d

CHAPTER 2

Quick Quiz #3 Answers

1. a, b, d
2. b
3. a, b
4. a

Quick Quiz #4 Answers

1. b, c, d
2. b
3. c
4. a

CHAPTER 3

Quick Quiz #5 Answers

1. b
2. b
3. c
4. b

Quick Quiz #6 Answers

1. b
2. a, b, c

3. b, c
4. a

CHAPTER 4

Quick Quiz #7 Answers

1. a, d
2. a
3. b
4. a

Quick Quiz #8 Answers

1. e
2. b
3. b, d
4. a
5. b

CHAPTER 5

Quick Quiz #9 Answers

1. a, b, c
2. b
3. f
4. a

Quick Quiz #10 Answers

1. a, b
2. a, b
3. b
4. b

CHAPTER 6

Quick Quiz #11 Answers

1. b
2. c

3. a
4. e

Quick Quiz # 12 Answers

1. f
2. b, c, d
3. d
4. a

CHAPTER 7

Quick Quiz #13 Answers

1. a, b, c
2. c
3. a
4. b

Quick Quiz #14 Answers

1. b
2. f
3. a
4. a
5. a, b, c
6. b, c, d

CHAPTER 8

Quick Quiz #15 Answers

1. b
2. e
3. a
4. b

Quick Quiz #16 Answers

1. a
2. a
3. c, d
4. b, c, d

CHAPTER 9

Quick Quiz #17 Answers

1. a
2. b, d
3. d
4. a

Quick Quiz #18 Answers

1. a, b, d
2. b
3. f
4. a

CHAPTER 10

Quick Quiz #19 Answers

1. a
2. e
3. a
4. b

Quick Quiz #20 Answers

1. a, b
2. c
3. b
4. b

CHAPTER 11

Quick Quiz #21 Answers

1. a
2. d
3. a, c, d
4. f

Quick Quiz #22 Answers

1. c
2. a
3. b
4. e

CHAPTER 12

Quick Quiz #23 Answers

1. b
2. b
3. c
4. c

Quick Quiz #24 Answers

1. a
2. b
3. b
4. a, c
5. b

CHAPTER 13

Quick Quiz #25 Answers

1. d
2. e
3. b, d
4. a

Quick Quiz #26 Answers

1. a
2. e
3. a
4. b

CHAPTER 14

Quick Quiz #27 Answers

1. a, c
2. b
3. e
4. a

Quick Quiz #28 Answers

1. b, c, d
2. b
3. a
4. a, b, c
5. b

CHAPTER 15

Quick Quiz #29 Answers

1. a, c
2. a
3. f
4. d

Quick Quiz #30 Answers

1. a, b, d
2. a
3. a
4. b

CHAPTER 16

Quick Quiz #31 Answers

1. a, b, d
2. e
3. b
4. b, d

Quick Quiz #32 Answers

1. a, c, d
2. a
3. b
4. e

CHAPTER 17

Quick Quiz #33 Answers

1. e
2. e
3. b
4. b
5. b

Quick Quiz #34 Answers

1. b
2. c, d
3. b, c, e
4. e

CHAPTER 18

Quick Quiz #35 Answers

1. c
2. b
3. d
4. c

Quick Quiz #36 Answers

1. c
2. b, d
3. c

Glossary

A

Acromion   Outer end of the scapula. The point where the scapula attaches to the clavicle.

Actin filament   A filament comprised of the protein *actin*. Together with myosin filaments, actin filaments make up the contractile units (sarcomeres) of muscle cells.

Active acupoint   Acupoints exhibiting pathology, including knots, tension, or focal points of pain.

Acupoint   Acupoints are points in the skin, muscles, and joints that commonly reflect pathology and are used to access the Qi for treatment. Categories of acupoints include active acupoints, traditional channel acupoints, classically effective acupoints, and Ashi acupoints.

Acute   A course of pathology which develops rapidly and/or is of short duration (as opposed to chronic).

Adhesion   A condition in which tissues (especially those found in the myofascia) that are normally separate become bound or "stuck" together. This can also refer to the area of tissue which is bound together by fibrous or so-called scar tissue.

Agonist   A muscle whose contraction is opposed by another muscle (the antagonist).

Anatomic barrier   The limit in the range of motion of a joint as determined by the shape and fit of the bones at the joint (AKA absolute end range).

Antagonist   A muscle that functions to oppose the action of another (the agonist).

Anterior superior iliac spine (ASIS)   The projection located at the anterior end of the iliac crest.

Antibody   A special type of protein molecule with many forms. Antibodies have the immune function of binding with and disabling viruses, bacteria, or other substances.

Archer stance   The main position for applying most massage techniques with a client on a table.

Armoring   A defensive covering. In bodywork, this refers to the severe muscular tension (as in chronic holding patterns) which causes an injury site to be isolated and less functional.

Ashi acupoints   Acupoints with no specific location. They may be located anywhere there is a painful spot on the body.

Associated channels   Acupressure channels which are not considered to be the primary location of injury or client complaint, but which contain pathology due to their close functional relationship with the primary area of complaint (frequently the mirror channel, the Yin/Yang complement channel, or channels in the sequence of the flow of Qi).

ATP (adenosine triphosphate)   ATP is the main energy storage and transport molecule within a cell. ATP provides energy for many biochemical reactions, including muscle contraction.

Atrophy   A decrease in the size of an organ or tissue due to injury, pathology, or lack of use (especially atrophied or atrophic muscles).

Axilla   The underarm or armpit. The area directly underneath the joint of the arm and shoulder.

B

Bradykinin   An inflammatory chemical that promotes vasodilation and induces pain.

C

Cell   The smallest functional unit of all known living organisms. Sometimes called "the building blocks of life," groups of many cells make up the different tissues and organs within our bodies.

Channels (aka meridians)   In traditional Chinese medicine these are pathways in the body along which vital energy (Qi), blood, and body fluids flow. Channels include all tissues such as nerves, blood vessels, muscles, connective tissue, and organs that lie along the pathway. Channels form a network that connects the various components of the body.

Chronic   A course of pathology which develops slowly and/or is of long duration (as opposed to acute).

Chronic holding patterns   A fixed position in the posture that has been present for a long time.

Circular strokes   Massage strokes applied in a circular motion.

Collagen/Collagen fibers   Bundles of the protein collagen found in connective tissue. These fibers are strong and add rigidity to the extracellular matrix.

Colloids   A type of mixture in which particles of one substance are evenly distributed within another substance. The ground substance of connective tissue is a colloidal solution.

Comfort barrier   The position just short of the physiologic barrier. This is the position used during the contraction phase of postisometric relaxation.

Compensation   The process where new muscles are recruited into assisting an injured muscle.

Complementary channels   The Yin/Yang pairs of channels located on opposing surfaces of the body.

Connective tissue   Tissue that includes an extracellular matrix made of collagenous, elastic, and reticular fibers, as well as ground substance. It forms the supporting and connecting structures of the body. Blood is sometimes considered to be a fluid connective tissue.

Contracture   A pathological chronic shortening of a muscle, often due to scar tissue, that results in restriction of a joint.

Contraindication   A factor that renders the application of a massage therapy technique inadvisable.

Controlling cycle (Ke cycle)   The cycle in the five element theory in which each element is said to control the action of another element.

Costal area   The area of the rib cage.

Cross-fiber strokes   Strokes that are performed across the grain of the majority of muscle fibers.

Cun   Also called "body inches"; units of measurement in acupressure for finding acupoints.

Cutaneous   Pertaining to the skin.

D

Dermatomes   An area of the skin that receives nerve supply from the spinal nerve of a single spinal segment.

Direct methods   Pertains to those techniques that are applied directly over the pathology.

Distant acupoints   Acupoints that are located away from the pathology. Distant points are combined in treatment with local points close to the pathology.

Dysfunctional endplate hypothesis   A proposed explanation for the formation of trigger points. The endplate is overwhelmed by excessive stimulation and depletes its store of ATP. This leads to chronic contraction and trigger point pathology.

E

Elastic fibers/Elastin   Bundles of the protein *elastin* found in connective tissue. These fibers add a flexible quality to the extracellular matrix.

Endocrine   An integrated system of organs that release hormones. The endocrine system helps to regulate growth, development, puberty, metabolism, and tissue function and also plays a part in determining emotions.

Endomysium   Meaning "within the muscle," this is the layer of fascia that wraps a muscle fiber.

Endplate   The flattened surface of the end of a nerve.

Energy crisis hypothesis   A proposed explanation for the formation of trigger points. Biomechanical disfunction in a muscle can deplete its store of ATP. When the muscle is low on ATP, it cannot perform the function of contraction and release properly. This results in the inability of the myofilaments to separate to release a contraction.

Epicranius   The muscle of the skull which consists of the frontalis on the anterior skull and the occipitalis on the posterior skull. These muscles are connected by a sheet of connective tissue called the *galea aponeurotica* that covers the top of the skull.

Epimysium   Layer of connective tissue which ensheathes the entire muscle. It is continuous with fascia and other connective tissue wrappings of muscle, including the endomysium and perimysium. It is also continuous with tendons.

Epithelial tissue   Pertains to a tissue that forms glands, covers the body surface, and lines the internal cavities.

External auditory meatus   The ear canal or auditory canal. The passage from the outer ear to the eardrum.

Extracellular matrix   The noncellular portion of connective tissue that provides structural support to the cells in addition to performing various other important functions. It is composed of collagen, elastin, and reticular proteins as well as ground substance.

F

Facilitated stretching   A group of techniques that lengthen and re-educate the muscle by stimulating or manipulating certain proprioceptors in the muscle.

Facilitation   The process by which neural signals travel faster each time they are sent through a nerve pathway.

Fascia   An uninterrupted, three-dimensional web of connective tissue that extends from head to toe, from front to back, and from interior to exterior. It interpenetrates and surrounds all structures. It is responsible for maintaining structural integrity, for providing support and protection, and to act as a shock absorber.

Fascicles   A bundle of skeletal muscle fibers surrounded by connective tissue.

Fibroblast   A cell that synthesizes and maintains the extracellular matrix of connective tissue. Fibroblasts provide the fibers and ground substance for the structural framework of connective tissue and play a critical role in wound healing.

Fibroclast   A type of cell found in connective tissue that breaks down fibers.

Fibrotic   Having an unusually high number of fibers or fibrous cells.

Five element theory   The theory that everything in the universe is the product of the continual changes among, and the interactions between, the five elements: wood, fire, earth, metal, and water. The five elements represent concepts rather than simple substances or objects.

Fixed spasm   A condition in which a muscle is undergoing a chronic spasm.

Flaccid paralysis   Paralysis characterized by limp, unresponsive muscles.

Fu   The term for one of two groups into which organs are classified (the other group being zang). The Yang organs: Gall Bladder, Small Intestine, Large Intestine, Stomach, and Bladder belong to the fu group.

G

Gait   The way locomotion is achieved. Gait describes how locomotion looks. It includes the swing of the arms, the movement of the hips, and the contact with the ground.

Generating cycle (sheng cycle)   The cycle in the five element theory in which each element is said to nourish or create the next element in the cycle.

Golgi tendon organ   A proprioceptor located within the tendons or musculotendonous junction. These receptors are responsible for the muscle-lengthening reaction.

Golgi tendon reflex   A reflex that causes relaxation in the local muscle as part of the Reciprocal Activation process.

Gross swelling   Any swelling which is visible to the naked eye.

Ground substance   The gel-like material in which connective tissue cells and fibers are embedded.

Guarding   A spasm of muscles that limits the ability to treat the affected area. This often occurs when a muscle is too tender to the touch or when a massage technique is applied too deeply and/or too quickly.

H

Health survey   Performed in the first (Subjective) step of the SOAP process. It involves making a list of the client's current and past health conditions and related habits.

Histology   The field of science concerned with the structure and function of the tissues of the body.

Holding pattern   An undesirable posture pattern that occurs when the client is compensating for an injury or pathology.

Holism   The theory that systems (biological, social, etc.) are made up of organic or unified wholes that are greater than the sum of their parts.

Hormone   Any of a number of chemical compounds produced in specialized glands, which are transported in the blood and body fluids and which have specific affects on receptive organs and tissues.

Hyperalgesia   An unusually high sensitivity to pain.

Hyperesthesia   A pathological increase in sensitivity to sensory stimuli.

Hyperkyphosis   Excessive anteriorly concave curvature of the thoracic segment of the vertebral column. Sometimes referred to as "dowager's hump."

Hyperlordosis   Excessive forward curvature of the lumbar segment of the vertebral column. Sometimes referred to as "swayback" or "saddle back."

Hypertonus   Muscles that have an excessive amount of continuous partial contraction (tonus, tension) are said to be hypertonic.

I

Ilium   One of the three bones that make up the pelvis. The ilium is the large flat bone that makes up the superior lateral portion.

Instep   The longitudinal arch of the foot.

Interneuron   An important component of neural pathways. Interneurons are neurons located in the central nervous system (especially the spinal cord) that connect neurons flowing in from the periphery with neurons flowing out to the periphery.

Interphalangeal joints   The joints in the fingers between the phalanges.

Interstitial fluid   A solution found in the tissue spaces, which bathes and surrounds the cells of the body.

Intrinsic reflex   A rapid response to a stimulus that is inborn, or part of the neural wiring. It does not have to be learned and is mostly involuntary.

Ischemia   A restriction in blood supply, generally due to factors such as injury or disease, which can cause damage or dysfunction to the tissues.

Isometric contraction   A contraction of a muscle where the muscle does not shorten. There is no movement, only an increase in internal tension.

Isotonic contraction   A contraction of a muscle where the muscle shortens and movement is produced.

J

Jing   The Chinese word for "essence." This is the pure physical substance that gives rise to the body. There are prenatal and postnatal forms of Jing.

Jing Luo   The acupressure channels, or meridians, that form a network of pathways through which the Qi flows and that link and balance the various body areas and organs.

Joint end feel   The way a joint feels when it is passively taken to the end of its range of motion.

L

Lateral malleolus   A boney landmark on the distal end of the fibula.

Lean and drag-back   A technique used in the application of DTM strokes where the therapist maintains contact with the client while returning to the starting position of the stroke.

Learned reflexes   Reflexes that are based on a person's experiences. This type of reflex is developed when a movement is repeated over and over.

Lengthwise strokes   Massage strokes that are applied along with the grain of the majority of muscle fibers.

Leverage   A factor that multiplies a force. Leverage increases a person's mechanical advantage so that a small force applied over a long distance uses the same amount of work as a large force applied over a small distance.

Local acupoint   An acupoint that is located close to the location of pathology.

M

Macrophage   A type of white blood cell which engulfs and then digests cellular debris and other pathogens and stimulates immune cells to respond to the pathogen.

Marked or pitted edema   Edema or swelling under the tissue. Pressing the area will leave a dent even after the pressure is released.

Mechanistic   A philosophy which asserts that wholes, such as living systems, function simply as mechanisms, or as a result of their relatively unchanging parts.

Mechanoreceptors   A sensory receptor that responds to mechanical pressure or movement of the body.

Medial maleolus   A bony landmark on the distal end of the tibia.

Medulla oblongata   The lower portion of the brainstem. It controls autonomic functions, such as breathing and blood pressure.

Mirror channels   There are 12 acupressure channels located on the right side of the body and 12 channels on the left side of the body, which mirror each other in location and function.

Muscle spindle cells   Specialized proprioceptors located in the bellies of muscles. They respond to a stretch by stimulating a contraction.

Muscle tissue   A tissue of the body made of long multinucleated cells that contain contractile filaments which attach to and move past each other to change the size of the cell.

Myofascia   The layers of connective tissue that cover and integrate with the muscles.

Myofascial holding pattern   An unbalanced posture pattern created by dysfunction in the myofascial structures.

Myogelosis   A condition in which there is abnormal hardening within the muscle tissue. Tissues containing such hardening are referred to as *myogelotic*.

Myosin filament   A filament comprised of the protein myosin. Together with actin filaments, myosin filaments make up the contractile units (sarcomeres) of muscle cells.

Myotatic unit   All the muscles that act on a joint. These include agonists, antagonists, synergists, fixators, and stabilizers.

N

Nerve plexus   A network of converging and diverging nerve fibers.

Nervous tissue   The tissue which makes up the central and peripheral nervous systems. Nervous tissue consists of neurons and other specialized or supporting cells.

Neurology   The field of science concerned with the nervous system.

Neuromuscular   Pertaining to both neural tissue and muscular tissue.

Neuron   Any of the conducting cells of the nervous system. A nerve cell. Sensory neurons (afferent neurons) carry information from receptors toward the central nervous system. Motor neurons (efferent neurons) carry information from the central nervous system toward effectors.

NMDA receptor   (N-methyl-D-aspartate receptor) A brain receptor which may sensitize the spinal cord when excessively stimulated.

Nociceptors   A group of cells that acts as a receptor for painful stimuli. Damaging stimuli from mechanical, chemical, and thermal stressors may prime these cells.

Nuchal line   One of the curved lines that extend laterally from the external occipital protuberance.

O

Occiput   The posterior bone of the skull.

Olecranon process   A bony landmark on the proximal end of the ulna. Forms the bony prominence of the elbow.

Osteoarthritis   Inflammation of the joint.

P

Pain reflex cycle (pathophysiological reflex arc)   The process occurring when a pain signal is sent to the spinal cord, which responds by sending a signal of contraction back to the site of pain. The contraction causes more pain, which causes further contraction, which then continues the cycle.

Pain threshold   The point at which a stressing stimulus (such as pressure or temperature) activates pain receptors, producing the sensation of pain. This is usually the point at which tissue damage has occurred.

Pain tolerance   The amount of pain that an individual is able to withstand. Pain tolerance is moderated by a variety of personal experiences such as lifestyle, age, history of injury, and mood.

Paraesthesia   A skin sensation, such as burning, prickling, itching, or tingling, caused by injury, compression, or entrapment of the nerves supplying the area.

Parasympathetic nervous system   The portion of the autonomic nervous system that innervates the heart, smooth muscle, and glands of the head and neck and thoracic, abdominal, and pelvic viscera. The parasympathetic nervous system is activated when the body is in a relaxed state.

Passive stretching   A form of stretching in which the therapist moves the client's body while the client's muscles are relaxed. This is used to test noncontractile structures such as ligaments and fascia and to gently re-educate the muscle.

Pathologic barrier   The point at which a muscle can no longer stretch due to injury or other pathology. This is usually short of the physiologic barrier.

Pathology   A structural and/or functional manifestation of disease.

Pathophysiological   Pertaining to the physiology of the disturbances of body function.

Perimysium   The sheath of connective tissue that groups skeletal muscle fibers into a fascicle.

Periosteum   Specialized connective tissue that wraps and covers all bones. The periosteum also has important bone-repair and regenerative properties.

Peripheral nerves   Nerves found throughout the body that carry information to and from the spinal cord.

Physiologic barrier   Normal end range for a particular joint.

Piezoelectricity   Electrical current produced by mechanical pressure on connective tissue as well as crystals such as quartz and mica.

Plasma cells   A type of white blood cell which produces antibodies.

Popliteal fossa   The depression in the posterior region of the knee.

Postisometric relaxation (PIR)   A form of facilitated stretching that manipulates proprioceptors in order to achieve a longer resting length in the muscle.

Postural analysis   The process of evaluating the positioning of the client's body and limbs to determine directly observable physical dysfunctions.

Primary affected channels   The acupressure channels that are directly affected by a particular pathology.

Prone position   Lying with the anterior side of the body toward the table or mat (face down).

Proprioceptor   A type of sensory receptor found in muscles, tendons, joints, and the inner ear that detects the motion or position of the body or a limb.

Proximal   Describing the location of some feature that is nearest to a particular point of reference, usually the center or midline of the torso. In reference to a limb, the proximal end is the end which attaches to the torso.

Pubis   The pubic bone.

Q

Qi   Basic life energy, or life force.

R

Range of motion (ROM)   The range, measured in degrees of a circle, through which a joint can be extended and flexed.

Reciprocal activation   A process moderated by the Golgi tendon organ in a muscle. It causes relaxation within the muscle where the Golgi tendon organ resides and causes contraction of the opposing (antagonist) muscle.

Reciprocal inhibition   A facilitated stretching technique that stretches the target muscle by contracting the opposing muscle against resistance.

Reductionist   A philosophical approach that attempts to explain complex systems (biological, social, etc.) by reducing them to simple interactions between their constituent parts.

Referral zones   Areas on the body that express referred phenomena or sensation from the activation of a trigger point.

Referred pain   Pain felt in a part of the body other than the area in which the cause of the pain is located.

Reflex arc   The neural pathway of a reflex action. An impulse is sent along a nerve fiber toward the spinal cord, and the response is sent outward to an effector organ or part.

Refractory state   A condition of relaxation following a period of excitation, such as when a muscle relaxes following an isometric contraction.

Release   The letting go of muscle tension and associated emotional stress.

Restriction   Lack of mobility in a muscle or tissue caused by injury, pathology, or emotional causes.

Reticular fibers   Small thin connective tissue fibers made of a modified form of collagen called *reticulin*.

Retinaculum (*pl.* Retinacula)   A band or structure made of connective tissue that wraps, stabilizes, or holds a body structure in place.

Rhabdomyolysis   An acute breakdown of skeletal muscle often accompanied by the excretion of myoglobin in the urine.

Rheumatoid arthritis   a chronic autoimmune disease that causes inflammation and deformity of the joints.

S

Saggital groove   The midline between the left and right gluteal muscles.

Sarcomeres   The contractile unit of a myofibril within a muscle.

Segment reflex massage   A therapeutic approach that incorporates connective tissue massage with theories of reflex zones and the segmentation of the nervous system.

Sensory adaptation   A decrease in the transmission of sensory information to the brain when a receptor is stimulated continuously and without a change in strength.

Sensory receptor   A structure that recognizes a stimulus in the internal or external environment of an organism.

Serotonin   A neurotransmitter commonly associated with feelings of well-being. It is synthesized in neurons in the central nervous system (CNS) and in the gastrointestinal tract. Serotonin is also found in many plants.

Shen   A concept in traditional Chinese medicine. The Shen represents a person's overall appearance and personal emotional expression.

Side-lying position   A common position in which the client is placed on their side during the application of massage therapy.

SOAP   An acronym for Subjective, Objective, Assessment, Plan. This is the proper medical procedure for analyzing a client's condition and making a plan for treatment.

Somatic pain   Pain located in the skin or myoskeletal system.

Somatic reflexes   Reflexes that activate skeletal muscles.

Spinal reflexes   A type of somatic reflex that is moderated at the spinal cord.

Splinting   A process in which pain causes tension in the muscles surrounding it. If the pain is prolonged, more muscles can be recruited into the process.

Stimulus   An internal or external factor or change that influences a neural receptor.

Stretch reflex   A muscle contraction that occurs in response to a stretch within the muscle or tendon. This type of reflex regulates skeletal muscle length, maintains upright posture, and protects against injury.

Stride   The coordinated movement of taking a step.

Subcutaneous   Referring to the area or tissues located beneath the skin.

Supine position   Lying with the posterior side of the body toward the table or mat (face up).

Sympathetic nervous system   The portion of the autonomic nervous system that becomes more active during times of stress. Its actions during the stress response comprise the fight-or-flight response.

Synergist   A muscle which assists the agonist in performing a joint motion.

Systemic postural dysfunction   A condition in which a myofascial holding pattern has led to dysfunctional patterns throughout the body.

T

Taiyang   An acupoint found on the sides of the face at the corner of each eye.

Tao   A concept in ancient Chinese philosophy. The character itself translates as "way," or "path." The Tao represents the fundamental or true nature of the world as an ever changing whole system. Taoism includes an active and holistic appreciation of the world.

Tapotement   A common Swedish massage technique. The body is tapped ryhtmically with short, rapid movements.

Tensegrity   Refers to the integrity of certain structures, including the body and body parts, as being based in a balance between tension and compression components.

Thixotropy   The property of some fluids to show change in viscosity due to heat or stress.

Tonus   The continuous partial contraction of a muscle that is maintained by unconscious nerve impulses. Sometimes referred to as "muscle tone."

Treatment plan   The result of the last stage of the SOAP process. A treatment plan includes which areas and structures will be treated, which techniques will be used, and may include recommendations for the client and for follow-up sessions.

Trigger point   Hyperirritable spots in skeletal muscle that are associated with knots and taut bands of muscle fibers. Compression of a trigger point may elicit local tenderness, referred pain, or local twitch response.

Trigger point pressure release   A technique used in the neuromuscular approach to release trigger points. It employs pressure applied directly to the trigger point.

Tui-na   A type of massage and body manipulation found in the traditional Chinese medical system.

V

Vasoconstriction   The narrowing of the blood vessels, which may restrict or slow the flow of blood.

Venous stasis   Any restriction or slowing of blood flow in the veins.

Visceral   Relating to, situated in, or affecting the internal organs.

Visceral pain   Pain arising from the internal organs.

Viscous   Commonly thought of as thickness or thinness of a fluid or gel. Viscosity is a measure of a liquid's or gel's resistance to flow.

W

White blood cells   Any of various blood cells that help protect the body from infection and disease.

X

Xiphoid   A process extending downward from the base of the sternum.

Y

Yang   The male cosmic principle in Chinese dualistic philosophy associated with day, warmth, action, function, exteriors, and rising.

Yin   The female cosmic principle in Chinese dualistic philosophy associated with night, coolness, rest, structure, interiors, and descending.

Yin/Yang complement   Refers to one of a pair of Yin and Yang channels on opposing surfaces of the body.

Z

Zang   The term for one of two groups into which organs are classified (the other group being fu). The Yin category of organs: Liver, Lung, Pericardium, Heart, Kidney, and Spleen belong to the zang group.

24-hour flow of Qi   The order in which Qi flows throughout the channels. The Qi is said to become full in each channel in two-hour increments. The flow of Qi system is helpful in diagnostics and tracing the path of injury along the channels.

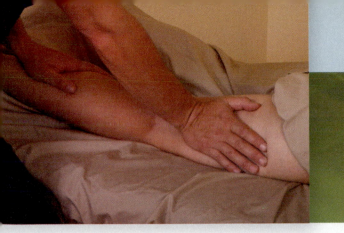

CHAPTER 1

Lai, M. Y., Yang, S. P., Chao, Y. Lee, P. C., Lee, S. D. (2006). Fever with acute renal failure due to body massage-induced rhabdomyolysis [Electronic version]. *Nephrology Dialysis Transplantation* 21(1): 233–234. Retrieved June 10, 2010, from http://ndt.oxfordjournals.org/cgi/content/full/21/1/233.

Marieb, Elaine N. (2004). *Human Anatomy & Physiology, 6th Edition.* San Francisco: Pearson Benjamin Cummings.

Lowe, Whitney, W. (1997). *Functional Assessment in Massage Therapy.* Bend, OR: Orthopedic Massage Education & Research Institute.

CHAPTER 2

Marieb, Elaine N. (2004). *Human Anatomy & Physiology, 6th Edition.* San Francisco: Pearson Benjamin Cummings.

Turchaninov, Ross (2006). *Medical Massage, Volume 1, 2nd Edition.* Phoenix: Aesculapius Books.

Werner, Ruth (2005). *A Therapist's Guide to Pathology, 3rd Edition.* Philadelphia: Lippincott Williams & Wilkins.

CHAPTER 3

Benjamin, Ben E. (1978). *Are You Tense? The Benjamin System of Muscular Therapy: Tension Relief Through Deep Massage and Body Care.* New York: Pantheon Books.

Marieb, Elaine N. (2004). *Human Anatomy & Physiology, 6th Edition.* San Francisco: Pearson Benjamin Cummings.

Riggs, Art (2007). *Deep Tissue Massage: A Visual Guide to Techniques, Revised Edition.* Berkeley: North Atlantic Books.

CHAPTER 5

Aetna InteliHealth, Inc. (1996–2010). *The Trusted Source: Complementary & Alternative Medicine—Index of Alternative Therapies and Modalities.* Retrieved June 24, 2010, from http://www.intelihealth.com/IH/ihtIH/WSIHW000/8513/34968.html #ab.

CHAPTER 6

Chaitow, Leon (2000). *Modern Neuromuscular Techniques.* New York: Churchill Livingstone.

Cohen, Barbara J., Taylor, Jason (2005). *Memmler's The Structure and Function of the Human Body, 8th Edition.* Philadelphia: Lippincott Williams & Wilkins.

Fritz, Sandy (2000). *Mosby's Fundamentals of Therapeutic Massage, 2nd Edition.* St. Louis: Mosby.

Goubet, N., Rattaz, C., Pierrat, V., Bullinger, A., Lequien, P. (2003, March). Olfactory experience mediates response to pain in preterm newborns. *Developmental Psychobiology* 42(2): 171–80.

Marieb, Elaine N. (2004). *Human Anatomy & Physiology, 6th Edition.* San Francisco: Pearson Benjamin Cummings.

Sayyah, M., Saroukhani, G., Peirovi, A., Kamalinejad, M. (2003, August). Analgesic and anti-inflammatory activity of the leaf essential oil of Laurus nobilis Linn. *Phytotherapy Research* 17(7): 733–36.

CHAPTER 7

Chaitow, Leon (1999). *Muscle Energy Techniques.* Edinburgh: Churchill Livingstone.

Chaitow, Leon (2000). *Modern Neuromuscular Techniques.* New York: Churchill Livingstone.

Fritz, Sandy (2000). *Mosby's Fundmentals of Therapeutic Massage, 2nd Edition.* St. Louis: Mosby.

Knott, M., Voss, D. (1968). *Proprioceptive neuromuscular facilitation: patterns and techniques.* New York: Hoeber Medical Division, Harper & Row.

McAtee, Robert E., Charland, Jeff (1999). *Facilitated Stretching: Assisted and Unassisted PNF Stretching Made Easy, 2nd Edition.* Champaign, IL: Human Kinetics U.S.

Muscolino, Joseph E. (2009). *The Muscle and Bone Palpation Manual: with Trigger Points, Referral Patterns, and Stretching.* St. Louis: Mosby Elsevier.

Simons, David G., Travell, Janet G., Simons, Lois S. (1999). *Travell & Simons' Myofascial Pain and Dysfunction: The Trigger Point Manual, 2nd Edition.* Baltimore: Lippencott Williams & Wilkins.

Turchaninov, Ross (2006). *Medical Massage, Volume 1, 2nd Edition.* Phoenix: Aesculapius Books.

Werner, Ruth (2005). *A Therapist's Guide to Pathology, 3rd Edition.* Philadelphia: Lippincott Williams & Wilkins.

CHAPTER 8

Chaitow, Leon (2000). *Modern Neuromuscular Techniques.* New York: Churchill Livingstone.

Simons, David G., Travell, Janet G., Simons, Lois S. (1999). *Myofascial Pain and Dysfunction: The Trigger Point Manual, 2nd Edition.* Baltimore: Lippincott Williams & Wilkins.

CHAPTER 9

Aetna InteliHealth, Inc. (1996–2010). *The Trusted Source: Complementary & Alternative Medicine—Index of Alternative Therapies and Modalities.* Retrieved June 24, 2010, from http://www.intelihealth.com/IH/ihtIH/WSIHW000/8513/34968.html #ab.

CHAPTER 10

Guimberteau, Jean-Claude (2005). *Strolling Under the Skin: Images of Living Fascia (Video).* English version. Centre de resources et d'information sur le multimedia pour l'enseignement superior/ADF Productions.

Marieb, Elaine N. (2004). *Human Anatomy & Physiology, 6th Edition.* San Francisco: Pearson Benjamin Cummings.

Myers, Thomas W. (2001). *Anatomy Trains: Myofascial Meridians for Manual and Movement Therapists.* Edinburgh: Churchill Livingstone.

Schultz, Louis R., Feitis, Rosemary (1996). *The Endless Web: Fascial Anatomy and Physical Reality.* Berkeley, CA: North Atlantic Books.

Turchaninov, Ross (2000). *Therapeutic Massage: A Scientific Approach.* Phoenix: Aesculapius Books.

Werner, Ruth (2005). *A Therapist's Guide to Pathology, 3rd Edition.* Philadelphia: Lippincott Williams & Wilkins.

CHAPTER 11

Ingber, Donald E. (1998, January). The architecture of life [Electronic version]. *Scientific American, Volume 278,* pp. 48–50. Retrieved June 10, 2010, from http://web1.tch.harvard.edu/research/ingber/PDF/1998/SciAmer-Ingber.pdf.

Myers, Thomas W. (2001). *Anatomy Trains: Myofascial Meridians for Manual and Movement Therapists.* Edinburgh: Churchill Livingstone.

Schultz, Louis R., Feitis, Rosemary (1996). *The Endless Web: Fascial Anatomy and Physical Reality.* Berkeley, CA: North Atlantic Books.

Simons, David G., Travell, Janet G., Simons, Lois S. (1999). *Myofascial Pain and Dysfunction: The Trigger Point Manual, 2nd Edition.* Baltimore: Lippincott Williams & Wilkins.

Turchaninov, Ross (2006). *Medical Massage, Volume 1, 2nd Edition.* Phoenix: Aesculapius Books.

CHAPTER 13

Myers, Thomas W. (2001). *Anatomy Trains: Myofascial Meridians for Manual and Movement Therapists.* Edinburgh: Churchill Livingstone.

Schultz, Louis R., Feitis, Rosemary (1996). *The Endless Web: Fascial Anatomy and Physical Reality.* Berkeley, CA: North Atlantic Books.

CHAPTER 14

Beissner, F., Henke, C., Unschuld, P. U. (2009). Forgotten Features of Head Zones and Their Relation to Diagnostically Relevant Acupuncture Points. *Evidence-based Complimentary Alternative Medicine, doi: 10.1093/ecam/nen088.* Retrieved June 17, 2010, from http://ecam.oxfordjournals.org/cgi/content/full/nen088.

Fritz, Sandy (2000). *Mosby's Fundmentals of Therapeutic Massage, 2nd Edition.* St. Louis: Mosby.

Marieb, Elaine N. (2004). *Human Anatomy & Physiology, 6th Edition.* San Francisco: Pearson Benjamin Cummings.

O'Connor, John, Bensky, Dan (Trans. and Eds.) (1981). *Acupuncture: A Comprehensive Text.* Seattle: Eastland Press.

Rosenberg, S. (2003, August). Rolfing, visceral manipulation and acupuncture. *Structural Integration: The Journal of the Rolf Institute* 31 (3).

Williams, Tom (1996). *The Complete Illustrated Guide to Chinese Medicine.* Shaftesbury, Dorset, GB: Element Books.

CHAPTER 15

Burmeister, Alice, Monte, Tom (1997). *The Touch of Healing.* New York: Bantam Books.

Huihe, Yin. (Translated by Xuezhong, Shuai) (1992). *Fundamentals of Traditional Chinese Medicine.* Beijing: Foreign Language Press.

Lao Tzu (n.d.). *Tao Te Ching* (Translated by Wu, J. C. H.) (1990). Boston: Shambhala Publications.

Maciocia, Giovanni (1989). *The Foundations of Chinese Medicine: A Comprehensive Text for Acupuncturists and Herbalists.* Edinburgh: Churchill Livingstone.

O'Connor, John, Bensky, Dan (Trans. and Eds.) (1981). *Acupuncture: A Comprehensive Text.* Seattle: Eastland Press.

Teeguarden, Iona M. (1978). *Acupressure Way of Health: Jin Shin Do.* Tokyo: Japan Publications.

Thie, John (1994). *Touch for Health: A Practical Guide to Natural Health Using Acupressure Touch and Massage (Original Work 1973).* Malibu, CA: Touch for Health Education.

Williams, Tom (1996). *The Complete Illustrated Guide to Chinese Medicine.* Shaftesbury, Dorset, GB: Element Books.

Ya-li, Fan (1994). *Chinese Pediatric Massage Therapy.* Boulder: Blue Poppy Press.

CHAPTER 16

Aetna InteliHealth, Inc. (1996–2010). *The Trusted Source: Complementary & Alternative Medicine—Index of Alternative Therapies and Modalities.* Retrieved June 24, 2010, from http://www.intelihealth.com/IH/ihtIH/WSIHW000/8513/34968.html\#ab.

CHAPTER 17

Aetna InteliHealth, Inc. (1996–2010). *The Trusted Source: Complementary & Alternative Medicine—Index of Alternative Therapies and Modalities.* Retrieved June 24, 2010, from http://www.intelihealth.com/IH/ihtIH/WSIHW000/8513/34968.html #ab.

CHAPTER 18

Benking, H., van Meurs, M. (1997). History, Concepts and Potentials of Holism. *Holistic Aspects in Systems Research,* InterSymp '97, Baden-Baden, August 18–23, 1997. Retrieved July 1, 2010, from http://www.ceptualinstitute.com/genre/benking/holismsmuts.htm.

Index